POTS
Together We Stand
Riding the Waves of
Dysautonomia

Jodi Epstein Rhum

Part I- Edited by Karen Timko

Part II- Medical Content Edited by Svetlana Blishteyn, MD

A portion of the proceeds will be donated to POTS research.

This book will serve as a lifeline in many ways. After reading this book, you will:

1. be cognizant of the most up to date POTS research from medical experts around the globe;
2. understand new ways to help lesson symptoms through proper exercise, nutrition and other non-pharmaceutical, as well as alternative therapies;
3. learn how to advocate for yourself or your loved one who has POTS (or any other chronic illness);
4. discover the secret of securing an IEP (individualized Educational Plan/Program) and getting your child's school on board with the diagnosis of POTS;
5. learn how to get the academic adjustments and accommodations you need;
6. understand pharmaceutical choices available to help reduce symptoms;
7. learn beneficial tips to help you ride the tumultuous waves of Dysatuonomia;
8. know how to help your doctors to better understand POTS;
9. figure out how to get social security benefits for you or your loved one;
10. discover how to secure a handicap sticker, if necessary;
11. learn how to get the accommodations you need in the work force to be successful in your career;
12. help your family and friends to better understand your syndrome;
13. learn how doctors treat POTS around the globe and,
14. realize you are not alone, for "Together We Stand."

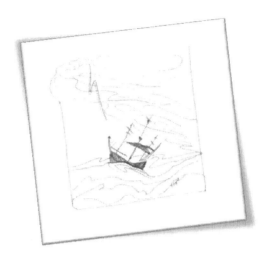

"I'm not afraid of storms for I'm learning to sail my ship."
Louisa May Alcott

Table of Contents

Part I.. **12**

Section 1. Introduction 13

About the Author... 14

About the Medical Content Editor and Co-author 15

Dedication Page 16

Introduction - *Jodi Epstein Rhum*................................. 18

Introduction - *Svetlana Blishteyn, MD*........................... 19

What is POTS? - *Svetlana Blitshteyn, MD* 20

Letter from Senator (now President) Obama about POTS 36

Being Nikki - Personal Story of a 14 Year - Old Girl Living with POTS.. 38

Section 2. Riding the Waves of Dysautonomia........................... 44

Chapter 1. Combating Insomnia 46

Chapter 2. Surviving Syncope 52

Chapter 3. Dysautonomia Don'ts- Things to Avoid 61

Chapter 4. Dysautonomia Q & A, a Mother's View 68

Chapter 5. Cosmopots; NASA and POTS Research 81

Section 3. Coping 85

Chapter 6. Impact on the Family-How Chronic Illness can Impact the Entire Family Unit.. 86

Chapter 7. POTS Storm - A Day in the Life of a Family Coping with POTS... 94

Chapter 8. Grief and Dysautonomia - *Michelle Roger, Psychologist* 98

Chapter 9. Changing for the Better: The Positive Aspects of Living with POTS – *Danielle Hines*... 104

Section 4. Other Syndromes.. 111

Chapter 10. Ehlers-Danlos Syndrome.................................... 112

Chapter 11 Physical Therapy in Children Presenting with Ehlers-Danlos Syndrome and Postural Orthostatic Tachycardia Syndrome -*Ashley Summers, PT, DPT*.................................... 123

Chapter 12. Familial Dysautonomia - *President of FD Now, Ann Slaw*... 127

Section 5. Surviving the Educational System............................. 134

Chapter 13. Dealing with Dysautonomia in the Classroom - Tips for Teachers 135

Chapter 14. Surviving High School - Helpful Hints to Make it Through Secondary School 171

Chapter 15. When It's Time for the Dizzy Bird to Leave the Nest- Going off to College. 190

Section 6. More Helpful Hints.. 214

Chapter 16. Securing a Handicap Sticker- *Jesse White, Secretary of State of Illinois* 215

Chapter 17. Assistive Devices - *Megan Ong, Ana Collins and Katie Ziegler - POTS patients*.. 219

Chapter 18. 25 Necessities for a POTS friendly life 222

Chapter 19. How to Get Job Accommodations in the work force - *Dr. Suzanne Gosden Kitchen, Senior Consultant for the Job Accommodation Network (JAN)* 227

Chapter 20. Dysautonomia and Disability Benefits - *Amy Michelle Krakower, Esq*... 238

Chapter 21. Tips for Vacationing with someone who has Dysautonomia... 244

Chapter 22. Finding a Physician that is right for you............. 258

Chapter 23. Going to the Dentist, Orthodontist or Oral Surgeon - *Jodi Rhum and Dr. Mark Cannon, DDS* 267

Chapter 24. POTS and Visual Disturbances 274

Section 7. Pass the Salt.. 279

Chapter 25. The Importance of proper Nutrition - *Darren Friedman, Nutritionist*... 283

Chapter 26. Nutritional Recipes Designed for POTS patients - *Created by Chef Randy Ordonio of San Francisco*.................. 290

Section 8. Alternative Therapies and Exercise 303

Chapter 27. Tips, Natural Supplements and Vitamins that May Help with Symptoms - *Co-written by Sharon Cini, M.D. Edited by Rosalee Jaeger* 304

Chapter 28. The Basics of Going Gluten Free 324

Chapter 29. Yoga, Meditation and Spirituality - *Lynda Dresher, Cantor* 334

Chapter 30. Home Workouts - *Dave Warren, personal trainer* 340

Section 9 - Inspiration.. 357

Chapter 31. Spreading Awareness... 358

Chapter 32. Poems and More Inspiration 363

Section 10. Personal Narratives... 365

Chapter 33. Inspirational Personal Narratives - *A variety of stories of people around the globe with varying degrees and types of Dysautonomia. Their journeys are filled with courage, strength and insurmountable inspiration.* 366

Section 11. Just For Fun... 382

Chapter 34. You Know You Have POTS When........................ 383

Chapter 35. Interesting Facts about Dysautonomia.............. 387

Chapter 36. Poem - "Fly Again"- *Jodi Rhum* 391

Part II - POTS; It's Real - Written by Medical Professionals .. 392

Chapter 37. Symptoms, Signs and Mechanisms of POTS. *Svetlana Blitshteyn, MD* 395

Chapter 38. POTS and Lifestyle - *Svetlana Blitshteyn. MD* 409

Chapter 39. The Tip of the Iceberg- Overview of Dysautonomia - *William Suarez, Pediatric Cardiologist*.. 430

Chapter 40. When to see a Gastroenterologist (GI Specialist) and what to expect- *John Fortunato, M.D.*.. 439

Chapter 41. POTS; Clinical, Pathophysiological Aspects and Treatment- *Raffaello Furlan- University of Milan* 448

Chapter 42. How to Know When to Seek Professional Help- *Dr. Neil Gordon, Licensed Clinical Psychologist, Harvard* 455

Chapter 43. Coping with POTS - *Svetlana Blitshteyn, MD.* 463

Part III – Patients' Experiences about Treatment Options that have Worked for them... 478

Chapter 44. Patient Story – *POTS Treatment Center – Dallas, Texas- Nikki Rhum* 479

Chapter 45. Mayo Clinic's Pediatric Pain Rehab Center - *Ellen Kessler*.. 484

Chapter 46. When POTS is More than Just POTS 490

About Dysautonomia International..................................... 498

Wrapping Up... 501

Forward to Reader

Dear Readers,

As you read this book, please keep in mind that I am not a doctor and as such this book was not intended to treat, diagnose, or offer professional services. The reader must consult his or her medical, health, alternative or other competent professional before adopting any of the suggestions in this book or drawing inferences from it.

This book is a collaborative effort of many doctors, teachers, counselors, parents, and patients who have come together to weave this tapestry. I am a mom of two children who have POTS as well as a former educator. I do not claim to be a POTS expert; I am simply giving practical tips that have worked for my family as well as other POTS patients that I have come to know over the past four years.

I wrote this book in response to the fact that when my children were first diagnosed, I felt overwhelmed, lonely and discouraged. I did not know where to turn. I was unable to find any comprehensive book on this syndrome that could answer the plethora of questions I had. That's when I decided to write this "survival guide" with the hope that it would help others who found themselves similarly situated.

I have asked many medical doctors to supplement this book. They have come together to help further educate the POTS population. These doctors hail from diverse fields to address the physiology, as well as the pathology, of POTS. I am confident that you will learn from their expertise as medical professionals.
It is my hope that this knowledgeable and experienced blend of various authors from all areas of expertise will provide you with clear-cut medical explanations about this syndrome, coping tech-

niques, helpful tips, educational considerations, inspiring narrative accounts and more.

From patients to providers to parents to educators, we join hands in this compendium to support the Dysautonomia community in its struggles, hopes, concerns and endeavors, indisputably serving as a living testament that "Together We Stand."

Sincerely, Jodi Epstein Rhum

How to read the book: This book was designed to encourage the reader to skip around and dig into the sections that they are most interested in. Just as each person with POTS is unique, so too is the concept of this book. The book was not designed to be read from front to back cover. It was specifically set up so the reader can skip freely around the book and pick and choose topics that are relevant to him or her. It is a survival guide and as such it is to be used as a resource. Many topics are introduced and later reintroduced. This redundancy was done on purpose as many people, for example teachers, school nurses, tutors and the like may only read one or two sections that are pertinent to them, and therefore I have explained things over again in various sections in full anticipation of this. Whether you decide to read every word of this book or just a couple of chapters, I hope you find it interesting, insightful and most of all, helpful.

Part I

Section 1. Introduction

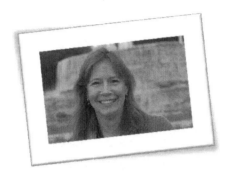

About the Author

Jodi Epstein Rhum was born and raised in Illinois. She received her degree in Education from the University of Illinois.

Jodi has four children, two of whom have POTS and one who has Ehlers-Danlos Syndrome. Having grown up with an undiagnosed mild case of POTS herself, she understands the complexities and frustrations of this syndrome, first hand. Jodi, who is a former middle school teacher, has devoted herself to POTS Awareness, since her children's diagnosis three years ago.

Jodi has spoken at various schools in the area advocating for POTS patients as well as educating staff members and school nurses on the syndrome. She has spoken with many doctors and attends conferences trying to further educate herself on the illness.

Jodi started a POTS Awareness Facebook Group, which now has over 3, 500 members. She has been on the news and has been interviewed for many newspaper articles trying to raise awareness. She consults with numerous patients on a daily basis giving advice and providing direction. This book *"Together We Stand; Riding the Waves of Dysautonomia"* is the culmination of her efforts to help others who suffer from POTS, to learn through her experiences as a mother, a teacher and patient.

About the Medical Content Editor and Co-author

Dr. Svetlana Blitshteyn is a board-certified neurologist who is a renowned specialist in POTS and other autonomic disorders. She is the Director and founder of the Dysautonomia Clinic located in Buffalo, New York, and a Clinical Assistant Professor at the University at Buffalo School of Medicine and Biomedical Sciences.

Dr. Blitshteyn completed her neurology training at Mayo Clinic. She received her Medical Doctor degree and Bachelor of Science in Biochemistry with Summa Cum Laude from the University at Buffalo School of Medicine and Biomedical Sciences, where she was also the valedictorian and an Honor's Scholar. Dr. Blitshteyn has been awarded numerous awards and honors, including the American Academy of Neurology Student Prize; a Research Award from the Florida Society of Neurology, a US Human Health Award from the American Headache Society and a Marquis Who's Who in Medicine and Healthcare.

Dr. Blitshteyn serves as a medical adviser for the Dysautonomia International and Dysautonomia Information Network (DINET) and has been a regular contributor to the DINET newsletter. She was also featured in the documentary "Changes: Living with Postural Orthostatic Tachycardia Syndrome". Dr. Blitshteyn has been the principle research investigator on several nationally acclaimed studies and has presented her research at various national and international meetings, including the American Academy of Neurology and American Autonomic Society scientific meetings. She published in many scientific journals on the topics of POTS after vaccination, POTS and pregnancy and others.

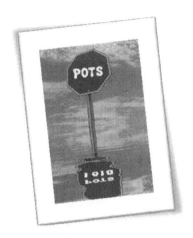

Dedication Page

"If children have the ability to ignore all odds and percentages, then maybe we can all learn from them. When you think about it, what other choice is there but to hope? We have two options, medically and emotionally: give up, or fight like hell." - Lance Armstrong

This book is dedicated to my dad, who suffered from a neurological illness called PPA, primary progressive aphasia. My father taught me many things. He taught me to never give up. He taught me that life is a rollercoaster. It is filled with many ups and downs and unpredictable and scary twists and turns, but in the end, even when you are down, you come back up and are all the better for having experienced the thrilling journey. I thank him for always providing me with unconditional love and teaching me so many valuable lessons along the way. Thank you for being my "ROCK" and always believing in me. I hope I can be as well respected in my lifetime as you were in yours.

A big thank you to my mom who always believed in me, even when I did not believe in myself.

To my children, those that have POTS and those that do not, you are all warriors. Never lie down to an illness and never let anything stop you from achieving your dreams. Don't ever give up the fight. I love you as much as a mother can love. Thank you for teaching me new lessons every day. Remember to LIVE, LAUGH AND LOVE, and Always Dance in the Rain!

To Debbie and Dynakids (Dysautonomia Youth Network of America) for guiding us through the most difficult time in our lives. Thanks for your caring, knowledge and support. You carried us when we could not walk. We will forever be grateful to you and DYNA.

To The Make-A-Wish Foundation and Gloria for being our Angels on Earth.

To Dr. Grubb, Dr. Suarez, Dr. Gilden, Dr. Lin, Dr. Berndtson, Dr. Berliant, Dr. Neuberger, Dr. Suleman, Dr. Kyprianou and Dr.Thoele for being great doctors and wonderful humanitarians.

A gigantic thank you to Stevenson High School, Helen Magid, my daughter's case manager, and the entire Stevenson staff, for believing my daughter's illness was real from the get go, providing her the services she needed to make it through high school, for being supportive, empathetic and accommodating. We are so lucky to live in the Stevenson district. It is apparent why Stevenson is among the top schools in the nation. Thank you for helping my daughter to fly, even when gravity was attempting to hold her down.

And finally, a colossal thank you to all of those doctors, specialists, experts and patients who contributed to this book. I could not have written this without you.

Jodi Epstein Rhum

Introduction - *Jodi Epstein Rhum*

Dear Readers,

I always wanted to write a book. Never in my wildest dreams did I ever think I would write about a word that three years ago, I had never even heard of: POTS, Postural Orthostatic Tachycardia Syndrome. POTS was as foreign to me as was riding California Screaming at California Adventure Park or kayaking over a school of sharks - both of which I have since done. But then again, when does life give you what you expect? There is a saying in Yiddish, "A mentsh tracht und Gott lacht" - a person plans and God laughs. God must be roaring with laughter now. I have the only eight year old twins in the country who can ramble off, "postural orthostatic tachycardia syndrome," as easily as someone can ramble off "Rice Krispies cereal."

Dan Millman, in his novel, *"The Peaceful Warrior"* alludes to the fact that life is a journey and what matters is the journey itself, not the final destination. I like to think of people who have POTS as warriors. They are strong souls who need to fight through every day battles. Just trying to stand up and get out of bed for them every morning is a small war, a war that they will eventually win if they hang in there.

This book is a cornucopia of inspiration; information and practical tips that will help you navigate your journey with Dysautonomia. It is a survival guide for all POTS warriors, their doctors, teachers, friends and families. It is my hope this book gives you strength, knowledge and courage to ride the Waves of Dysautonomia.

My favorite quote of all times is, "Life is not about waiting for the storm to pass, it's about learning to dance in the rain." I hope that through reading this book you will be inspired to dance even in a torrential downpour.

Jodi Epstein Rhum

Introduction - *Svetlana Blishteyn, MD*

If you are a patient, a family member or a health care provider who wants to learn about POTS, you are probably aware that information about this disorder is extremely scarce and often confusing. What is POTS? Is it a real medical condition? Is there a cure? Can it be diagnosed objectively or is it a non-specific diagnosis?

If you tell your family or friends that you have POTS, you will probably be faced with strange looks and many questions. Recognition of the acronym, or the full name of Postural Orthostatic Tachycardia Syndrome, is limited in the general public and in the medical community. Many patients resort to explaining their illness through other related, yet completely separate, conditions. For example, when describing POTS to other people, including physicians or nurses, some patients may say, *"It's like orthostatic hypotension, without the orthostatic hypotension,"* or, *"It's like mitral valve prolapse syndrome, without the actual mitral valve prolapse."*

It can be very frustrating when your disorder is not recognized or validated like other medical conditions. POTS should be recognized and viewed as a unique and distinct medical condition, a form of Dysautonomia, which is a term used to describe a dysfunction of the autonomic nervous system.

This book is devoted entirely to POTS, its symptoms and signs, proposed mechanisms and causes and available treatment options, as well as its relationship and associations with other medical conditions. Coping strategies and various lifestyle modifications will be discussed in detail in order to educate, empower and reassure those who have POTS that, despite this chronic disorder, living well and feeling good is possible.

Svetlana Blitshteyn, MD

What is POTS? - *Svetlana Blitshteyn, MD*

Postural Orthostatic Tachycardia Syndrome (POTS) is a syndrome. A syndrome is defined as a collection of symptoms and signs that tend to occur together. A disease is defined as a set of symptoms and signs with identifiable cause, mechanisms or anatomical location. POTS is a syndrome and not a disease because it is not characterized by one cause, mechanism or location. Examples of other well-known syndromes include Irritable Bowel Syndrome, Down Syndrome and Fibromyalgia, while thyroid disorders, asthma and Alzheimer's dementia are examples of diseases.

POTS is a form of Dysautonomia, which is a term used to describe any dysfunction of the autonomic nervous system (ANS). The hallmark of POTS is orthostatic intolerance. Orthostatic intolerance means an inability or intolerance of the body to withstand gravity, whether in the standing or sitting position. It is important to note that in patients with POTS, the ANS does not function properly in any position, but the dysfunction is more apparent and unmasked in the standing, and sometimes, sitting position. This in turn causes one to have more symptoms in the standing position than in the sitting position, and sitting more than lying flat, or supine position.

Tachycardia simply means rapid pulse or heart rate. Normal heart rate in humans ranges between 60 to 100 beats per minute, regardless of the position, and normally increases with exercise. In POTS, the heart rate is inappropriately increased in response to standing, but can also be increased in the sitting or supine positions. Patients with POTS also have intolerance to exercise, partly because their heart rate increases even higher with physical activity. As you can imagine, if your heart rate becomes inappropriately high just from standing, you would get tired easily just by standing or walking for a few minutes. Similarly, people with POTS may feel exhausted after routine activities where standing or walking is required because, as if continuously exercising, their body is working hard and expending energy constantly to maintain an upright posture.

Criteria for POTS

If you are wondering why you never heard of POTS or if POTS is a new medical condition, you are asking the right questions. POTS is not a new medical condition and has been around for centuries under different names. These include "effort syndrome", "neurasthenia", "irritable heart", "soldier's heart", and "DaCosta Syndrome." Other names that have been used for this condition are Mitral Valve Prolapse Syndrome, Idiopathic Postural Tachycardia, Idiopathic Hypovolemia, as well as Chronic Fatigue Syndrome. Some of these conditions and their relationship to POTS are described in greater detail later in the chapter, but it is important to emphasize that POTS is a distinct medical condition, regardless of its similarities to other disorders.

Although the syndrome has been around for a long time, it is only within the past 20 years that POTS has been more specifically defined and investigated through research studies. POTS is a syndrome of orthostatic intolerance and orthostatic tachycardia, and its name is based on the diagnostic criteria that characterizes this disorder. In 1995, Dr. Philip Low and colleagues from the Mayo Clinic proposed a specific set of criteria for diagnosing POTS, along with a system that grades severity of orthostatic intolerance [1]. Criteria for POTS include the following:

- Increased heart rate of 40 beats per minute (or 30 bpm for adult patients) or more within 5 minutes of standing or tilt table test
- Heart rate equal or greater than 120 beats per minute within 5 minutes of standing or tilt table test
- Orthostatic symptoms consistently develop

The above criteria is generally used by most physicians to

diagnose POTS. Additionally, it is important to note that the presence of orthostatic symptoms is one of the main criteria for diagnosis. Some people may experience a 30 beats per minute elevation of heart rate when being upright, but do not have any symptoms of orthostatic intolerance. In fact, they may not even know that their heart rate is high when they stand, because they do not experience any problems when being upright, walking or exercising. By definition, these patients do not have POTS since they do not have orthostatic intolerance.

The Autonomic Nervous System

As humans had evolved to walk upright, so did the mechanisms that allowed a person to counteract the effects of gravity. The autonomic nervous system, in combination with the heart, blood vessels and skeletal muscles, plays a major role in the ability and tolerance to withstand orthostatic stress.

The ANS is a vital component of the human nervous system and is very complex. It consists of structures in the brain, spinal cord and peripheral nerves that run through the major organs of the body. There is a very elaborate communication system between the brain, the spinal cord, the peripheral nerves and the organs that it innervates. In addition, there is also a complicated communication system between the external environment and the internal environment of the body.

The ANS is an "automatic" system, which means that you do not have to think about major processes in the body, such as, for example, the heart rate and blood pressure control, digestion, and body temperature regulation, for these to occur. In contrast, you have to think about grabbing a penny with your fingers before executing the task.

The ANS plays a major role in regulating the heart rate, blood pressure, gastrointestinal and urinary bladder function, body temperature, sweating and the size of the pupil in the eye. Not surprisingly, when ANS malfunctions, any or all of its major functions can be affected.

The ANS consists of two major divisions: the Sympathetic Nervous System and the Parasympathetic Nervous System. Each organ is innervated by nerve fibers from both systems, and their effect on an organ is usually opposing. Each system has a unique organization and function, but in simple terms, the Sympathetic Nervous System is an activating system, preparing the body for the "flight or fight" response, while the parasympathetic is a calming system and is concerned with conservation and restoration of energy.

The sympathetic system increases heart rate and blood pressure and diverts the blood flow away from the skin, stomach and intestines to the skeletal muscles, all in preparation for "flight or fight" response. In contrast, the parasympathetic system decreases heart rate and blood pressure and promotes digestion and waste excretion, all in the attempt to restore balance and conserve energy.

For a complete list of sympathetic and parasympathetic nervous systems function, please see the table.

Table 1.1 The Autonomic Nervous System

Structure	Sympathetic Stimulation	Parasympathetic Stimulation
Iris (eye muscle)	Pupil dilation	Pupil constriction
Salivary Glands	Saliva production reduced	Saliva production increased
Oral/Nasal Mucosa	Mucus production reduced	Mucus production increased
Heart	Heart rate and force increased	Heart rate and force decreased
Lung	Bronchial muscle relaxed	Bronchial muscle contracted
Stomach	Peristalsis reduced	Gastric juice secreted;

		motility increased
Small Intestine	Motility reduced	Digestion increased
Large Intestine	Motility reduced	Secretions and motility increased
Liver	Increased conversion of glycogen to glucose	
Kidney	Decreased urine secretion	Increased urine secretion
Adrenal medulla	Norepinephrine and epinephrine secreted	
Bladder	Wall relaxed Sphincter closed	Wall contracted Sphincter relaxed

Fainting and POTS

Fainting, or syncope, is defined as a sudden, temporary loss of consciousness. It is estimated that up to 30% of healthy adults may experience fainting during their lifetime. Occasional fainting may not be harmful, but repeated episodes of fainting need to be investigated by a doctor.

Fainting occurs because of the temporary loss of blood supply to the brain. Fainting has many causes and can be associated with different medical conditions, but the most common cause is vasovagal syncope, also known as the neurocardiogenic syncope and the "common faint". The mechanism of vasovagal syncope includes an abnormal circulatory reflex where the blood vessels dilate causing an abrupt decrease in blood pressure, but the heart rate does not compensate enough to maintain adequate blood flow to the brain. As a result of this temporary loss of blood flow to the brain, fainting, or syncope, occurs. The common causes of vasovagal syncope include the following:

- Temperature – heat, whether outside, or indoors, espe-

cially when not drinking enough water
- Strong emotions – whether it's fear, excitement or stress
- Sight of blood – especially during blood draws
- Standing in one place for too long and not moving
- Getting up too quickly from lying to a standing position
- Dehydration – whether from not drinking enough water or having severe vomiting or diarrhea
- Low blood sugar – whether from skipping meals, extreme dieting, or illness that prevents you from eating.

Situational syncope means that fainting occurs in the context of a particular activity or situation. It can happen in healthy people, but also in serious medical conditions. Causes of situational syncope include the following:

- Cough syncope occurs when coughing forcefully.
- Swallow syncope occurs upon swallowing in some people. (Remember President George W Bush fainting after eating a pretzel?)
- Micturition syncope occurs when a susceptible person empties an overfilled bladder.
- Defecation syncope occurs in the context of having a bowel movement, particularly when straining.
- Carotid sinus hypersensitivity occurs in some elderly people when turning the neck, shaving, or wearing a tight collar.
- Postprandial fainting is common in elderly people when their blood pressure falls about an hour after eating a heavy meal.

Syncope can also be caused by heart disease, and this type of syncope can be dangerous and even life-threatening. Heart problems that can cause syncope include the following:
- Cardiac rhythm abnormality or arrhythmia: Electrical

problems of the heart can sometimes impair its ability to pump blood to the body. This causes a decrease in blood flow to the brain. The heart rate may be either too fast or too slow to pump blood well. This condition usually causes fainting without any warning symptoms.

• Cardiac obstruction: Blood flow can be obstructed within the blood vessels in the chest. Cardiac obstruction can cause fainting during physical exertion. Many disorders can cause obstruction, including heart attacks, diseased heart valves, pulmonary embolism, cardiomyopathy, pulmonary hypertension, cardiac tamponade, and aortic dissection.

• Heart failure: The heart's pumping ability is impaired, which may lower the force with which blood circulates through the body and decrease blood flow in the brain.

Syncope can also occur in many other medical conditions, including anemia, various electrolyte abnormalities, or hormonal disorders. It is also more common in people who have migraines.

Recurrent syncope can be a sign of the ANS dysfunction. In fact, some physicians erroneously assume that syncope has to be present in any disorder of the ANS. This could not be further from the truth. In fact, most patients with POTS do not faint. It is estimated that syncope occurs only in about 30% of those with POTS. Furthermore, recall from the criteria for POTS that syncope is not a part of the diagnosis. Thus, the absence of syncope does not exclude a diagnosis of POTS.

Presyncope is a term used to describe an episode that does not result in loss of consciousness, but that has all other characteristics of a syncope. Presyncope simply means "near fainting." In presyncope, the blood flow to the brain is decreased, but not enough to result in a complete loss of consciousness. Presyncope is very common in patients with POTS, it is one of the main features of the disorder.

Blood Pressure and POTS

Blood pressure is defined as the force of blood exerted on the walls of the blood vessels. It is expressed as a ratio between systolic pressure, which is the pressure when the heart pumps the blood out to the arteries, and a diastolic pressure, which is the pressure when the heart rests. Blood pressure changes throughout the day, depending on the activity or time of day. It is higher when you exercise or work and lower when you rest or sleep. Normal blood pressure falls within a range and is not one set of numbers.

Hypertension, or high blood pressure, affects approximately 25% of adults in the United States and is a major risk factor for stroke and heart disease. Major public awareness and research initiatives have been launched to address recognition, treatment and prevention of hypertension. Numerous medications, approved by the Food and Drug Administration, are available to treat people who have hypertension.

Hypotension, or low blood pressure, on the other hand, is a very different problem than hypertension. Unlike high blood pressure, which is defined by the American Heart Association as a blood pressure measurement above 140/90, low blood pressure is not defined by a number, but rather the presence of signs and symptoms of hypotension. For example, some people may have a blood pressure of 90/50 and feel great, with no signs or symptoms of hypotension, while others may experience dizziness or weakness with the same blood pressure reading, and, therefore have hypotension.

POTS may occur more often in those with low blood pressure, but people with normal or high blood pressure can also have POTS. POTS can also result in greater variability of blood pressure than in healthy people, whereas blood pressure can rise and fall abruptly, resulting in different symptoms and signs associated with these sudden blood pressure changes. It is generally believed that unlike hypertension, chronic hypotension and POTS are not known to be associated with increased risk of stroke or heart disease.

Orthostatic Hypotension and POTS

When a person stands up, as much as 25% - 30% of blood volume may pool in the legs as a result of gravity. To counteract the effect of gravity on the body, the blood pressure, heart rate and tone in the blood vessels have to adjust in order to maintain an upright posture. As stated before, the autonomic nervous system plays a major role in the body's ability to tolerate upright posture and therefore, in regulating blood pressure, heart rate and tone in the blood vessels during standing.

Normally, when a person stands up, the systolic blood pressure remains the same or slightly decreased while the diastolic blood pressure is slightly increased compared to laying down. In people with an impaired autonomic nervous system, or Dysautonomia, both systolic and diastolic blood pressure may fall abnormally when standing. Sometimes, the fall in blood pressure is substantial enough to cause the temporary loss of blood flow to the brain and result in syncope, or fainting. Orthostatic hypotension is defined as blood pressure drop of more than 20/10 mmHg on assuming an upright position. Orthostatic hypotension is also known as postural hypotension or neurally-mediated hypotension.

Orthostatic hypotension (OH) has many different causes and can occur in people of all ages, but especially in the elderly. OH is a common side effect of many drugs, including those that are used to treat hypertension. Some of the drugs that can cause OH are summarized below:

- Antypertensive medications
- Beta blockers
- Diuretics
- Insulin
- Nitrates
- Narcotics
- Tranquilizers
- Tricyclic antidepressants
- Viagra

Some common neurological conditions that can cause OH include:
- Dysautonomia
- Parkinson's Disease
- Spinal cord problems
- Conditions of the peripheral nerves, also known as neuropathy
- Multiple Sclerosis
- Certain types of stroke

Heart problems can also cause OH:
- Heart failure
- Cardiac arrhythmia
- Heart attacks

Hormonal problems, infection, dehydration, diarrhea, bleeding and burns are other common causes of OH.

When caused by dysfunction of the autonomic nervous system, OH by itself can be considered a form of Dysautonomia. However, OH can also be a sign of more serious types of Dysautonomia, such as Progressive Autonomic Failure or Multiple System Atrophy.

OH is different from POTS because criteria to diagnose OH includes a fall in blood pressure while criteria to diagnose POTS is an increase in heart rate upon standing. Thus, OH and POTS are separate medical conditions, although both can be viewed as different forms of Dysautonomia.

Some patients who have POTS also have OH. Additionally, some researchers believe that if patients with POTS are allowed to stand long enough, a proportion of these patients will eventually develop OH. When that happens, the term "delayed orthostatic hypotension" is used.

OH is more common in elderly men, while POTS typically affects young women between ages 15-50. There is some evidence that when OH occurs in men, age 45-64, it may be a risk factor for stroke [2]. At this time, based on the available research, POTS is not known to be associated with such a risk.

Mitral Valve Prolapse Syndrome and POTS

It was once thought that mitral valve prolapse, an anatomical malformation of the valve located between the left atria and left ventricle of the heart, is the cause of a wide range of seemingly unrelated symptoms in young women. When these symptoms accompanied the finding of Mitral Valve Prolapse, the condition became known as Mitral Valve Prolapse Syndrome.

There have been many misconceptions and misinterpretations about the Mitral Valve Prolapse Syndrome over the years, from its frequency in the general population to its diagnosis and association with symptoms of ANS dysfunction, to its risks of serious complications. Currently, it is felt by many researchers that Mitral Valve Prolapse Syndrome is, in fact, a form of Dysautonomia which is not caused or influenced by the actual finding of mitral valve prolapse.

A landmark study published in one of the most premier medical journals, the New England Journal of Medicine, provided much needed data on mitral valve prolapse [3]. The researchers studied 1845 women and 1646 men by echocardiogram, a test that is used to evaluate the structure and function of the heart. Using special criteria to diagnose mitral valve prolapse on echocardiogram, the authors found that only 2.4% of people had mitral valve prolapse, whereas previous studies reported numbers as high as 5-35%. In addition, the study published in the New England Journal of Medicine showed that people with mitral valve prolapse are not at higher risk of heart disease or stroke compared to people without this finding.

Another interesting study, published in the American Journal of Medicine, examined patients who had Dysautonomia with and without the accompanying mitral valve prolapsed [4]. They studied the results of the autonomic function tests in 118 people with Dysautonomia, 78 of whom had mitral valve prolapse and 40 of whom did not. What researchers found is that there was no significant difference in the test results between the two groups. They concluded that abnormalities in the autonomic function tests occur in patients with Dysautonomia regardless of the presence or absence of mitral valve prolapse.

Furthermore, these researchers found that the most common abnormality in autonomic function tests in patients with or without mitral valve prolapse was an increased heart rate. Therefore, it is probable that POTS and Mitral Valve Prolapse Syndrome is the same disorder. Specifically, people with Mitral Valve Prolapse who demonstrate an increased heart rate of 30 beats per minute (adult patients) or more within 10 minutes of standing have POTS rather than the Mitral Valve Prolapse Syndrome.

If the above explanation has been confusing, consider thinking of Mitral Valve Prolapse Syndrome as the wrong name for the right syndrome. The syndrome, with its many symptoms and signs, is characteristic of a form of Dysautonomia. When a person with Mitral Valve Prolapse displays the diagnostic criteria for POTS, that person has POTS, not Mitral Valve Prolapse Syndrome. If a person with Mitral Valve Prolapse Syndrome displays the diagnostic criteria for orthostatic hypotension, she/he has orthostatic hypotension, not Mitral Valve Prolapse Syndrome.

Chronic Fatigue Syndrome and POTS

Despite various causes proposed for Chronic Fatigue Syndrome (CFS), such as viral, bacterial, autoimmune and autonomic, the precise causes and mechanism of CFS remain unknown. CFS is characterized by severe and persistent fatigue lasting six months or more and causing significant functional impairment and disability. The Center for Disease Control includes eight primary symptoms in the diagnosis of CFS [5]. These include:

- cognitive dysfunction, including impaired memory or concentration
- post - exertional malaise lasting more than 24 hours (ex-

haustion and increased symptoms) following physical or mental exercise
- unrefreshing sleep
- joint pain (without redness or swelling)
- persistent muscle pain
- headaches of a new type or severity
- tender cervical or axillary lymph nodes
- sore throat

In addition to the eight primary defining symptoms of CFS, a number of other symptoms are common. These include:

- irritable bowel, abdominal pain, nausea, diarrhea or bloating
- chills and night sweats
- brain fog
- chest pain
- shortness of breath
- chronic cough
- visual disturbances (blurring, sensitivity to light, eye pain or dry eyes)
- allergies or sensitivities to foods, alcohol, odors, chemicals, medications or noise
- difficulty maintaining upright position (orthostatic instability, irregular heartbeat, dizziness, balance problems or fainting)
- psychological problems (depression, irritability, mood swings, anxiety, panic attacks)
- jaw pain
- weight loss or gain

The relationship between CFS and POTS is complex and is not entirely understood. Some physicians suggest that CFS is caused by an autonomic dysfunction and thus is another form of Dysautonomia [6,7], while others believe that only a percentage of patients with CSF have abnormal function of the autonomic nervous system [8]. One study reported that approximately 25% of adult patients with CFS have evidence of POTS [7].

Fatigue is a common and often the most disabling symptom of POTS, with some patients qualifying for both POTS and CFS diagnoses. Recently, however, it has been suggested that fatigue is the final common pathway of many illnesses and disease processes, which are themselves unrelated (like Multiple Sclerosis, Parkinson's Disease, and Primary Biliary Sclerosis) but which ultimately result in fatigue. [9-11]

Autonomic dysfunction may be associated with mechanisms or causes in the final common pathway resulting in fatigue, but at this time, more research is necessary to precisely define the role Dysautonomia plays in fatigue or CFS.

Anxiety and POTS

One of the major frustrations for patients with POTS is that they are commonly misdiagnosed with anxiety disorders by their doctors. In fact, most patients have been erroneously diagnosed with anxiety at some point in the course of their illness prior to receiving a correct diagnosis of POTS. Even more worrisome and counterproductive is when patients are told that their physical symptoms are "psychological," after which they are sent to a psychiatrist or a psychologist, without proper investigation, diagnosis and management of POTS. Sometimes, an astute mental health professional is able to correctly identify that the patient has an undiagnosed medical condition and refers them back to the referring physician or consults another physician for further evaluation. Lack of knowledge and recognition of POTS in the medical community is a major obstacle to the proper diagnosis and treatment of patients, often resulting in delay of diagnosis, sometimes by as long as decades, financial and psychological burdens on the patient, mistrust of health care providers, strained doctor-patient relationships and non - compliance with doctor's recommendations.

POTS is not a form of anxiety disorder, nor is it caused by anxiety. [12, 13] POTS and anxiety disorders may share common physical symptoms and signs, such as racing heart, palpitations, light-headedness, sweating and trembling, but POTS and anxiety disorders have different mechanisms and causes. Nevertheless, anxiety can be a symptom of POTS in the same fashion as it can be a symptom of thyroid disease. Thus, it is important for health care providers to review the diagnostic criteria for both POTS and anxiety disorders in order to be able to differentiate between the two conditions. Anxiety and its relationship to POTS are also discussed in the chapter, *"Coping with POTS."*

References

1. Low PA, Opfer-Gehrking TL, Textor SC, et. al. Postural Tachycardia Syndrome (POTS). Neurology 1995; 45: S19-S25.
2. Eigenbrodt ML, Rose KM, Couper DJ, Arnett DK, Smith R, Jones D. Orthostatic hypotension as a risk factor for stroke: the atherosclerosis risk in communities (ARIC) study, 1987–1996. Stroke 2000; 31: 2307–2313.
3. Freed LA, Levy D, Levine RA, et. al. Prevalence and clinical outcome of mitral-valve prolapse. NEJM 1999; 341: 1-7.
4. Taylor AA, Davies AO, Mares A, et al. Spectrum of Dysautonomia in mitral valvular prolapse. American Journal of Medicine. 1989;86(3): 267–274.
5. Center for Disease Control
    http://www.cdc.gov/cfs/cfssymptomsHCP.htm
6. Rowe PC, Calkins H. Neurally mediated hypotension and chronic fatigue syndrome. Am J Med 1998; 105:15–21S.
7. Freeman R, Komaroff AL. Does the chronic fatigue syndrome involve the autonomic nervous system? Am J Med 1997; 102: 357–364.
8. Jones JF, Nicholson A, Nisenmaum R, et al. Orthostatic instability in a population-based study of chronic fatigue syndrome. Am J Med 2005; 12: 1415.
9. Newton JL, Allen JA, Kerr S, Jones DEJ. Reduced heart rate variability and baroreflex sensitivity in primary biliary cirrhosis. Liv Int 2006; 26:197–

202.

10. Flackenecker P, Rufer A, Bihler I, Hippel C, Reiners K, Toyka K, et al. Fatigue in MS is related to sympathetic vasomotor dysfunction. Neurology 2003; 61:851–853.

11. Chaudhuri A, Behan P. Fatigue in neurological disorders. Lancet 2004; 363: 978–989.

12. Raj V, Haman KL, Raj SR, et al. Psychiatric profile and attention deficits in postural tachycardia syndrome. JNNP 2009; 80: 339-344.

13. Blitshteyn S. Postural tachycardia syndrome and anxiety disorders. Journal of Neurology, Neurosurgery and Psychiatry, April 8, 2009. http://jnnp.bmj.com /cgi/eletters/80/3/339

Letter from Senator (now President) Obama about POTS

BARACK OBAMA
ILLINOIS

COMMITTEES
HEALTH, EDUCATION, LABOR AND PENSION
HOMELAND SECURITY AND
GOVERNMENTAL AFFAIRS
FOREIGN RELATIONS
VETERANS' AFFAIRS

United States Senate
WASHINGTON, DC 20510-1306

October 28, 2008

Ms. Jodi Rhum

Dear Jodi:

Thank you for contacting me to express your strong support for adequately funding postural orthostatic tachycardia syndrome (POTS) research.

I cannot pretend to understand the pressures that come with having a child with POTS, but I am touched that you thought to write me in support of your daughter, Nikki, and increased funding measures for this disease.

The National Institutes of Health and the Centers for Disease Control and Prevention do excellent work researching many diseases. I agree that we must strengthen the federal commitment to the vital research efforts of both the NIH and CDC. Spending on such medical research is absolutely necessary for the health care community to improve treatments and find cures for the diseases ailing our nation. I have previously requested additional funding to support these federal public health service agencies, above the President's budget request, and I plan to continue to do so. We should devote the highest level of funding possible in support of our federal medical research endeavors.

As you may know, the President's proposed budget for Fiscal Year (FY) '09 would maintain funding levels for the NIH at the same amount as FY '08 at $29.3 billion. In addition, the President's budget proposed cutting funds to the CDC by 7.1%, or $433 million, from $6.1 billion to $5.7 billion. By not increasing the budget level to take into account the rate of inflation, let alone providing new funds, the President's request is inadequate to address our research needs.

Hope is about understanding possibilities, not probabilities. If you leaf through history books, you'll quickly come to see that the true achievers are those who are driven by possibilities, not guided by probabilities. But wishing isn't enough to get there. To make the impossible possible, and the possible probable, we all must keep on fighting and believing. In saying that, during Senate debate on the budget resolution (S. Con. Res. 70) this Spring, I was proud to be an original cosponsor of an amendment by Senators Arlen Specter and Tom Harkin to add $2.1 billion for health programs, including a funding increase to the National Institutes of

WASHINGTON OFFICE   CHICAGO OFFICE   SPRINGFIELD OFFICE   MARION OFFICE   MOLINE OFFICE

Health. For families such as yours living with POTS, I am pleased that this amendment passed the Senate by a vote of 95-4.

Jodi, I see that your strength is a hope to others and that although you have got a difficult set of circumstances to deal with, there are many great things for you to do.

I wish you, Nikki, and the rest of your family strength, hope and love.

Sincerely,

Barack Obama
United States Senator

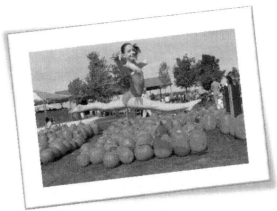

Nikki Rhum

Being Nikki - Personal Story of a 14 Year - Old Girl Living with POTS

My name is Nikki. I am 14 years old, and I live in a suburb of Chicago. The actress Whoopi Goldberg once said, *"The only normal is a setting on my washing machine."* If we are comparing life to washing machines, I would have to say that I have always been on the spin cycle. From as early as I can remember, I would always experience bouts of dizziness. I also had lots of headaches and stomachaches. Strangely, I always felt better when I was upside down. Perhaps that is why I gravitated towards gymnastics. I began doing gymnastics when I was four years old. By the time I turned eight; I was competing and working out in the gym some twelve plus hours a week. My joints always ached, and my mom would put ice packs all over my body. Of course, we always attributed the joint pains to typical gymnastic aches. As the years went on, and I competed more, I began to have more aches and pains, my lower back, neck and wrists hurt, in particular. I began to get more migraines. With more symptoms, I began to have more doctor appointments. I had MRI's and CT scans. Other than a sinus infection, all the tests came back normal. I then began to experience more chest pains (these started when I was six years old). The cardiologist explained that these were normal growing pains (ha, ha) and not to worry. She made me wear a holter monitor for a month and sure enough, the results were normal. At age nine, my foot began to hurt terribly, but I continued to do gymnastics on it. Finally, after a month of being in pain, I went for an X-Ray. It turns out I had a stress fracture in the navicular bone, a bone the orthopedic doctor said he had never seen broken in his 20-year career. I was placed in a cast for six weeks and could not do gymnastics. I was so scared my foot would break again that I didn't want to go back to the gym. My parents forced me back to the gym to at least say goodbye to my team. They knew how much gymnastics meant to me and did not want me to quit on a negative note. It took all my strength and courage to walk back into the gym, but when I did I was so happy that I didn't give up. So I began working out harder than ever. I started competing again and three months later took first place all-around in the state of Illinois for my level.

Over the years, I began to do more complex skills and work out harder and more often. At age 11, I was averaging 17 hours per week working out. My headaches worsened. I went to a neurologist who diagnosed me with migraines and put me on a drug called Periactin. I gained ten pounds in three months (I found out later that this drug is also used to treat anorexics to make them put on weight). The weight gain changed my center of gravity and within three months of beginning the drug therapy, I broke both of my feet at the gym. Two months later, after my feet should have healed, I was still in excruciating pain. The doctor X-Rayed my feet, and proclaimed that they were still broken. Now I was placed in hard casts. After the casts came off, the pain was no better. My feet, especially my left one, burned even upon touch. I had shooting pains and was having a hard time concentrating at school. I was diagnosed with RSD, Reflex Sympathetic Dystrophy, a chronic pain syndrome. I was sent to a pain clinic and was put on lots of drugs that seemed to make all of my symptoms worse instead of better. I began to have problems sleeping. I missed gymnastics and my friends at the gym. I began to go to physical therapy three times a week, had water therapy once a week and went back to the chiropractor. My feet were still killing me. Now I was sent to a psychiatrist, as a few doctors could not understand why I was still in so much pain. It must surely be in my head, so they thought. The psychiatrist immediately reassured me that she did not think it was in my head, at all. She felt strongly that we were missing something medical. She even called my pediatrician to tell him so.

Several months later an article came out about two local girls that had POTS. The article was called POTS, a Life Interrupted. My Nonie found the article. A light bulb went off. The girls' symptoms were identical to mine. My mom called the author of the article and our suspicions were confirmed. We went to see Dr. Blair Grubb, in Toledo, Ohio, where I was officially diagnosed with POTS. I was terrified and relieved at the same time. I now had a real diagnosis, but what now? I cried because I knew I could probably never do gymnastics again.

My symptoms got worse and extreme fatigue set in. I went from getting straight A's in school to barely passing. I cried myself to sleep every night, because I missed the old me. Many friends, family members and teachers questioned my illness. They could not understand how I could look so healthy. Sometimes they saw me at the mall on the weekends and they could not understand how I could be so sick and yet be able to shop. My good friends stuck by me, but I was feeling more and more down and lonely. My Mom took me to healers: massage therapists, chiropractors and acupuncturists, just to mention a few. I was getting more frustrated and mad at her, as nothing seemed to help my symptoms. Some made them worse.

A typical day in my life started with my Mom attempting to wake me up at 6:30 AM. We both knew this was a joke. My head ached, and I was too dizzy to lift my head off of the pillow, let alone attempt to dress myself. I would roll over in protest. *"Give me five more minutes."* This went on over and over again for the next several hours. "You have to take your medicine and go to school," she would yell. "Five more minutes," I would reply. Didn't she realize that I had only fallen asleep two hours earlier? I spent the hours watching TV, chatting on Facebook, and staring at the ceiling. I prayed I could fall asleep, knowing I had to be up in a few hours to go to school. Thinking about getting up for school made me more anxious and made it three times harder to fall asleep. How could I possibly wake up when I just fell asleep? My eyes could not stay open if I pried them open with a pencil. This would continue until noon, when my mom would finally give up and let me sleep; yet another missed day of school. I would take my medicine, roll over and go back to sleep. I would usually sleep until 4:00 P.M., just in time for another round of my medicine. On the rare occasion that my mother's threatening words could get me up, I would go to school and go straight to the nurse's office. One day after my mother forced me to go to school; I ended up on the floor in the hallway. I was too dizzy to walk and my head felt like someone was hammering the inside of my skull. My heart was racing and the walls felt like they were closing in on me. Everything went black. I could not stand any longer. Some of my friends ran for the nurse. My pulse was so weak she could barely feel it. My mother came to get me. I told her that I knew I could not make it. She needed to listen to me. After all, I knew my own body. We decided at that point, that I needed to be home tutored. This took some pressure off, but I still yearned to be with my friends and lead a normal life.

The next year, in seventh grade, I made a new friend at school who was having her own medical issues. Some of them seemed similar to mine. As it turns out, she was diagnosed with POTS too. Finally, I had someone who totally understood how I was feeling. We hung out all year and helped each other through many tough times. A third person in my grade was diagnosed shortly after.

By the end of seventh grade, I was feeling worse and had to

once again be home tutored. I kept in touch with friends via Facebook. I was getting more down. My blood pressure was so low; it was too dangerous for me to exercise. I was put on Midodrine to raise my pressure. This was one of the first drugs that really seemed to help. I felt a bit more like myself. My mom sent me to an herbalist and made me work out with a trainer two times a week. This combination seemed to make a difference. I slowly began to feel a bit better and was able to exercise without too much difficulty. After two years of not being able to do gymnastics, I was finally able to go back to the gym a couple of times. It made me feel so good to be back. To my surprise, I found that I had not lost all of my skills!

Having POTS has taught me a lot. I am more sympathetic toward other people and know firsthand how bad it feels to be stared at or judged. I now know that I have to appreciate every good moment, and I need to live in the present. I am a stronger person, as I have to face so many obstacles every day. I know I can never give up, and I can never give in to my illness. I have had to redefine myself. I used to always be known as "the gymnast." POTS forced me to recreate myself. I began to have more friends outside of the gym, and I learned to discover new and hidden talents that I had. I discovered that I loved to write. It really helped to get my emotions out on paper. Now that gymnastics was out of the picture, I began to have more free time with my friends to go to movies, the mall and play on my computer. I learned that an illness cannot define you. You are the driver of your own vehicle, and you can take it anywhere you want to go.

Because of my illness, I also got to meet many wonderful people. After being diagnosed in the sixth grade, I wrote a paper about a book I read called, *"The Peaceful Warrior"*. This book paralleled my injury and my gymnastics career. I won first place in the state of Illinois for writing this paper and I got to meet and spend time with Jesse White, the Secretary of State. Through Chai Lifeline, a Jewish Organization that supports kids with chronic illnesses, I got to go to an overnight camp for two weeks in New York. I met so many terrific people at this camp.

I also got the opportunity of a lifetime when I was granted a wish from an incredible organization. They sent my whole family and me to the Beijing Olympics to watch women's gymnastics. We got to meet the entire US Olympic Gymnastics Team. They were so nice to me. Chellsie Memmel, one of the gymnasts, even gave me her winning bouquet of flowers. We met other wonderful people in China too. Our translator, named Pongo, carried me all the way up to the Great Wall on his back, because I was too dizzy to walk and my wheelchair could not make it up the cobblestone path. I met a volunteer at the Olympic Stadium who wrote and sang a song for me, the first song he had ever written in English. The person who granted my wish still calls me every day to see how I am feeling.

I would never have met any of these people, if it had not been for my illness. I now try to think of all of the positive things in my life and try not to dwell on the bad things I have been given. I have great friends, great family and great doctors. Despite my condition, I feel I am truly blessed. I know I will get through this, and I will be a better, stronger, and kinder person because of it. I will not let my illness stop me from living the life I want to lead. I am even planning on trying out for the high school gymnastics team next year. My mom always loved the quote, *"Do not wait for the storm to pass, learn to dance in the rain."* I am sick of being sick, and I am ready to dance again.

Nikki Rhum

**Section 2. Riding the
Waves of Dysautonomia**

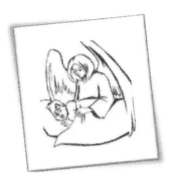

POTS Lullaby

Now I lay me down to bed, I pray the Lord to fall asleep.
Angels watch me through the night, and wake me with the morning light.
I count sheep, I count shepherds, and I sing lullabies,
I text, I watch reruns of Nick at Night,
Still no sleep is in sight
I pray if I ever do fall asleep that when I wake,
The Earth will not spin and the ground will not shake.
I pray that if I can rise, my heart will not race, my chest will not pound and my head and joints will not ache.
I pray to the Lord that when I get out of my bed, I won't feel nauseous,
Please allow me to run, skip and play like the other kids on my block, without having to be so cautious.
I want things to be the way they were before,
when I could go all day and not be so exhausted,
I pray to the Lord, they will once more.
Now I lay me down to sleep,
I pray the Lord, my energy to restore.

Written by: Jodi Rhum

Chapter 1. Combating Insomnia

"A flock of sheep that leisurely pass byone after one; the sound of rain, and beesmurmuring; the fall of rivers, winds and seas, smooth fields, white sheets of water, and pure sky - I've thought of all by turns, and still I lie Sleepless." - William Wordsworth

"If a man had as many ideas during the day as he does when he has insomnia, he'd make a fortune." - Griff Niblack

Sleep is almost as vital to the body as is breathing. Sleep restores energy to the body, especially to the nervous system. Sleep allows the body to repair itself. During sleep our heart rate and blood pressure fall, our muscles relax and our body rebalances itself. Despite its importance, most people take sleep for granted.

Insomnia is often a common complaint among those who have Dysautonomia. Insomnia often not only affects the patient, but also can affect the entire family unit. Anyone who suffers from insomnia knows firsthand how horrific of a problem this is. Not being able to fall asleep or having interrupted sleep is one of the most frustrating and anxiety provoking things a person can experience. As a matter of fact, sleep deprivation has long been used as a wartime torture. Those of you who suffer from insomnia live this on a daily basis. Insomnia is one of mankind's oldest complaints. It affects one in ten Americans and about 30 percent of seniors. Insomnia is such a major issue among people who suffer from Dysautonomia, that I have devoted an entire chapter to it.

First, it is prudent to investigate why you are having insomnia in the first place. Sometimes the sleep disturbance may be due to extreme dizziness, migraine headache, effects of the medications you are on, intolerable pain, etc. In some cases, the person who has Dysautonomia has increased levels of adrenalin in the blood stream due to orthostatic stress, the stress of standing upright. These elevated adrenalin levels often make optimum sleep difficult to achieve.

It is also imperative to rule out sleep apnea. Sleep apnea is a condition whereby the person actually stops breathing while they sleep. Sleep apnea is one of the major causes of insomnia, affecting about 20 million Americans. This can happen repeatedly up to 200 times a night and keeps a person from entering REM (Rapid Eye Movements or REM is the fifth stage of sleep, where dreaming occurs and is the most important stage of sleep). Sleep apnea occurs more frequently in those people who snore. A formal sleep study can be conducted to rule sleep apnea out.

Once underlying issues of insomnia have been dispelled, there are many natural aids as well as pharmaceutical medications available to help achieve a normal and healthy sleep cycle. Whether or not you choose to alleviate your symptoms of insomnia by going the natural route or taking pharmaceutical drugs, you should first discuss your plan of action with your team of physicians. Below are some helpful hints that may help you to combat insomnia.

Turn your bedroom into a Sleep Haven
Your room should be kept completely dark. The temperature should be kept at 70 degrees or less. A fan is often helpful to help keep the temperature cool. Playing soft music or nature sounds can be very calming. Do not watch TV, text friends or work on the computer before going to sleep; instead, read a good book or write in a journal. Bright lights and stimulating activity, before bedtime, should be avoided at all cost.

> *Note: Alarm clocks and cable box lights may prohibit sleep.*

Melatonin

Melatonin is a neurohormone that is released from the pineal gland during sleep. Throughout our life, melatonin is produced in abundance but begins to decrease after puberty and throughout the rest of our days. This may account for the fact the older we get, the harder it is to fall asleep.

Melatonin helps produce a substance called argine vasotocin, which inhibits an adrenal gland stress hormone called cortisol. Scientists have discovered that there are increased levels of stress hormones with people that have chronic insomnia. Melatonin helps induce sleep by providing arginine vasoctin to inhibit cortisol production. Melatonin may also help regulate REM sleep and as it is an antioxidant, may be helpful in warding off certain types of cancers.

Melatonin is most effective when taken one hour before your desired bedtime. Always begin with a small dosage (1mg or less). Melatonin can lower blood pressure, so it is important, especially if you already have low blood pressure, to speak with your physicians before taking any dosage of Melatonin.

> *IMPORTANT: It is critical that if you are taking Melatonin, you sleep in total darkness. Natural Melatonin production can only take place in total darkness. A nightlight, closet light or even an alarm clock light can interfere with natural Melatonin Production. If you do not like to sleep in total darkness, "eye pillows" can provide a good alternative.*

Avoid Caffeine

Avoid all forms of caffeine after 3:00 PM, or at least six hours before you plan on going to sleep. Avoid coffee, tea, soda, chocolate, and antihistamines. All forms of caffeine remain in your system for up to six hours and may prevent you from falling asleep.

Avoid late night snacking

Try to avoid eating snacks or heavy meals for up to two to

three hours before bedtime. Digestion places heavy energy demands on the body, especially for someone who has Dysautonomia, and can interfere with deep sleep. If you wake up in the middle of the night and cannot fall back to sleep, try to avoid eating. If you cannot, try to eat something very light.

Excessive fluids before bedtime should be avoided

This can help prevent late night bathroom runs. If you feel the need to drink before bedtime try a warm liquid like warm milk (this contains tryptophan, an amino acid, that helps induce sleep) or chamomile tea.

Do not participate in any vigorous activities one to two hours before bedtime

Although POTS patients often feel better at night and are usually more apt to want to exercise after dinnertime, exercising heavily too soon before bedtime is not a good idea.

Avoid taking medications before bedtime that contain alcohol and or caffeine

Many over the counter cough syrups, pain relievers and headache medications contain alcohol and or caffeine. Be sure to read all labels carefully.

Avoid mid-day naps

This can really throw off your sleep cycle; throwing your body into a nocturnal pattern. Will yourself to stay up and attempt to go to sleep for the evening a few hours earlier.

Wear warm socks to bed or consider soaking your feet in warm water for ten minutes before bedtime

Keeping the feet warm has been known to induce restful sleep.

Calcium and Magnesium Supplements

Using a magnesium supplement could be your best natural bet for insomnia relief. Because magnesium relaxes your body's muscles and has a calming effect, it will help bring you insomnia relief by reducing stress and anxiety, as well as calming jumpy legs and jerking during sleep. In many, cases, after taking magnesium supplements, people have woken up less and have slept for longer periods of time through the night, giving them their much needed deep sleep, which is imperative for the body to regenerate itself. They also found that they were much more relaxed, which helped them to fall asleep faster. Unfortunately, over the years, our soil has become more and more depleted of magnesium. Our surface water supply is also low in magnesium, and on top of that, our process of preparing food by way of steaming, boiling and broiling, further removes magnesium from our diets. Magnesium is the 4th most abundant mineral in our bodies and is necessary for over 350 different bodily processes, including digestion, energy production, muscle function, bone formation, creation of new cells, activation of B vitamins, relaxation of muscles, as well as assisting in the functions of the heart, kidneys, adrenals, brain and nervous system. Lack of sufficiently available magnesium in the body can interfere with all of these processes, including sleep.

Magnesium depletion can be caused by a variety of physical factors, including over-training, surgery, sweating, consumption of caffeine, alcohol, tobacco, certain medications, increased perspiration, low thyroid function, diabetes, chronic pain, and a high carbohydrate, high-sodium or high-calcium diet.

Many people do not realize that Calcium and magnesium have some polar opposite functions in the body. Calcium excites nerves while magnesium calms them down. Calcium makes muscles contract, while magnesium is necessary for muscles to relax. Calcium is also needed for blood clotting, whereas, magnesium keeps the blood flowing freely. It is vital to keep these minerals in balance. Too little magnesium to balance calcium can be unhealthy. Also, to ward off the negative effects of stress, calcium needs to be balanced with adequate amounts of magnesium.

Calcium and magnesium supplements should be given with dinner and before bedtime. One can also take more in the night if one wakes up and cannot fall back asleep. It could take 15-30 minutes for a calcium tablet to dissolve in the stomach. For a more rapid effect during the night, chew or grind up a tablet, or use a liquid preparation. Speak to your doctor before using any supplements.

Morning awakenings should be firmly fixed:

Awakenings should not vary for more than one and a half hours on weekends, school days and holidays. Sticking to a schedule can help your body get into a healthy routine.

Chapter 2. Surviving Syncope

According to Blair Grubb, MD, syncopal episodes account for 6% of ER visits and 3% of hospital admissions in the U.S.

As stated earlier on the book, syncope, or fainting, is a medical term used to describe a brief loss of consciousness caused by a sudden lack of blood (oxygen) supply to the brain. It is estimated that about 30% of people who have Dysautonomia faint. Many people, who have POTS, experience presyncope. During presyncope episodes, symptoms are similar to a faint but no loss of consciousness is experienced.

My 14 year old daughter, who has POTS, describes episodes where everything in her vision will turn black or white. She will then get so dizzy, she will go to the ground, but does not lose consciousness. Eventually, the spell will pass and she is able to stand upright again.

Roughly half of all humans will experience syncope at least once during their lifetime. There are many types of syncope but the most common type is known as Vasovagal Syncope, also called Reflex Syncope or Neurocardiogenic Syncope. This type of fainting, known as the "common faint," is not caused by a problem with the rhythm or structure of the heart. Neurocardiogenic syncope is the most common type of fainting that is associated with POTS. In Vasovagal Syncope, the heart rate goes down or may even stop for a second (bradycardia) and the blood pressure drops severely (hypotension). This mechanism happens in all humans but in some, those with autonomic dysfunctions, it happens in a more exaggerated form. In people who experience syncope, this reflex will slow down the blood circulation. As a result not enough oxygenated blood gets to the brain resulting in dizziness and finally syncope.

Many syncope sufferers will experience a simple faint. This is a faint where you have a warning before becoming unconscious. Common warnings signals may include: going pale, feeling dizzy, cold sweats, feeling nauseous or visual disturbances. With a common faint, loss of consciousness will be brief and a full recovery will be made. Complex fainting, on the other hand, may involve a far more dramatic set of circumstances. Complex faints often have no precursors or warnings. They may appear to come out of nowhere. There may be jerking of the limbs and in some cases there is incontinence. Complex fainting often may look like a seizure, and may have a longer unconscious and recovery period than the simple faint. It is important to get this checked out, as you need to rule out epilepsy as the root of the syncopal episode. In either case, the act of fainting can be very scary and traumatic, not just for the person fainting but also for everyone who witnesses the faint.

Common Triggers of Fainting Include:

- Anxiety
- Stress
- Warm environments
- Positional changes (i.e. from lying to standing)
- Loud noises
- Traumatic events

- Migraines
- Site of blood or blood draws
- Blood loss (menstruation)
- Bowel movement or urination
- Standing still for long durations of time (blood   pooling)
- Dehydration
- Flashing light

Syncope Tips

- Drink lots of water. Never let yourself become dehydrated.
- Increase your salt intake to keep up blood volume.
- Avoid large meals. Instead, eat six small meals a day.
- Try to avoid straining when making bowel movements.
- After necessary blood draws, eat a salty snack and drink some juice. Have this with you on hand as not all labs will provide this for you.
- Eat salty snacks throughout the day.
- When it is necessary to stand, do not stand perfectly still. Move when you can to maintain better blood flow.
- Change positions slowly. Do not get out of bed or rise from a sitting position too quickly. Dr. Grubb advises to first sit on the side of the bed for a few minutes before you try to stand up. If dizzy, sit back down for another few minutes.
- Sit down in a squat like position or lie down with your legs up in the air as soon as you feel dizzy, your vision dims, you have cold sweats or notice any other sign of a faint to come.
- Keep yourself cool. Avoid allowing yourself to become overheated.
- Exercises that use the calf muscles such as walking, climbing stairs, squats and lunges may improve your symp-

toms.

- Try to get enough sleep whenever possible.
- If you feel faint, never take the stairs. You are not only putting yourself at risk, but you are putting those around you in danger as well.
- "Tilt-training" will build your endurance. Stand at a slight angle with your back against the wall, heels twelve inches away, for 30 minutes twice a day. In some people, this results in a complete disappearance of the fainting episodes.
- Be extra vigilant in following these recommendations during menstruation. Some individuals experience an increase in syncope during this time.

A fabulous organization known as STARS, (Syncope Trust and Reflex Anoxic Seizures) is a great resource for those POTS sufferers who also have syncope. They are based in the USA and England. Their web address is *www.stars.org.uk* Stars has published a "blackout checklist" to aid you and your doctor in finding the correct diagnosis for your syncope.

A blackout is a temporary loss of consciousness, If someone loses consciousness for a few seconds or minutes, they are often said to have had a blackout.

Every patient presenting with an unexplained blackout should be given a 12-lead ECG (heart rhythm check). It is important that the ECG is passed as normal.

Most unexplained blackouts are caused by syncope. Many people, including doctors, assume that blackouts are due to epileptic seizures, but much more commonly, they are due to syncope (pronounced sin-co-pee), a type of blackout which is caused by a problem in the regulation of blood pressure or sometimes with the heart.

Syncope can affect all age groups but the causes vary with age, and in older adults multiple causes often exist.

There are three major reasons for why people may experience a fainting episode:

1) Syncope: a medical term for a blackout that is caused by sudden lack of blood supply to the brain. Syncope is caused by a problem in the regulation of blood pressure or by a problem with the heart.

2) Epilepsy: an electrical 'short-circuiting' in the brain. Epileptic attacks are usually called seizures. Diagnosis of epilepsy is made by a neurologist. It is important to rule out seizures as the cause of syncope.

3) Psychogenic blackouts: resulting from stress or anxiety. Psychogenic blackouts occur most often in young adults. They may be very difficult to diagnose. 'Psychogenic' does not mean that people are 'putting it on'. However there is often underlying stress due to extreme pressure at school or work. In exceptional cases it may be that some people have experienced ill treatment or abuse in childhood.

Misdiagnosis is common but avoidable:

- Many syncopal attacks are mistaken for epilepsy.
- However epilepsy only affects slightly less than 1% of the population.
- UK research has shown that approximately 30% of adults and up to 40% of children diagnosed with epilepsy in the UK do not have the condition.
- Many elements of a syncopal attack, such as random jerking of limbs, are similar to those experienced during an epileptic seizure.
- It can be difficult to tell the causes of the blackout apart.

Syncope causes falls:

- Syncope causes a significant number of falls in older adults, particularly where the falls are sudden and not obviously the result of a trip or slip.
- Many older adults will only recall a fall and will not realize they have blacked out.
- Greater awareness of syncope as a cause of falls is key to effective treatment and prevention of recurring falls.

STARS Blackouts Checklist

The Blackouts Checklist was prepared under the guidance of STARS' expert Medical Advisory Committee. Its principal aim is to help you and your doctor reach the correct diagnosis for any unexplained loss of consciousness (fainting).

The Checklist gives you information and advice on the major reasons for experiencing a faint, helps you prepare for a doctor's appointment, and provides information on what to expect if you have to attend a hospital appointment.

CHECKLIST: Preparing for an appointment with your Doctor

o Before visiting your doctor, it is important to write down what happens before, during and after a faint or fall, including any symptoms you may experience.

o Try to take along a family member or friend who has seen your blackout(s) or fall(s) to your appointment. If they cannot accompany you, ask them to write down exactly what they saw in the Checklist or ask them how the doctor could contact them if necessary. If they can video an attack this is often very helpful.

o Family history; check with relatives whether there is any family history of blackouts, faints, epilepsy, or sudden/ unexplained deaths. This is important as it can often provide a clue to the possible cause of your fainting.

o If there are any questions you want to ask your doctor or specialist, make a note of them on the Checklist as it can be easy to

forget to ask them during the consultation.
o   Check that both syncope and epilepsy have been considered.
    Ask for referral to a syncope expert, if possible, or to both a
    cardiologist and a neurologist if you are not sure that the diag-
    nosis is accurate. You could ask about possible referral to local
    rapid-access clinics for fainting, falls or arrhythmias.
o   Make detailed notes.

Take the Checklist and your notes with you to your appointment.

CHECKLIST: Questions to ask your Doctor

o   Can I still go to school or work while I am waiting to see the
    specialist?
o   Can I go to the gym/play sports while I am waiting to see the
    specialist?
o   Can I still drive while I am waiting to see the specialist?
o   What is the likelihood that a diagnostic test will deliver a defini-
    tive result?
o   What will the treatment involve? Do you think I will have to visit
    the hospital frequently or stay overnight?

CHECKLIST: Preparing for specialist tests at the hospital

Following your appointment with the doctor you may be
referred for some tests with a specialist to discover the cause of
your fainting. Being prepared for these can significantly reduce the
anxiety of a hospital visit. Try to learn about these tests in advance
at www.stars.org.uk

The latest guidelines on the diagnosis of syncope state that
patients suspected of having syncope should receive one of the following tests. Make sure that you receive the right test based on the
nature of your symptoms.

There are information sheets on the following diagnostic

tests available from www.stars.org.uk

Every patient presenting with an unexplained blackout should be given a 12-lead ECG.

If there is uncertainty about diagnosis the ECG should be reviewed by a heart rhythm specialist (Electro physiologist).

Tests aimed at syncope:

o Lying and standing blood pressure recording - Drops in blood pressure with changes in posture can cause dizziness, falls and blackouts, particularly in older patients and those on blood pressure and water tablets.

o Tilt Table Testing - This procedure can be used to induce a syncopal/fainting attack while connected to heart and blood pressure monitors.

o Heart Monitor - This is used to record heart rhythms whilst away from the hospital or to activate during an episode. A 24-hour/7 day heart rate monitor is very unlikely to identify any problems if you experience fainting episodes once a week or less, so do not be afraid to ask about other options.

o Implantable Loop Recorder (ILR) - This device should be used to monitor heart rhythms for months at a time if the episodes are less frequent than every 4 weeks. The device can remain in place for up to 3 years.

Tests aimed at epileptic seizures:

o Electroencephalogram (EEG) - For brain activity analysis to check for epilepsy. The EEG cannot be used to diagnose epilepsy, but it is helpful to neurologists to decide which type of epilepsy is happening. The EEG is much less useful over the age of 35 years.

o MRI or CT- scan - These are not aimed at showing that someone has epilepsy, but are used to seek the cause when epilepsy is likely.

Visit www.Stars.og.uk for more valuable information on syncope and a very helpful checklist that you can bring to your doctors' appointments.

Chapter 3. Dysautonomia Don'ts- Things to Avoid

Alcohol
Can cause dehydration. It can also enhance venous pooling, which will exacerbate symptoms.

Anesthesia
When anesthesia is necessary an arterial line should be inserted to monitor blood pressure. Pulse should be monitored constantly and extra IV fluids should be considered, before, during and after anesthesia.

Bed Rest
Keep the body moving to prevent atrophy of the muscles and deconditioning of the heart. Bed rest, in the long run, will make a person with Dysautonomia more symptomatic. On days when it is impossible to get out of bed, consider doing some simple exercising in bed. For example, lifting small hand weights, squeezing a stress ball, tightening and releasing your thigh and buttocks muscles, and writing the alphabet in the air with your toes.

Bending at the waist
When bending is necessary, be sure to bend at the knee and squat down rather than bending at the waist.

Blowing up Balloons
Hyperventilation can cause extreme dizziness in certain individuals with Dysautonomia.

Climbing Stairs
Though climbing stairs is great exercise, it can cause fatigue in some patients for the rest of the day. Avoid climbing stairs unattended when feeling dizzy.

Caffeine

Caffeine can trigger migraines in some people, while it can abort a headache in others. It is important to know your own body and the unique sensitivities you may have. Caffeine acts as a diuretic and may lead to dehydration. It may also cause an increase in heart rate. Instead of caffeine, try an apple. Apples have 20 grams of carbohydrates and can give you as much energy as a cup of coffee without the inevitable crash.

Carbohydrates

Excessive carbohydrates can cause a rise in sugar (glucose) levels. This in turn increases insulin levels, which may exacerbate POTS symptoms.

Chocolate

Chocolate contains caffeine and can trigger migraines.

NOTE: My friend, who is extremely sensitive to chocolate and suffers from migraines, says the only chocolate that does not affect her is SEE'S CANDIES. If you are a chocoholic, it is worth a try.

Co - Q10

This supplement can lower blood pressure by up to 30% in some people. This could potentially interfere with other blood pressure medications you may be taking.

Dairy Products

Dairy products increase symptoms in some people with Dysautonomia.

Disbelieving Doctors

If your doctor tells you this illness is all in your head, or due to anxiety, run as quickly as you can and do not stop until you find a doctor that, knows about Dysautonomia or is willing to research it and learn more about it.

Energy Drinks
Large amounts of caffeine can cause tachycardia and dehydration. Red Bull, an energy drink, actually triggered a case of POTS, in a volleyball player, who drank an excessive amount.

Epinephrine
This is sometimes found in Lidocaine based numbing agents like those used at the dentist or for biopsies. This can stimulate the heart and cause an increased pulse rate. Ask for a stimulant free numbing agent like plain Lidocaine.

Fatigue
Make it a priority to get enough sleep. Do not attempt to "catch up" on days you feel well. Don't try to cram a month's worth of activities into one day. It is critical to stay well rested and avoid the notorious "crash."

Fried Foods
Fatty food can worsen delayed gastric emptying. Fried foods also often times contain MSG, which can cause headaches in many people.

Garlic
In large amounts, garlic can lower blood pressure.

Ginseng
This herb can stimulate adrenalin.

Giving Blood
Most people with POTS need to continually increase fluid and salt intake to maintain blood volume, and thus, blood pressure. Giving blood may lower blood volume and exacerbate symptoms.

Gluten
Many people have gluten sensitivities. Try taking gluten out of your diet for several days. You may be surprised that some of your symptoms may improve. If so, you can be tested for a gluten sensitivity or Celiac Disease. It can take a few weeks to notice an improvement.

Heat
Heat causes capillaries to dilate in the largest organ of the body - your skin. The result is peripheral venous pooling and reduced blood flow back to the general circulation. Avoid being outside on hot days. Avoid hot showers, hot baths, Jacuzzis, steam rooms, saunas, or crowded spaces.

High Elevation
Barometric pressure is lower at high altitudes. Low barometric pressure exacerbates symptoms in some people who have Dysautonomia. Planning a vacation in the mountains, for example, may be inviting more symptoms.

Holding Your Arms above Your Head
By raising your arms and working with your hands over your head, you require your heart to work extra hard to counteract the effects of gravity. The result can be tachycardia and fatigue.

Large Meals
A large meal requires a lot of work to digest! Blood flow must be shifted to the abdomen and away from the general circulation. The effect is lower blood volume available to the brain, a situation that is similar to peripheral blood pooling or dehydration. Instead, eat smaller amounts more frequently, such as six small meals a day. Give yourself snacks often. Avoid getting too hungry so you are not tempted to eat a large meal.

MSG (monosodium glutamate)

MSG can aggravate POTS Symptoms. MSG is found in a myriad of foods. Some of the top offenders are: Doritos, Cheetos, soy sauce, bouillon cubes, most salad dressings, seasoning salts, powdered cheeses (Mac & Cheese), flavored chips, gelatin, processed meats, diet drinks, and others.

> *Note: NATURAL FLAVORS- food labels that say their product contains "natural flavors" may contain up to 20% of MSG.*

Nitrates

Found in almost all processed lunchmeats and hot dogs, nitrates can cause migraines in many people.

Over Stimulating Environments

Many people who have Dysautonomia are sensitive to light and noise. Avoid over stimulating situations whenever possible.

Pharmaceutical drugs can lower your blood pressure.

Be wary of the following drugs and be sure to consult your physician before starting any of these medications:

A-Receptor blockers
Angiotensin-converting-enzyme inhibitors
B-Blockers
Bromocriptine
Calcium channel blockers
Diuretics
Ethanol
Ganglionic blocking agents
Hydralazine
Monoamine oxidase inhibitors
Opiates
Phenothiazines

Viagra
Tricyclic Antidepressants
Salt containing aluminum

Many salts and salt products can contain aluminum. Aluminum is usually added as a drying agent to keep the salt from clumping. A deficiency of trace minerals and the addition of aluminum are both detrimental to one's health. Aluminum is a toxic metal, which is considered by some researchers to be linked with Alzheimer's disease.
Be sure to read all salt labels. Many holistic practitioners recommend Celtic Salt or Sea Salt, because it is aluminum free. Morton Salt says that they also no longer use aluminum in their product.

Straining
Avoid straining such as when lifting or making a bowel movement. Straining can raise cerebral spinal fluid pressure. Straining too much during a bowel movement can cause lack of blood to the brain, causing syncope or near syncope.

Standing Too Quickly
This is never a good idea for anyone but is especially not a smart idea for the person who has Dysautonomia. Be sure to get up slowly. You should sit at your bedside for at least 12 seconds before rising to a standing position.

Interesting fact: The Modeh Ani is a Jewish prayer that is recited every morning upon waking up. It should be said while sitting on the bed before standing up in the morning. It is a prayer that gives thanks to the Almighty for allowing us to wake up healthy and whole. The Modeh Ani is made up of 12 words. If said slowly this prayer should take precisely 12 seconds to recite.

Mode Ani Lefanecha Melech Chai VeKayam, Shehechezarta Bi Nishmati Bechemla Raba Emunatecha - 'I thank Thee, O living and eternal King, because Thou hast graciously restored my soul to me; great is Thy faithfulness.'

Professor Linda McMaron of Great Britain studied the subject of syncope. She came to the conclusion that fainting is caused by a sharp transfer between laying and standing up. Professor McMaron said that it takes precisely 12 seconds for the blood to flow from the feet to the brain. She said that when this process happens too quickly the blood get "thrown" to the brain too quickly and may result in syncope. She suggested that all people, even those that do not have a tendency to faint, should sit on the bed and count to 12 to avoid dizziness, weakness and or fainting. Jewish people have recited this prayer for centuries. The 12 seconds that the Modeh Ani takes to recite provides a poetic 12 seconds not only to help the blood to properly get to the brain but to also take time to give thanks for the gift of the day to come.

Vinegar

Any product containing vinegar, especially apple cider vinegar, can lower blood pressure by up to 30%. Most condiments contain vinegar so be sure to check all labels.

White Sugar:

Too much white sugar can cause increased venous pooling in the gut, which may cause hypotension.

See Dinet.org for a more expansive list.

Chapter 4. Dysautonomia Q & A, a Mother's View

This section is not endorsed by any of the medical doctors, who have written in this book. This is solely the view of the author and various healthcare professionals.

Frequently asked questions

Over the years, I have asked doctors a myriad of questions about Dysautonomia. I have also been asked many questions. Below are some of the common questions I have been asked and explanations that I have researched. Perhaps they can alleviate some of your concerns.

Q. How did I get POTS?

A. They say doctors practice medicine for a very valid reason. The practice of medicine is just that, a practice. The autonomic nervous system is a very complex system that doctors seem to know little about. In some cases, POTS may be hereditary. It lays dormant until it is triggered. Many things can trigger Dysautonomia. The most common triggers are as follows:

1. **A viral or bacterial infection** - Many people told me their illness was triggered after strep throat, the flu or mononucleosis.
2. **Diabetes** - Uncontrolled diabetes can cause neuropathy which can cause POTS
3. **Toxic chemicals** - Some Gulf War Veterans developed POTS after being exposed to pesticides and nerve gas.
4. **Adverse reactions to prescription drugs**
5. **Growth spurt during puberty**
6. **Trauma** - My daughter became ill after breaking both of her feet, doing competitive gymnastics. This seemed to trigger it.
7. **Pregnancy** - possibly due to increased hormones and

changes in blood volume.

8. Norepinephrine transporter deficiency - a genetic neurotransmitter disorder that affects catecholamine production and release.

9. Vagus nerve damage (cranial nerve 10) or spinal cord

10. Rapid weight loss

11. Alcoholism

12. Ehlers-Danlos Syndrome, a connective tissue disorder,
which allows veins to dilate excessively. Most people who
have this are very flexible, double jointed and have stretchy
velvety skin.

13. Spinal cord stenosis in the upper cervical spine.

14. Chiari 1 malformation - a condition in which brain tissue
protrudes into the spinal canal, trapping cerebral spinal fluid. It occurs when part of your skull is too small or crowded;
pressing on your brain and forcing it downward. The hallmark symptoms of Chiari include severe headaches, (especially in the back of the head) fatigue, dizziness, vertigo,
light sensitivity, neck pain, etc. A MRI (Preferably in a
standing or sitting position) can rule this out.

Q. Who gets POTS?

A. Anybody can get POTS, but it's more common in:

- High achievers (successful in school, athletics, Etc.)
- Females
- People who are flexible or double jointed.

Autonomic dysfunction can occur at any age. For teens, it is often
within a year of starting puberty. Teens can often connect their
symptoms with a specific event or trigger:

- Acute illness such as a respiratory infection (cold virus),
intestinal viral infection, or "mono" or a "mono-like" infec-

tion
- Injury
- Major surgery or a stay in the hospital
- Weight loss

Q. Am I lazy?

A. This could not be further from the truth. Most people, who have Dysautonomia, are quite the opposite. They push themselves beyond their limits. They are typically strong bodied and willed. Many were former athletes and most are high achievers. Upon standing, an individual's heart rate goes up. The heart rate of a person who has Dysautonomia goes up excessively high in an attempt to bring the blood pressure back to a more normal level. This process is extremely taxing on the body. Dr. Blair Grubb says that the heart of a person that has Dysautonomia has to work three times as hard as a person that does not have this illness. That means that everything the person with Dysautonomia does, takes three times more energy than that of an average individual. This is extremely stressful on the body and can cause unremitting fatigue.

Q. Why do I have such poor balance?

A. This may be caused by decreased blood flow to the brain and other vestibular system disturbances. Orthostatic intolerance and the feeling of always being dizzy, may contribute to poor balance, as well. Patients with Dysautonomia often have an abnormal gait and may walk with their legs wide apart and feet flared to the side to compensate for their poor balance. Patients are often unable to walk in a straight line placing one foot in front of the other, making it almost impossible for some to pass a drunk driving test, even when totally sober.

Q. Why did I have to go to so many doctors before I could be diagnosed?

A. Most doctors have little experience diagnosing and treating POTS patients, because many did not study this syndrome in medical school.

A person who has Dysautonomia usually has normal (to a bit low) blood pressure when in a sitting position. This is normally how blood pressure is taken in the doctor's office, so it can be misleading. Also, symptoms are so all encompassing and seem disconnected that doctors often pass them off as anxiety, hypochondria, or depression. Patients are sent on a medical scavenger hunt, often having to put the pieces together themselves. Many patients, who complain of headaches and dizziness, are sent to a neurologist, who may tell them they suffer from migraines or vertigo. After experimenting with various pharmaceutical drugs, their symptoms fail to disappear and often become more pronounced. Tell the doctor you are having joint pain and you end up at the rheumatologist. Mention frequent urination, you are at the urologist; mention feeling bloated, go straight to the GI specialist. Visual disturbances lead you to the ophthalmologist. Mention loss of appetite, anxiety, heart palpitations, fatigue, or insomnia, and you have now been sentenced to a dozen sessions with the psychiatrist, with a possible diagnosis of depression, hypochondria, anxiety, or an eating disorder. Of course, this is not a real diagnosis and you end up as sick as ever. The only exception is now you are filled with self-doubt, and begin wondering if you really are going crazy. Could all of these symptoms just be a figment of my imagination? Am I hyper sensitive? Do I have an extremely low pain tolerance? With such a disconnected healthcare system one hand does not know what the other hand does. Each doctor fits your symptoms into his or her own specialty and does not see the whole picture, the gestalt. Nobody bothers to connect the dots; often leaving the patient frustrated and without answers. It is therefore prudent to find a doctor, and there are plenty great doctors out there, who does understand the complexity of POTS.

Interesting Fact: Animals can get Dysautonomia too. My friend, who is a veterinarian, knew more about Dysautonomia, than my former pediatrician. Animals get Dysautonomia less frequently than humans, yet veterinarians study the illness in veterinarian school!

Q. I often see tiny black spots or squiggly lines floating in my eyes. Is this normal?
A. It is normal for the person with Dysautonomia to see black spots in their vision. It is due to fluid in the eyes, which can happen when your autonomic nervous system is deregulated. This happens naturally in aging individuals but is common among POTS patients and patients with CFS, chronic fatigue syndrome.

Note: When I was a little girl, I thought these black dots were gumballs falling from the sky. I used to try to catch them in my hands. I always thought I was crazy, I am relieved to learn 40 years later, that I am not as nuts as I thought.

Q. Why can't I remember things? Am I suffering from early onset Alzheimer's?
A. Memory impairment, or brain fog, as we refer to it in the POTS world, is a common complaint among Dysautonomia patients. It is due to lack of adequate blood flow to the brain.

Q. I have never fainted. Do all people with POTS faint?
A. It is said that about 30% of people who have POTS faint. Many others will experience pre-syncope symptoms, but remain conscious.

Q. Why does the heat always make me feel worse?
A. Heat dilates blood vessels and diverts blood to the skin. This process reduces blood flow to the key arteries that feed the brain. When the brain does not receive enough oxygen, many things can

occur ranging from severe dizziness to headache or even syncope (fainting).

Q. Why can't I sleep at night?
A. Most patients with POTS have trouble falling asleep. This is often due to high adrenaline levels caused by increased orthostatic stress (the extra stress on the body to remain upright). Some people's circadian rhythm is off, and they sleep during the day and are up all night.

Note: I joke with my daughter and tell her she must have been an owl in a former life. She is nocturnal. Some people with POTS also have central sleep apnea or damage to the medulla, the part of the brain that controls cardiac and respiratory functions. A sleep study can rule out some of these possibilities.

Q. I am always so tired during the day, is it a good idea for me to take naps?
A. As a rule, naps should be saved for those rare occasions when you will be up late. And even then, limit naps to no more than 45 Minutes.

Q. Why does my stomach hurt so much after meals?
A. Many POTS patients suffer from delayed gastric emptying. Also, when the brain does not receive adequate blood circulation, it will shunt blood away from the stomach, creating digestive difficulties and pain. At other times, there may be too much blood flow or venous pooling to the digestive tract. Either way, the result is stomach or intestinal discomfort.

Q. Why do I always feel bloated?
A. Most people who have Dysautonomia have low motility in the intestines. Slow movement of the intestinal tract creates the bloating. Many also have IBS, irritable bowel syndrome, which is a form

of Dysautonomia itself. IBS causes the intestines to feel raw and painful.

Q. Why am I having problems with bedwetting?
A. Dr. William Suarez, pediatric cardiologist at the Northwest Ohio Congenital Heart Center, explains that enuresis (bed wetting) can frequently come into play with patients being treated for Dysautonomia. One explanation for this is that they are salt and fluid loading during the day to help with their blood pressure. The kidney senses this extra fluid and the tendency is to relieve the body of this extra fluid by triggering a response to go to the bathroom. However once the patient finally falls asleep, they are so tired they are unable to wake themselves up to use the toilet. Bladder control is also under Autonomic control and some patients will have difficulty sensing when they have to urinate and can even have difficulty with bladder spasms. In some cases, bedwetting could be a sign of more serious neurological involvement. Discussing this issue with an urologist is suggested.

Q. I have been experiencing a lot of twitches in my arms, eyelids, and various other body parts. Why is this happening?
A. A doctor that I asked this question to explained that this twitching might be caused by the muscles not having the oxygen they need. He said it was nothing to be alarmed by; just another symptom of a deregulated autonomic nervous system.   It is possible that this could be caused from a vitamin deficiency. Ask your doctor to check.

Q. It seems like my stomach hurts every time I take salt tablets. Can the salt tablets be causing this?
A. Yes, some people tolerate salt tablets with no problems. For others, salt tablets can irritate the stomach and even cause vomiting. Salt tablets accumulate body fluids in the digestive tract, which is not good for blood pressure or blood volume. If the tablets bother

your stomach, switch to sea salt. Sea salt mixed with food tends to be easier on the stomach.

Q. Is it possible to take in too much sodium?
A. According to Mayo Clinic (MayoClinic.com) the average amount of sodium intake per day should be between 1,500 to 2,400 for a person who is free of illness. A person who has Dysautonomia should consume as much salt as possible, providing that their blood pressure is not elevated. POTS specialists, usually suggest that a person with POTS takes at least 3,000 – 10,000 mg per day. (Check with your doctor) Blood pressure should, of course, be closely monitored. If the blood pressure begins to exceed the normal limits (130/90), salt intake should be cut back. Swollen hands or feet are red flags to look for. This is usually a sign of high blood pressure and fluid retention. If this happens, you should immediately contact your doctor and cut back on your salt intake.

Q. Should I go on the birth control pill?
A. This is a very complex and personal issue that should be thoroughly evaluated by your family and your team of doctors. I always like to ask the doctors this question, "*If she was your daughter, what would you do?*" This always gets them to give you a well thought out response. Potential for a blood clot always is a concern when beginning oral contraceptives, especially if there is a personal or family history. If deciding to go on oral contraceptives, Dr. William Suarez, POTS specialist believes that typically low estrogen preparations would likely be of more benefit since estrogens have a vasodilatation property to them. The risk benefit ratio should always be measured before starting oral contraceptives or any other medication.

Q. Can I have a mild case of POTS?
A. Yes, you can. The spectrum of POTS symptoms can range from mild to debilitating. You can think of the range of POTS symptoms

as analogous to the range of asthmatics. Some people have asthma so mild that they only need an inhaler every once in a while. Others are so severe that they are in and out of hospitals.

Q. Should I quit my sports activities?
A. Not necessarily. If you cannot make it through the school day or do not have enough energy to complete your homework at night, then you have to weigh the pros and cons. Leading an active life-style and staying physically fit will definitely help reduce your symptoms in the long run and help you to lead a more normal and fulfilled life. It will keep your body in condition and may keep you from becoming more severe. Exercise, if you can tolerate it, is one of the best ways to ensure a quicker recovery. It is critical to keep muscles conditioned as they produce the hormone norepinephrine, a natural vasoconstrictor. It is suggested by most cardiologists that you perform 25 to 30 minutes a day of aerobic exercise. Of course, this is not possible for all people who suffer from Dysautonomia, due to exercise intolerance. See Chapter on exercising with Dysautonomia.

Q. Why does my chest hurt all of the time?
A. It is believed that the left-sided chest pain associated with POTS patients is due to differences in the heart chamber pressures, abnormal heart wall motions and or nerve damage. The pain normally lasts from 30 seconds to a few minutes and is sharp and often debilitating. The pain usually occurs while the patient is at rest. If this pain occurs during exercise, it is imperative to mention this to your cardiologist. Although very uncomfortable, these chest pains are not believed to be life threatening.

Q. Why does my heart feel like it is skipping beats?
A. Sometimes POTS and NMH patients experience what feels like a skipped heart beat or a feeling that their heart has stopped and re-started again. When you are under orthostatic stress the small

blood vessels in the brain constrict. This cuts off blood supply to the brain cells. At the same time this is occurring, the veins in the legs and splanchnic bed (internal organs) are dilating and pooling away from the heart. With inadequate filling of the left ventricle of the heart and abnormal function of the alpha and beta-adrenergic systems, it causes irregular heartbeats. These irregular heartbeats are known as ectopic heartbeats or premature heart beats. Frequent premature heartbeats are a common hallmark of this illness. Justifiably these heartbeats can be quite scary and produce severe anxiety. Luckily, they are almost always benign, but you should still inform your doctor of these episodes. Most people experience premature heartbeats, even those without Dysautonomia. Some people have no symptoms and the premature heartbeat goes unnoticed. Premature heartbeats can be made worse by alcohol consumption, caffeine, dehydration, electrolyte imbalance or certain medications that are stimulants such as Sudafed.

> *Note: My daughter gets a lot of premature heartbeats. When this happens I try to reassure her that it is normal for her. This reduces her anxiety. I then give her lots of fluids that contain electrolytes. This almost always reduces the frequency of the attacks.*

Q. Why do I feel so much worse in the mornings?

A. Your blood pressure is naturally lower in the morning. As the day goes on and you drink an ample amount of fluids, the blood pressure naturally rises. Also, once out of bed, the blood has a better chance to circulate.

Q. Why do I feel so bad before it rains?

A. According to Mike Caplan, weatherman at Channel 7 (ABC) in Chicago, rain and snow are accompanied by low barometric pressure. Before a storm comes in and as it leaves, there is low barometric pressure. Most people who have Dysautonomia fair better in environments with high barometric pressure. When the barometric pressure is high, the atmosphere presses down on our bodies and helps the blood to circulate more efficiently. It is analogous to wearing invisible compression stockings.

Q. Should I avoid caffeine?
A. All substances that contain caffeine such as chocolate, coffee and tea can potentially aggravate Dysautonomia symptoms. Try taking them out of your diet and see if your symptoms abate. For other people caffeine can help alleviate headaches.

Q. I always seem to have a low-grade fever, is this a symptom of POTS?
A. Many people who have POTS have low-grade fevers, chills and flu-like symptoms. This could be due to many factors. The Autonomic Nervous System (ANS) controls body temperature. When the ANS is not working properly many things, like body temperature control, may be out of sync. These symptoms could also be caused by an overactive immune system or abnormally elevated adrenalin levels that effect the body's heat production. Many POTS patients also have positive ANA (anti-nuclear antibody tests). This may be because high adrenalin levels can activate the immune system and can cause the aforementioned symptoms. Some doctors believe that the positive ANA results may be due to an autoimmune disorder.

Q. I recently took Sudafed and my heart started to race. Should I stay away from certain medications?
A. Many over the counter drugs such as sinus and cold medications can exacerbate your symptoms. Use them with caution. You will need to weigh the benefits verses the potential side effects. For sinus issues, first try a Neti Pot or a natural saline spray.

Note: A Neti Pot should be used with warm filtered or distilled water.

Q. What percent of the population has POTS?
A. Mayo Clinic believes that 1 in 100 people have some form of Dysautonomia. That equivocates to 1% of the population. It is also shown that girls get it 5 to 1 over boys.

Q. Why do I have so many symptoms?
A. Dysautonomia affects the blood supply to the brain. The brain requires a sufficient amount of glucose and oxygen to insure healthy function. The brain only represents 1% to 2% of the body's mass, yet is responsible for 20% of the body's oxygen consumption and 15% of cardiac output. The brain depends on proper circulation for healthy and normal functioning to occur. So many of our autonomic (involuntary) functions are impaired when the brain does not receive enough oxygen (blood). Inadequate blood flow to the brain affects the ability to think, stabilize body temperature, and regulate hormones and blood pressure. When the brain does not get what it requires, it causes problems with the body's involuntary actions (autonomic functions) such as: digestion, blood pressure, vision, temperature, etc. This is why the patient with Dysautonomia experiences such a multitude of symptoms.

Q. What are my chances of recovery?
A. There is limited information about the prognosis of the patient with POTS. Some studies have indicated that about half the patients who have post-viral forms of POTS will improve over a two to five year period. It seems the younger the patient, the better the prognosis. About 70% of youth with the developmental form of POTS will significantly improve by their mid-twenties. About 90% of patients will respond to a combination of physical therapy and pharmacotherapy. (Grubb)

Q. Why do so many doctors say that people with POTS tend to outgrow these symptoms in their mid - 20's? Why is the mid - 20's the magic number?

A. I researched this question as it has always baffled me. Most doctors I talked to were perplexed, as well. Two cardiologists suggested that this might be due to the fact that by your mid-twenties, you no longer have as many hormonal fluctuations. This sounds reasonable to me since POTS can show up again during pregnancy and menopause – also times of fluctuating hormones.

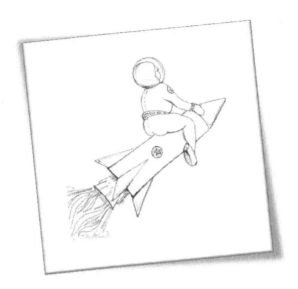

Chapter 5. Cosmopots; NASA and POTS Research

"That's one small step for man, one giant leap for mankind."
- Neil Armstrong

What do astronauts and people who have POTS have in common? Believe it or not, this seemingly odd combination of people have a lot in common. Researchers have found that many astronauts, mostly those who are on prolonged space flight missions (three to six months), experience orthostatic hypotension (a drop in blood pressure) upon reentering Earth's atmosphere. According to one NASA doctor, astronauts that are on prolonged space missions are not allowed to walk from the space shuttle to the awaiting helicopter. Protocol demands that they must be carried to the helicopter, as a safeguard to ensure their safety. Most are too dizzy to make the journey themselves.

In an article entitled, *"When Space Makes you Dizzy"* (Science and NASA) Dr. Richard Cohen of Harvard, the head of the cardiovascular Alternations Team at the National Space Biomedical

Research Institute, explains that on Earth gravity pulls blood toward the lower body, but in space, because of lack of gravity, blood that normally pools in the legs collects in the upper body instead. He said that is why astronauts come back to Earth having puffy-looking faces and spindly "chicken legs." [1]

Astronauts do not experience orthostatic hypotension in space; they begin to feel it during reentry and after landing. When they reenter Earth, because of gravity, blood returns to the lower body and blood pressure to the brain is suddenly reduced, thus dizziness sets in. [1]

Astronauts, according to several doctors from NASA, experience orthostatic intolerance after returning to Earth, although only temporarily. Their body seems to readjust to Earth's atmosphere after a few weeks and their symptoms of OI disappear.

Astronauts as well as us Earth bounders, experience the old adage, "*use it or lose it.*" On Earth, veins in the legs contain tiny muscles that contract when the veins fill with blood. They send blood up towards the heart to maintain a stable blood pressure. In space however, there is no up or down, so the muscles in the legs veins are used less often. This is a normal adaptation to weightlessness. [2] "*During reentry those muscles are needed again, but they have temporarily "forgotten" how to contract. They fail to push blood back toward the heart and brain.*" Says Dr. Richard Cohen. This same use it or lose it concept seems to apply to those who have orthostatic intolerance on Earth. Many people who have Dysautonomia seem to get it after being injured or getting a virus that left them bed bound.

During space flight, there is a loss of body fluids and many astronauts become dehydrated. To counteract the dehydration, which we all know can lead to worsened orthostatic hypotension astronauts are told to increase their water and salt intake. Sound familiar? Astronauts also wear "G-suits," a rubberized full body suit that can be inflated with air. This action squeezes the extremities and raises blood pressure, [3] probably similar to what compression stockings do for us COSMOPOTS. As a matter of fact, one woman with orthostatic intolerance uses a G-suit to stand long enough to wash dishes.

Midodrine is a drug that is used for many people who have POTS. This drug helps to raise blood pressure. As it turns out, Astronauts are given this same drug before reentry into Earth's atmosphere to help constrict their blood vessels and prevent dizziness - yet another similarity.

Dr. David Robertson of Vanderbilt University's Autonomic Dysfunction Center has been studying the genetic component of orthostatic intolerance (OI) on Earth bounders. He wanted to find out the cause of OI in astronauts. He designed several experiments for the Neurolab Space Mission in April of 1998. He hoped that his finding would help both astronauts and chronic OI sufferers from experiencing this disorder. In particular, he wanted to find out what these two subsets of people have in common. Dr. Robertson's studies revealed that orthostatic intolerance (the O in POTS) was caused by elevated levels of the neurotransmitter, norepinephrine in the blood. He explains that too much norepinephrine in the blood can raise the heart rate and cause constriction of all of the blood vessels. As a result, there is a secondary loss of blood volume to the brain, which will in turn cause dizziness and other complications. The higher levels of norepinephrine cause the blood vessels to constrict too much with the same results, insufficient blood supply to the brain.

For astronauts, the increase in norepinephrine appears to be caused by decreased blood volume that normally occurs in space. *"Low blood volume can make the sympathetic nervous system work harder. When the sympathetic nervous system works harder, the plasma (blood) norepinephrine level goes up because sympathetic nerves release norepinephrine,"* says Robertson. Robertson was able to deduct from his experiments that there could only be two causes for the excess in norepinephrine levels. One, that the body was producing too much norepinephrine, or two that the body was not able to eliminate the extra norepinephrine at the normal rate. The latter, appeared to have possibly been caused by a defect in the norepinephrine transporter function, or NET. The NET'S job is to remove excess norepinephrine from the blood. With this information under his belt, Robertson was able to locate the abnormal gene. This was the first time a genetic defect has been linked to a disorder of the autonomic nervous system. [4]

NASA is continuing to do research on orthostatic intolerance and its effects on astronauts. It is our hope that one day soon they will figure out how to alleviate this condition, so that astronauts can come back to Earth symptom free. Hopefully, added research will help figure out the connection between orthostatic intolerance and its role in POTS. It would be "out of this world" if NASA could help eradicate this syndrome, helping millions to lead more normal, healthy and productive lives.

Reference 1-4:
Science @ NASA Headline News. "When Space Makes You Dizzy." 25 March 2002.

Section 3. Coping

Chapter 6. Impact on the Family-How Chronic Illness can Impact the Entire Family Unit

"In some families, please is described as the magic word. In our house, however, it was sorry." - Margaret Laurence

They say you can lead a horse to water but you cannot make it drink. This saying certainly is pertinent when trying to explain POTS to family members. Sometimes, when dealing with this illness, you cannot even lead the horse to the water. When my children were first diagnosed with POTS, I took on the role of POTS advocate. I decided to be a POTS spokesperson extraordinaire, telling anyone, who could breathe (and some that could not) all about POTS. I wanted to convince the world that POTS was real. I wanted everyone to know my family's plight. I even had to convince the chef at the Japanese restaurant and the woman with Alzheimer's at my dad's nursing home. In my head, I was tallying everyone I convinced. I got more points for those that had never heard of the illness and even more points for every medical doctor I told. I was on a roll. I got good at telling who believed me and who did not. Body position always gave it away. I tried harder to convince those who gave me a negative body response. I got triple points for convincing them. I was diagnosing people left and right. My kids joked with me and told me that I could diagnose a rock with POTS, and I was proud to say I could. I was talking about it so much; I even started to annoy myself.

I was so elated that my children's school, family and doctors all supported us. I had heard so many horror stories about families not talking to each other anymore, because some family members were not on board with the POTS diagnosis. But not me, I was the lucky one, the chosen. Everyone in my family whole - heartedly supported me, or so I thought. Until one day, my bubble burst. It was revealed to me that one of my immediate family members (I will not say which one, to protect the innocent) did not believe my daughter was sick at all. He was convinced this whole POTS thing was just a cry for attention. I was fuming. I cried for two days. I called him up and called him every swear word I could think of. I disowned him in my head, and I think out loud too. How dare him! The summer prior we had gone to the Beijing Olympics and met the entire gymnastics team. We had been on the news several times talking about the trip and trying to spread awareness about POTS. I was doing everything I could to educate people about POTS and my own family member was a disbeliever.

I soon came to find out, that he was not the only one in my family, who did not believe that POTS was a real diagnosis. I wanted to run away and join a new family, one that would understand and support us through this horrific time in our lives. I was so disappointed, disheartened and disillusioned. He hurt me even further by telling me that his family observed that whenever we were at a family gathering my kids would be laying around complaining of not feeling well, until dessert was served. He said he joked with his family that dessert was the cure for POTS. Now I was really irritated. How was that funny (even though it was true)? This put me over the edge. I felt that we as a family were going through the biggest challenge of our lives, and my family was not there to support us through it. I was beyond hurt.

I decided to step back, where I could see things more clearly. After days of dwelling and fuming and perseverating and more perseverating, I came up with some profound realizations. First and foremost, I realized, I do not have to convince anyone of my children's illness. All that arguing with my family only got me more aggravated, but I was still left with sick children. What anyone thinks does not matter, all that matters is getting your loved one(s) well again. It always confused me that people could fully comprehend that a little innocent peanut could kill someone or that we had the capability of producing humans in test tubes and sending people to the moon; why can't these same people believe that one can have a problem with their autonomic nervous system?

People by nature only tend to believe what they know or what is in their comfort zone. Why is it that many people question how Moses supposedly opened the gates of the Red Sea, or that the sacrament is the true blood and body of Jesus. If we all believed the same way, we would all be the same religion. I found that many of my friends were more supportive during this time than were my own family members. Then it dawned on me, my family does not want to believe that my kids are sick. It is too painful of a thought for them. They would rather slough it off on anxiety or attention seeking behavior. This is easier to handle than acknowledging they have an illness. Whether this is the case or not, it is insignificant. I finally confronted my family members and told them that it is irrelevant what they believe or do not believe; the focus here should be on getting these kids better. We decided to go by the *"do not ask do not tell policy"*. I now tell my family very little about my children's health issues. In some ways, it is a shame, but I feel a lot less stress that way. I have different expectations of my family and what I can and cannot get from them. I know I can no longer use them as a sounding board; I no longer try. My family has always been too important to me to just write off. I love them dearly and did not want this illness to ruin yet another thing in my life. It was better for me to alter our relationship rather than destroy it. In retrospect, my oldest brother, who is a doctor himself said, *"It took me a long time to understand the true complexity and dynamics of this illness."*

You will come to know rather quickly through this illness who will listen without judgment. I have found that one of the worst aspects of this illness is how people come to judge you. *"Well if she was MY child, I would certainly not let her go out on the weekends, when she hasn't been to school all week."* All of a sudden, everyone around you becomes the perfect parent. Your life becomes filled with what they would or would not do. The truth is no one else lives in your shoes, so no one but you, could know what is best for your child, spouse, etc.;   As their father once said, *"This is all unchartered territory and we are all just trying to do the best we can do to make the right decisions for our family."* Since each person with POTS is unique, so too, are all decisions that are made. I have learned that judging others is one of the most painful things that you can do to another person. No one can stop others from judging you, the only thing we can do is learn from it and try not to judge others ourselves. I truly believe I have become a better person from this, and I can walk away from this syndrome knowing that it has somehow made me a better, more understanding human being. I can also reassure myself that my immediate family members are better people because of the lessons we have all learned via POTS.

This is a very typical scenario from everyone I have spoken with who has a family member with POTS. You are not alone. Whether it be a sibling, a sister, a nephew or even your husband who does not believe the diagnosis, your goal is to do whatever possible to help your loved one suffering from POTS. You do not have to convince anyone that POTS is real, it is. You can show family members this book or have them Google "POTS" to see the thousands of articles out there written about POTS from doctors at Mayo to Vanderbilt. You can shout until you are blue in the face, but those who are not going to believe you, are still not. One suggestion I can offer you is to ask the family member what it is about

POTS that they do not understand. After I did this with one family member, and I explained it again, he said he finally got it. He then even joined my POTS Awareness Group. I realized months later, that through this illness, my family has learned to be a lot more forthright with each other (something we could not seem to manage before) and because of that we have grown a lot closer as a family unit.

In further defense of those family members that are non-believers, this illness does look strange. One minute my daughter could be unable to sit up in her bed, because she is so dizzy and the next day, she could be well enough to be shopping at the mall. Each day and each minute with this illness is different. You never know what you are going to get, and it does look odd. It is episodic, invisible and unpredictable. If I were to be 100% truthful with myself, I am not sure that if I did not live with this syndrome on a daily basis, that I would believe it myself.

In 10 to 15 years, when POTS becomes a household name like autism or epilepsy, your non-believing family members will most likely beg for your forgiveness. In many ways, POTS is where autism was 15 years ago in terms of awareness. Many people believed that autism was due to the coldness of the mothers who raised the autistic child, thus the term *"refrigerator mothers"* came to be. We all know how ridiculous that statement sounds now. So many friends, doctors and family members want to believe that POTS is all in the person's head. Now instead of getting upset, I chalk it all up to pure unadulterated ignorance. Many people are just plain ignorant. They want to judge and psychoanalyze but are unwilling to search the truth. It would be so easy to say, *"just look up POTS on the internet and do some research for yourself."* Wouldn't that make sense? It is not worth ruining a relationship over an illness. There is already so much stress in the person's life who has POTS. Relationship issues are a stressor that should be avoided at all cost. We already know that stress makes the individual who has POTS more symptomatic. We need to try to make as little extra stress for them as possible. Losing an uncle or an aunt, etc... because this person does not believe in POTS, only creates more stress for them as well as the entire family unit.

POTS impacts siblings, as well. They feel very left out, as their sick sibling(s) seems to get all of the attention. Sometimes they behave inappropriately, as they are crying out to get attention in any way they can. My 8-year-old daughter seeks attention by constant complaining. She has become a hypochondriac and complains every few minutes about one thing or another. At least 20 body parts ail her daily. It has made it impossible to distinguish between when she is really sick versus just wanting attention. It is important to remember that everyone in the family is affected by a sibling or parent who has POTS, not just the one with the diagnosis. When one person in the family suffers, everyone suffers with them, though the suffering may be experienced differently. The stress in the family with a child or parent who has a chronic illness is high and must not be ignored. Each child is begging for attention and wants their needs to be met, too. Most children, though not intentional, will feel a sense of jealousy over the child who is sick. My 12-year-old son confessed to me that he often wishes he were as sick as his sister so he could get special accommodations and more time with me and his father. This is typical and normal. Do not berate your child for having these feelings; instead be glad that you have the kind of relationship where they can be forthright with you. Reassure them that their feelings are normal. The children in the family may see it as unfair that the ill sibling gets special attention. They often seek inappropriate and unconventional ways of getting this attention. They may not be able to articulate this to you; however, they feel a sense of loss. Children, no matter how young, can sense that their parents are sad, and they too can feel the stress. They are often reacting to what they feel. It is important to give the other children special attention, when you can. Taking the well child out alone and giving them special one - on - one time, can really help. This of course, is easier said than done, especially because having a sick child is mentally and physically exhausting. It often feels like there is no energy left to take care of the others. When it is physically impossible to take the well child out, spend some time at home alone with this child, just playing a card game or reading them a book. Most nights I let my children lay in bed with me, while we watch a special TV show. At 9:00 PM my older son, (after I put my younger kids to sleep) knows he gets to watch his favorite show with me. This has become our special show and our special time together. Your children need your undivided attention now more than ever.

Sometimes it's the parent who suffers from this syndrome. Being a parent is difficult to begin with, but unbelievably more difficult when dealing with a chronic illness. Parents with Dysautonomia often cannot perform the basic household duties such as cooking and cleaning let alone take care of the more complex demands of their children. They often miss out on mile marker events. The lack of ability to fulfill the parental role is heart - breaking enough but also leaves a huge feeling of guilt.

The stress that parents can experience at this time is beyond belief. There are so many emotional and financial stresses that go with having a sick child. It is said that a parent is only as happy as their unhealthiest child. If this is true, then the parent is often not in good shape. Having a child with POTS changes the whole dynamics of the family. Everything changes from daily living to family vacations. It is hard to make plans, as it is impossible to know what each day will bring with the POTS child. Every day seems to bring new challenges and obstacles. Plans constantly change depending on what kind of a day the child is having and sometimes it feels as if you are living by the moment. Planning is no longer part of the family vocabulary. I used to be an avid planner. Though, I have more of a B Type personality, I planned everything out from when I would go to the grocery store to what time I would be in bed every night. My husband, on the other hand, has always been a type A personality. There was no room in his life for anyone being late. We had to arrive at all of my kids sporting events, at least ½ hour early, and we had to be the first to arrive at every party and family gathering. There was no excuse good enough to be late. There was plenty of screaming and yelling to encourage promptness. Chaos often ensued as everyone scrambled to meet the imposed deadline. Stress was a thick fog that encompassed us like a corset. This had to STOP. After many talks with my husband, he began to compromise his ideal of being prompt. He came to realize that this couldn't exist when you live with someone who has POTS. Planning now just becomes an idea. Being late is now an everyday occurrence. It has really stretched my husband, but he has become a better person and dad because of it. It is frustrating for everyone, but can also be looked at as a sign of growth.

Financial issues also become heightened, as bills from tests and doctor visits come pouring in. During one bad week, we had to call the ambulance three times. Imagine that bill. More often than not, parents also see their child's road to recovery differently. One parent may tend to be more doting and less pushy with the sick child. The other parent may want to push their child to do as much as possible. Many spouses have different ideas regarding what is best for their child and this alone can cause terrible tension. It is important for both parents (divorced or not) to be on the same page and discuss all-important issues behind closed doors. You must keep the stress levels to a minimum. If you cannot agree, a third party may be necessary to intervene.

The impact that POTS has on each family member should not be disregarded. More stress will only make the sick child more symptomatic. It is important to address each family member's issues and not sweep them under the carpet. Stress has to be kept to a minimum for the good of the entire family. Time constraints have to become more relaxed and everyone in the family has to become more flexible. When this cannot be achieved on your own, it is best to seek professional help.

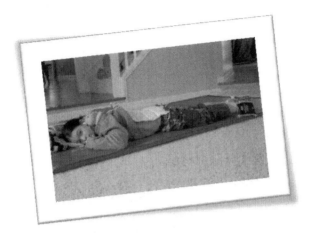

Chapter 7. POTS Storm - A Day in the Life of a Family Coping with POTS

"POTS STORM" is a phrase I coined to explain a rather typical day in the life of a mother whose children have POTS. "POTS STORM" is a day when nothing seems to go right and everything that can go wrong does. This is an actual day that happened in the life of my family.

I wake my 12-year-old son, who has many symptoms of POTS but does not have a diagnosis, at 6:40 A.M. He tells me to go away. He has a headache and stomachache and needs at least ten more minutes to sleep. I give him ten more minutes and try again. He refuses to get up. I turn on the lights and threaten to take away his sports, his computer, and his baseball collection. He finally takes me seriously. He gets up. I give him a handful of medicines, make sure he drinks at least eight ounces of water, and eats something salty. I rush him out the door to catch his school bus.

Next, I wake up my eight-year old twins. My son, who has POTS, complains of being dizzy and having a headache. I give him ibuprofen. He takes it with his beta-blocker and Florinef and gets ready for school.

The other twin, says she has a headache, a stomachache, chest pains, and a list of numerous other complaints, ranging anywhere from teeth pain to leg pain. Sarah has not been diagnosed with POTS and it's often difficult to know whether her symptoms are real or merely pleas for attention. One time I lied and told her if she had POTS her tongue would hurt her, she then looked at me very seriously and said that it did.

I feed both twins breakfast. I give my daughter special vitamins, because she is the only one not on any prescription drugs and she feels left out. I make my son drink 8 ounces of water and salt his scrambled eggs.

I now run upstairs to my 13 - year - old, Nikki, to give her the first batch of her many medications that she takes throughout the day. Nikki was diagnosed with POTS a year ago. She yells at me and refuses to sit up to take her medications. After she realizes I am not going to leave until she takes them, she reluctantly starts to swallow them. She takes two at a time to speed up the process. I tell her to take one at a time; she refuses to listen, like the typical teenager and chokes. Not learning from her mistake she takes two more at a time and chokes again. I then bring her miso soup to get her salt in. She complains again and drinks three tablespoons, wasting the rest. I tell her she has one more hour to sleep and then she has to get ready for school, or at least try. It is about to rain outside, so I have little hope that she actually will make it to school.

I get a call from the school counselor. She says the teachers are concerned that Nikki has missed so much school. They suggest full home - bound tutoring. We are presently doing partial home - bound tutoring. If she goes on full homebound tutoring, she will not be able to go to school at all. That means no socialization. What to do? If this is the case, I worry she will sleep all day having no reason to wake. Not getting up means no exercise, which equals no getting better. On the other hand, if I do not agree to full time homebound tutoring, they may hold her back a grade, because she has missed so much school. She loves school and seeing her friends. How can I take this away too? I am in a quandary. I decide not to decide.

I go to wake her up again sharing with her the threat that the counselor just laid on me. I am frustrated and want her to share in my misery. She could care less. All she wants to do is go back to sleep. I gently pull her by the legs. She shows no reaction. Now I pull her legs harder, feeling like the mother from "Freaky Friday." She grabs the headboard; with the little strength she has and fights me off. She puts her head back down on her pillow. I reiterate the importance of getting her to school. She reiterates how sick she feels. She is dizzy, tired and has a major headache. She tells me that she did not fall asleep until 6:30 A.M. She screams. *"Go Away!"*

I go away, write some more of my book, take the dog for a walk, visit my dad at the nursing home and come back for more abuse. *"Please wake up!"* Still, I get no response. The phone rings. It's the bad number. The school nurse says my eight-year-old son is in her office with a migraine. Can I bring some Motrin for him to take? I run to school, give him Motrin and beg him to try to make it through the day. I race home. It is now time to give my daughter her afternoon Proamatine. She is feeling a little less dizzy. She takes a shower and gets ready for school.

I walk her arm in arm to the front door of the school. We do this when she is feeling dizzy. I pray she will make it through her short day without ending up in the nurse's office.

I run to Whole Foods to buy groceries for the week. I am on a health kick to try to get the kids better with organic foods. I figure it cannot hurt. My shopping basket is filled to the brim with groceries. I am standing in line when I get the dreaded call again; the school nurse informs me that Nikki only made it to one class. Her pulse is at 140 and her blood pressure is 88 over 60. Sullenly, I pay for my groceries and go to school to collect her. My mind is clouded with a tornado of emotions. Why can't I keep these kids healthy? Am I doing something wrong? Am I a horrible mother? How is she going to make it through high school when she can't make it through seventh grade? I am becoming more and more disheartened. The silver lining is becoming more impossible to find.

Nikki is in a reclining chair fast asleep by the time I get to her school. The nurse helps me take her out in a wheel chair, because she is too dizzy to stand on her own. The nurse says with a smile; *"Hopefully tomorrow will be a better day."* I want to cry, knowing that it probably won't. I am beginning to lose all hope.

We go home. My daughter falls asleep for a few hours before her tutor comes. Today she is too sick to work with the tutor. She cannot lift her head off of her bed. The tutor accepts this and kindly says she will come back tomorrow to try again. Thankfully, she is empathetic and kind. She does not add to my stress.

My other kids come home from school. I make dinner, take them to their respective sports, give them their medications, baths and then I crash from exhaustion.

I get woken up in the middle of the night twice. Nikki cannot fall asleep. She has slept all day and is now ready to have an adrenalin rush. She is ready to compete in a triathlon. "Go watch T.V. I suggest a bit too harshly." Just as I fall back to sleep, Sarah wakes me up. She has a headache and needs Motrin. I get it for her, reluctantly, and fall fast asleep only to do the same thing all over again tomorrow, when I can experience yet another POTS STORM!

Chapter 8. Grief and Dysautonomia - *Michelle Roger, Psychologist*

I remember reading an article early on in my studies about a woman who was grieving the loss of her husband; only her husband was still alive but had developed Alzheimer's disease. Everyday this woman was mourning the loss of the man she loved. The man, whose mind was disappearing day-by-day, week-by-week, but was still physically sitting there in front of her. I found this article the other day and something in it hit me hard. This scenario is played out every day for people living with chronic illness although in our case the person mourning the loss is you, and the person you are grieving for is yourself.

It sounds strange to say you are grieving yourself. Grief is traditionally related to the loss of a loved one. But what we often forget is that grief is about loss, any loss. When we lose a job or perhaps a relationship we talk about anger, feeling upset or perhaps betrayed. What we don't realize is that we are actually grieving. There are different types of grieving and grief events. Grief, when you lose a loved one, has a sort of built in time limit. It's not that you actually stop loving or grieving for the person but that the grief becomes a little bit easier to bear with each passing day. There is truth to the old adage time heals all wounds. We need to be able to do this to be able to cope in the here and now. To sustain that initial grief over time can become debilitating and destructive to a person on many levels. It's not to say that you don't become upset at certain times, the holidays in particular can be tortuous, but the overall level of grief diminishes and becomes manageable.

But what do you do when the event that brought about the grief in the first place never leaves? How do you deal with something that can cause little losses (and sometimes big) every day, such as a chronic illness like Dysautonomia? Living with Dysautonomia you are constantly reminded that you are no longer the person you once were. From the moment you wake up, each and every morning is a struggle. Just to get out of bed and dress you are reminded every step that you aren't like other people. Like it or not, you are sick and to differing extents, perhaps even disabled. Each day you are reminded of your loss. It's almost as if you just get that wound to your spirit to heal over and someone comes along and rips the scab right off, leaving it raw all over again.

With chronic illness you may lose many things: your job, your friends, your house, your financial independence, but perhaps the biggest loss living with chronic illness is the loss of you. By that I mean the you, who you once were before you became ill; the picture you had in your head of you and where you fit in the universe.

It's your own personal picture not the one other people have, which can sometimes be dramatically different to our own. It's often not until you are faced with something like illness, that you realize that you did indeed have such a picture, one to which you were particularly attached.

I know this only too well. I had developed a nice little picture of me, which I rather liked. I had finally come to a place in my life where I was happy with my career, my family and life in general. I knew who I was, where I fit in and where I was going in the future. Other people had pictures of me too, wife, mother, daughter, sister, friend, etc. Then along came Dysautonomia, and the Michelle I was died. I know that sounds rather melodramatic, but it's how I felt at the time and to a certain extent even now. That person I was six years ago is gone. I catch glimpses every now and then but the me I thought I liked, the me I thought I was, the me I thought I wanted, is long gone.

We hear about the stages of grief: Denial, Bargaining, Anger, Depression and perhaps the most elusive, Acceptance. The funny thing about grief is that it is not a nice clean process: step 1 denial, step 2 anger...step 5 acceptance. Instead it's: step 1 anger, step 2 sadness, step 3 ticked off, step 4 really ticked off, step 5 denial, step 6 immerse yourself in Bold and the Beautiful (denial in any other language, or insanity), step 7 bargaining, step 8 depression, step 9 chocolate binging...and so on. It's a messy process and it's even messier when there is no finality to the loss. When you think you are finally getting a handle on what has happened to your life, Dysautonomia can jump up with a sucker punch, to remind you that the loss is still there and the process begins again. There can be many losses when you are ill. Loss of self, loss of friends, loss of family, loss of work, loss of financial security, loss of place, to name but a few, and it can often feel overwhelming. It doesn't help that you are ill and exhausted and have very few reserves left to deal with these changes.

For me, it was like someone was taking little bites out of me each day: reliability gone, independence gone, punctuality gone, intelligence gone, privacy gone, mothering skills gone, wife, (who's that?) driving gone, coffee with friends gone, dignity gone... and on, and on, and on. Each of these losses seemed insurmountable at the time. I had the tears, the anger, the swearing at the universe, I had it all. I'd always been in control, I'd always been independent, I was always the one other people came to for advice and support, be it professionally or personally. I could juggle it all with ease. So who the heck is this pasty-faced, fog brained woman in the mirror I see staring vaguely back at me every day?

What can be particularly hard is that other people are often unable to understand our level of grief. Heck, often we don't understand it ourselves. I often feel whiney, even now, when I complain about my lot in life. When someone makes one of those comments like "well at least it's not cancer," or "I'd love to not have to work," it undermines our right to feel what we are feeling. We are not asking for pity, and it's not about whose experiences are more worthy or legitimate. We are entitled to feel angry, upset, lost. It is completely normal to feel whatever you are feeling when you experience such a life changing event. We are NORMAL!

So what do you do? I hate those saccharine sweet lines like "When Life Gives You Lemons Make Lemonade." Do they realize the steps involved in making the lemonade? First, get the energy to get up out of bed. Second, get the energy to care that you have to make lemonade. Third, try and find a recipe book. Fourth, get your brain together to remember why you have the recipe book. Fifth, grab a coffee to get your brain going. Sixth, forget the reason you had the recipe book out again and tidy up the kitchen. Seventh, remember something about lemons. Eighth, remember obscure fact that Liz Lemon is a character on 30 Rock, and sit down to watch tapped program, forgetting lemonade completely. Making that darn lemonade is a Herculean task and often you need someone to hold your hand and guide you to the 7- Up.

Talk. Talk. Talk. Talk. Talk. We all need to let it out. Being a psychologist myself, I'm obligated to say find a psychologist to talk to about what has and is happening in your life. Being a human being as well, I know that not everyone is comfortable with this option. Heck, I was rather offended when my cardiologist suggested it to me. I'm a psychologist; I know the drill. Why would I need to talk to anyone? But I did talk to someone, and I'm really glad I did. You don't have to see a psychologist per se (although we do have many, oh so many, long, years of training), but there are great social workers out there, or some people may prefer to talk to their clergy. Maybe you have a great friend who has the knack, or you can go on the many available Dysautonomia support sites or blogs. What you do need to do is get it out before it begins to stew and ferment. Talking to a professional outside your family and friends is a great idea, because they don't know you; you can talk freely, and they have no stake in things, other than to help you find a path through the maze. You can't often talk about the issues you are having with your family members as they play a much larger role in the game, and may have a strong reaction to your illness in the first place. And we often don't want to burden our loved ones with our own issues, particularly the darker emotions and thoughts that can arise. Finding support, be it through the Internet or a group you meet with in person, can also help. It's nice to know you are not alone and that there are others who are having, or have had, the same experiences.

Letter writing is a really useful technique to help organize your thoughts and get out a lot of what can build up inside. You can do it anywhere, any time, and you can do with it whatever you want. The idea is that you write yourself a letter about what you are feeling. It was a technique I often used with family members of my patients with Alzheimer's. The patient never saw the letter; it was for the families to express what they felt, to let out that raw emotion. Some would come in and read it to me, because they just needed to share and to know if what they felt was normal. Others simply did it for themselves and then either put it away or destroyed it in a symbolic freeing of those burdens. A letter can be used to help family members understand what you are feeling or just to let you lighten the load. There's no right or wrong. I wrote a letter myself last year. I kept it hidden for a long time, believing others would think I was completely insane. But then I gave it to my immediate family to read, and it helped them understand. Then I gave the letter to a close friend, and eventually I posted it on my blog, which was freeing and probably the scariest thing I have done in my life. It's like those dreams where you find yourself stark naked in a crowd. I've never been as naked as I was the day I posted it on my blog.

There are a number of other ways to manage grief and stress that really deserve their own chapters. There are many great outlets: art, writing, painting, music, yoga, meditation, gardening, relaxation techniques, etc. can all serve as great coping tools as well as wonderful distractions. It's about finding what works for you.

Developing a new picture of you is important. Accepting what you can't do and embracing what you can, is imperative. Allow yourself to grieve. It's okay to need someone to hold your hand as you navigate along that path. I am a work in process, and I still have those days when I want to crawl into my bed and cry. Being a mum and wife doesn't often give you that opportunity, so you have to find a way through. Sometimes you just need someone else to give you a reality check and point out what you do have. For me, that happened a few years ago. I saw leaving work, in particular, as a huge loss at many levels. Then my youngest son turned to me one day and said, "I'm so glad you are home all the time, Mum. It's way better." He liked that part of the new me, and I've decided to embrace it too. I may not be able to bring in an income, but I get to spend time, all my "good" time with my kids and family now. And that's a much, much bigger payday.

In embracing the new me, life is easier. Being ill has given me a freedom that I wouldn't have experienced should I have remained in my former non-ill life. I don't have the time or the resources, emotional or physical, to worry about the perceptions of others. Instead, I find joy and take chances that I normally wouldn't have, be that to create a pair of completely impractical Dorothy heels, write a blog, or to dress up and be photographed as a zombie. I find joy in the small things and find laughter in the absurdity that is now my life. I appreciate and make the most of my good days and know even when the inevitable bad day(s) come I will make it out the other side and find the joy again. Some days I still grieve my old life and my old me. Some days I grieve the new losses that occur as my illness progresses. But it is easier now than it was in those initial days. I allow myself to feel the emotions as they arise rather than fight them and that removes a lot of the stress. Life is complicated, unpredictable and downright hard at times, but I choose to be happy when I can. Because happy or sad my health issues remain the same. And frankly, I'd rather break out some very bad Vogue moves while stuck lying on my bathroom tiles than waste time on wishing my life were otherwise.

Michelle Roger- Author of the popular "Living with Bob (Dysautonomia)" blog
http://bobisDysautonomia.blogspot.com

Chapter 9. Changing for the Better: The Positive Aspects of Living with POTS – *Danielle Hines*

My personal journey with chronic illness began eighteen years ago, at age twelve. It was at that time that I developed fibromyalgia, digestive issues and costochondritis, which was later diagnosed as asthma. The POTS diagnosis didn't actually come until this past autumn, though I realize now that I have battled the symptoms of it for much longer. Looking back at my life, it is difficult to remember a time when I felt physically strong, healthy or "normal." There have been days, months, perhaps even years, where I have been angry that this is my lot in life.

Then there are the moments when I am calm enough to stop being upset, and I can see that I have grown, not in spite of my limitations, but directly because of them. Though we each have our own distinctive path in life, the more I reach out to others dealing with Dysautonomia and other chronic illnesses, the more I realize that the strength and insight that comes from this daily battle is not unique to me. While I may never be happy that I have a chronic illness, I can at least be grateful for the life lessons I have learned because of it. Giving attention to the aspects of Dysautonomia that are difficult and negative is easy; however, reflecting on the ways in which it has changed me for the better is one way for me to focus on the positive.

These are the ways I have matured and the lessons I have learned during my journey. Some of them may seem familiar to you, others may not - we each have our own path. I believe that it is through struggles that we become stronger and that wisdom is gained through experience.

1.   I grew in perseverance. Every day is an opportunity to persevere when you live with Dysautonomia. Simply getting out of bed each morning and telling yourself you will make it through another day is an act of pushing through the pain

and fatigue. Yet, I also learned to persevere in greater ways. If someone had told me back in junior high that it would take me 11 years to earn my college degree because of my health, I would have laughed and called them a liar. But having a college degree was a goal I wasn't willing to give up. So, yes, it was difficult. Eleven years is a really long time to pursue something that most individuals accomplish in four or five, but today I can be proud of that achievement. I believe that when you know what it is like to really have to fight for something and to work harder than most to achieve it, the sense of triumph you gain in the end is all the greater.

2.   I learned the importance of taking care of myself. POTS has forced me to slow down and start assuming responsibility for my health. As someone who likes to constantly be taking care of everyone and everything, living at a slower pace has been a big adjustment. Experience has taught me that I will crash if I push myself too much, so I am learning to do what I can and to relinquish control of the rest. I have learned to be kind to myself and to appreciate my body for what it can do, not hate it for what it cannot. I have changed my eating habits by switching to mostly gluten-free foods and cutting down on caffeine and heavily-processed items. I see a physical therapist to work on my strength and balance, and I go to a psychotherapist every two weeks to deal with the emotional ups and downs of life with a chronic illness. I wish that it didn't take an illness like POTS for me to wake up and recognize the need to care for my body and mind, but I am content with the fact that I am now making strides in the right direction.

3.   I began offering more compassion and empathy toward others. This one took a while for me, and I still have room to grow. There are days when I look around at seemingly healthy people, and I can't help but feel a ping of jealousy.

There are moments when a friend will lament over a cold that has lasted a week, and it takes everything in me not to offer a snarky reply. However, I am learning to offer compassion instead. The majority of my struggles are almost invisible for an outsider to see and, yet, I know how to difficult they are to endure. When I acknowledge that I want to be treated with consideration and kindness, I am able to see that although another individual's journey may not involve dealing with a chronic illness, it is only because life has presented him or her with other challenges. The truth is - no one gets through life without fighting a hard battle. Living with Dysautonomia, we face judgment and misunderstanding from so much of the outside world; my goal is to do what I can to bring comfort and understanding to the lives I touch.

4.   I started accepting my limitations and learned to ask for help. Recognizing that I can't do everything I used to do and acknowledging that I need help from others does not make me weak; it means I am being smart. By allowing my friends and loved ones to help me when I need it, I am taking better care of myself and, ultimately, ensuring that I have more good days than bad. Letting go of some of my independence (and the pride that goes along with it) is not easy, but it allows me to conserve the limited amount of energy I have for the things that are most important. Asking for help is humbling, but I have found that if I try to do it all on my own, I end up frustrated and push people away as a result. Conversely, when I allow my friends and family to offer care and support, it gives those individuals an opportunity to learn more about my illness. Extending kindness and service to another person always makes me feel closer to that individual, and I find that a lot of my friendships today are stronger because of my willingness to let friends assist me.

5.   I saw the importance of nurturing and strengthening the supportive relationships in my life. Life with a chronic illness can be lonely and frustrating, especially if it causes you to be housebound often. I have found that I need supportive friendships to get me through the tough times and to help me celebrate the good times. Some friendships, and some people, are not strong enough to deal with the challenges associated with a chronic illness. While I have mourned those relationships at times, it makes me all the more grateful for the people in my life who stick around. I surround myself with people who bring me joy, and I don't waste time on those who bring me down. I have a small but steadfast group of friends that I can call on to cheer me up, to help take my mind off of things, to make me laugh, or to just listen during the hard times. I have learned that even wonderful friendships are not without effort. Relationships require maintenance and nurturing to survive, so I make phone calls and invite people over even when I don't feel like it. I also find comfort in online support groups for people dealing with POTS or fibromyalgia. There is nothing like bonding with individuals who are going through the same thing.

6.   I began setting small goals and taking pride in their accomplishment. There was a definite stage of grief that came with my fibromyalgia and POTS diagnoses, a time where all I could focus on was the dreams I would have to give up or change. While my life altered dramatically because of these illnesses, I am learning to find a new normal and to set new goals for myself. Given my current health, these goals are very small but manageable. For instance, I will give myself a few small tasks to accomplish each day: ride the recumbent bike for five minutes and sharpen the kitchen knives. Tomorrow's goals might be to clean out a dresser drawer, call a good friend or go grocery shopping with a family member.

While these goals may seem insignificant to some, I knew I needed to start small and that I should not diminish the value of, at least, accomplishing something. I need a sense of purpose every day and, honestly, I need activities to keep me from being bored. These small tasks offer something tangible to work toward and a sense of achievement on a daily basis. The bigger life goals are still in the works, but if I can manage the smaller goals day by day, I will be better equipped to handle the larger ones down the road.

7.   I no longer take the good times for granted. One of the advantages of feeling sick a good majority of the time is that you sure do appreciate those days when you feel better. I went to a local Spanish tapas restaurant with my husband recently, and I honestly felt like the happiest girl in the place. It was a day when my pain level and dizziness were minimal, and I actually felt somewhat normal. I took extra pleasure in getting dressed up. I relished in the ability to order whatever we wanted from the menu, selecting tried-and-true favorites and exciting new dishes. I savored my food. I laughed with my husband. I did not undervalue how good it was to feel well and to be out celebrating life. If I didn't have so many hard days, I am not sure I would appreciate the good days as much. Moments like these are rarer than I'd like. I think they are too infrequent for most of us with Dysautonomia; that's why it is best to make the most of them when they happen.

8.   I became my own advocate. I was very shy as a child and really struggled with standing up for myself. I remember an incident when I was around nine years old: a girl in my Sunday school class told me that she and I would bleed different colors and, to prove her point, she pinched me really hard causing me to bleed and leaving a nasty bruise. Although I knew she was wrong both in her thought process and later in her actions, I lacked the confidence to do any-

thing about it. I can't imagine responding that way today. One of the things I discovered early on was that there will be many situations where no one else is going to fight for me; I am going to have to buckle up and do it myself. In my life the capacity to not back down has been especially necessary when it comes to dismissive doctors, insurance companies and employers. I have had to learn to trust my body and not be afraid to voice my opinion. Having to stand up for myself has made me aware of just how courageous and determined I can be.

9. I matured more quickly than I would have otherwise. I think most individuals with a chronic illness are very aware of how different they are from their peers, especially during the teenage and college years. I hated being labeled the "sick" girl, but I didn't recognize at the time all of the ways in which being sick helped me mature. Living with a chronic illness, your life starts centering on bigger issues than what someone is wearing or what the girl who sits behind you in class thinks of your hair. Of course, these are silly examples. However, the truth is having a chronic illness throughout most of schooling and beyond taught me to focus on what is important. I learned not to judge too harshly. Because I had to fight to get through high school and college, I was excited when I could go to school and, thus, I developed a love of learning that has stuck with me to this day.

10. I learned to fill my days with things that make me happy. In my quest to find a new sense of normalcy, I not only uncovered new interests, I also learned to not feel guilty for pursuing things that bring me pleasure.   For me, these activities include listening to musicians, such as Otis Redding and Sam Cooke (It's summertime, and the living is easy...); eating sushi on a regular basis; talking on the phone to a compassionate and understanding friend; searching through cookbooks, magazines and Pinterest for new reci-

pes; getting out the house whenever I can, whether for a short trip to the grocery store or a dinner out with friends; and playing board games and cards with my husband. Yes, these activities are quieter and simpler than my favorite activities of the past, like ice skating or an all-day shopping excursion, but they are small moments in my day that bring me joy. And when you are stuck feeling miserable a lot of the time, finding things that you still enjoy becomes even more necessary.

One of the most inspiring aspects of human life is that growing and learning are continual. If I fall, I can pick myself back up, dust off and try again. When I reflect on my journey thus far, I am encouraged by the knowledge and strength I have gained through my battle with POTS and other illnesses. Living with Dysautonomia means accepting that much of what I deal with is beyond my control, but I take satisfaction in knowing that I can choose what I mentally and emotionally take away from the experience.

Section 4. Other Syndromes

Chapter 10. Ehlers-Danlos Syndrome

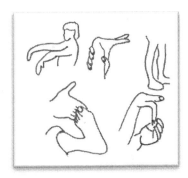

Ehlers - Danlos Syndrome is sometimes an underlying cause of POTS. Ehlers - Danlos Syndrome, or EDS, is a hereditary connective tissue disorder. There are many different types of EDS, but I will focus here on Ehlers - Danlos Syndrome Type III, often referred to as the Hypermobility type. This is one of the most common of the EDS types that occurs in POTS patients.

Individuals with EDS have a defect in their connective tissue, the tissue that provides support to many body parts such as the skin, muscles, ligaments and other organs. The fragile skin and unstable joints found in EDS are the result of faulty collagen. Collagen is a protein, which acts as a *"glue"* in the body, adding strength and elasticity to connective tissue.

Hypermobility is relatively common among children and affects more females than males. Symptoms may include a dull but intense pain around the knee and ankle joints and also on the soles of the feet. Using insoles in the footwear, which have been specially made for the individual after assessment by an orthopedic surgeon, can alleviate the condition affecting these parts.

In 1993, Dr. Beighton discussed the history of Ehlers-Danlos syndrome (EDS); beginning with a description of it in the fourth century BC. The first detailed clinical description of the syndrome is attributed to Tschernogobow in 1892. The syndrome derives its name from reports by Edward Ehlers, a Danish dermatologist, in 1901 and by Henri-Alexandre Danlos, a French physician with expertise in skin disorders.

The incredible, almost unnatural, positions that some patients with Ehlers-Danlos syndrome can perform often provoke curiosity. Many are extremely flexible and "double jointed (not all people who are flexible or who are double jointed have this syndrome.) People who have Ehlers-Danlos Type III frequently overextend their joints. *"Over extension"* is the ability to flex the joints beyond their normal limits.

Historically, some patients with Ehlers-Danlos Syndrome displayed contortionist maneuvers in circuses, shows, and performance tours. Some achieved fame and had titles such as *"The Elastic Lady," "The Human Pretzel"* and *"Rubber Band Man."*

> *Note: Many former gymnasts and dancers have Ehlers-Danlos Type III. They may have been drawn to these sports due to the extreme flexibility of their joints. However, talented they probably are, participating in these sports is very hard on the body and may lead to further complications of this disorder down the road.*

People with hypermobility syndrome may develop other conditions caused by their unstable joints. These conditions include:

- Joint hypermobility
- Loose/unstable joints which are prone to frequent dislocations and/or subluxations
- Joint pain (especially in the lower back, neck and wrists)
- Hyper extensible joints (they move beyond the joint's normal range)
- Frequent sprains, tendinitis, or bursitis
- Early-onset osteoarthritis
- Knee pain
- Back pain, prolapsed discs or spondylolisthesis
- Flat feet
- Joints that make clicking noises
- Susceptibility to whiplash
- Temperomandibular Joint Syndrome also known as

TMJ
- Increased nerve compression disorders (i.e. carpal tunnel syndrome)

Cardiovascular symptoms are also common. Approximately one-third to one-half of people that have EDS report chest pain, palpitations and or orthostatic intolerance. Holter monitoring often shows normal rhythm but sometimes will reveal premature beats or extra beats. Those that start in the upper chambers (atria) are called premature atrial contractions or PACs. Premature ventricular contractions or PVCs start in the ventricles. Many people with EDS and various forms of Dysautonomia have the feeling that their heart has "*skipped a beat*," it was probably from this type of arrhythmia. The heart really doesn't skip a beat. Instead, an extra beat comes sooner than normal. Then there's usually a pause that causes the next beat to be more forceful. The more forceful beat is the one you will feel.

Premature beats are very common in normal children and teenagers. Most people have them but do not always realize they have occurred. Usually no cause can be found and no special treatment is needed. The premature beats may disappear later. Even if they continue, your child will probably not need any restrictions. Occasionally premature heartbeats may be caused by an underlying condition. Your child's doctor may recommend more tests to make sure your child's heart is okay.

Many people who have EDS also suffer from gastrointestinal issues such as: functional gastritis, Irritable bowel syndrome, and delayed gastric emptying to name a few. Seeing a GI specialist may help rule out some other related issues and may be helpful in putting together a treatment plan to help lessen potentially painful symptoms.

EDS patients also may have very unique skin features. Their skin tends to be soft and stretchy. When grabbing the forearm of someone who has EDS, the skin feels loose and doughy. The skin may tear or bruise easily (bruising may be severe). Severe scarring; slow and poor wound healing; and development of molluscoid pseudo tumors (fleshy lesions associated with scars over pressure areas) are also hallmarks of people who have EDS.

At this time, there is no definitive blood test for Ehlers-Danlos type III. Diagnosis is made by family history, symptoms and clinical observation by a physician who specializes in EDS. (often a geneticist)

There is no cure for EDS. Having strong muscles that can support the joints is key to controlling EDS symptoms. It is imperative that the individual with hypermobility remain extremely fit (even more so than the average individual) to prevent recurrent injuries. Regular exercise and physical therapy or hydrotherapy can reduce symptoms of hypermobility, because strong muscles help to stabilize joints. These treatments can also help by stretching tight, overused muscles and ensuring the person uses joints within the ideal ranges of motion, avoiding hyperextension or hyperflexion. Low-impact exercise such as Pilates or Tai Chi is usually recommended for hypermobile people, as it is less likely to cause injury than high-impact exercise or contact sports.

Moist hot packs can relieve the pain of aching joints and muscles. For some patients, ice packs also help to relieve pain.

Note: If using a physical therapist, it is important that you find a manual therapist who is familiar with EDS and joint laxity.

Medications frequently used to reduce pain and inflammation caused by hypermobility include analgesics, anti-inflammatory drugs and tricyclic antidepressants. Some people with hypermobility may benefit from other medications such as steroid injections or gabapentin, a drug originally used for treating epilepsy. Europe is far ahead of the United States in terms of EDS recognition and its knowledge of how to treat it. Tramadol, a non-narcotic pain reliever that is nearly as effective as narcotics, has been used in England to treat EDS joint pain, and it is available by prescription from a doctor in the United States. Benzodiazapines are also used for EDS sufferers who experience painful muscles spasms around loose joints.

Dr. Brad Tinkle, a geneticist in Cincinnati, Ohio, a leading expert in the country on EDS, recommends that most of his patients take Ibuprofen daily to help reduce inflammation in the joints. Caution must be taken to avoid gastrointestinal side effects from long term Ibuprofen use, such as stomach ulcers. Dr. Tinkle also suggests that patients take Glucosamine and Chondroitin. See your doctor for appropriate dosing.

Life Style Modifications

For some people with hypermobility, lifestyle changes decrease the severity of symptoms.

For example if your hand is cramping or becoming weak after writing for long periods of time, there is a great writing apparatus, called PenAgain. They come in pens and mechanical pencils. The apparatus holds your fingers in a perfect position and will help avoid cramping and overextending the finger joints.

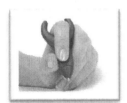

If writing is still painful, people may be able to reduce the pain by typing.

If typing is painful, they may try voice control software for their computer or a more ergonomic keyboard.

Avoid activities that can bring on symptoms, such as standing, stretching the joints (such as in some forms of yoga), and lifting heavy objects or weights.

A decrease in heavy exercise, such as lifting heavy weights or competitive running should be avoided. Instead, consider running on an elliptical machine.

Swimming is a wonderful activity for those with EDS. Try using a kickboard to exercise in a pool but be careful not to hyperextend your knees while kicking the water and keep a bend in your elbows. If you swim; if you have weak shoulders then avoid "arms-only" "pull" exercises in the water and try to focus on kicking without hyperextension while keeping a relaxed pace with your arms.

Posture should be closely monitored. Weakened ligaments and muscles contribute to poor posture, which may result in numerous other medical conditions. Isometric exercises and attention to where joints are (avoid crossing legs for example if you have hip problems) are helpful to keep posture from leading to more pain.

Bracing to support weak joints may be helpful when joints are injured or painful, but caution must be used not to weaken the joints further. Those who are overweight should lose weight. The extra weight puts additional stress on the already weakened ligaments, making them more susceptible to injury.

Individuals with EDS should wear sunscreen and avoid activities and sports that place too much stress on the joints. Contact sports, gymnastics and other sports that will cause the joints to go beyond their normal range of motion, may cause more complications and chronic pain for the person who has EDS in the future. Low impact sports are best but each person must weigh the pros and cons of all activities. They must find an activity that will allow them to keep their muscles fit (this will help hold the joints in place) while at the same time keeping their joints happy. If a sport or activity is causing too much pain, consider modifying the activity or choosing another one that is easier on the joints.

Patients with the hypermobility type of EDS can have an increased risk for pregnancy complications, including prematurity due to cervical incompetence and to premature rupture of membranes. Patients with EDS should demand the clinician's alertness for possible signs of this under diagnosed type of EDS and recommend the collaboration between the obstetrician and the medical geneticist in the obstetrical management of these patients.[1] During pregnancy certain hormones alter the physiology of ligaments making them able to stretch to accommodate the birthing process. For some women with hypermobility pregnancy related pelvic girdle pain can be debilitating.

Breech presentation, potentially related to hypotonia, is also more common with an affected infant. Other fetal malpositions (face and brow) as well as growth restriction have been reported with hypermobility-type EDS.

> *Note: I have a mild case of EDS that I carried on to my offspring. I had no major complications during any of my pregnancies. I had three pregnancies that resulted in four healthy babies. (One set of twins) All of the births were just slightly premature; none before 36 weeks.*

The outlook for individuals with EDS depends on the type of EDS with which they have been diagnosed. Symptoms vary in severity, even within one sub-type, and the frequency of complications changes on an individual basis. Some individuals have few symptoms while others are severely restricted in their daily life. Extreme joint instability and scoliosis may limit a person's mobility. Most individuals will have a normal lifespan.

Although individuals with EDS Type III face many challenges, it is important to remember that each person is unique with their own celebrated qualities and extraordinary potential. Persons with EDS go on to raise families, to have successful careers, and to be well accomplished, despite the challenges of their syndrome. It may be helpful to always keep life in perspective and to remember that *"You are not your illness."* Your syndrome can only win, if you decide to let it.

The Beighton scale a modification of the Carter & Wilkinson scoring system has been used for many years as an indicator of widespread hypermobility. A high Beighton score by itself does not mean that an individual has EDS. It simply means that the individual has widespread hypermobility. Diagnosis of EDS Type III is often made using the Beighton Criteria as well as through clinical observation by a trained medical professional.

The Beighton score is calculated as follows:

Score one point if you can bend and place your hands flat on the floor without bending your knees.	
Score one point for each knee that will bend backwards.	
Score one point for each elbow that will bend backwards.	
Score one point for each thumb that will bend backwards to touch the forearm.	

Score one point for each hand when you can bend the little finger back beyond 90°.

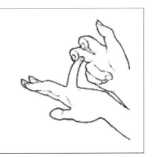

If you are able to perform all of above maneuvers then you have a maximum score of 9 points. [2]

More information go to http://www.hypermobility.org

Resources:

Ehlers-Danlos National Foundation (EDNF)
3200 Wilshire Blvd.
Suite 1601 South Tower Los Angeles, CA 90010 USA
Tel: (213)368-3800 Fax: (213)427-0057 Tel: (800)956-2902
Email: staff@ednf.org
Internet: http://www.ednf.org

NIH/National Arthritis and Musculoskeletal and Skin Diseases Information Clearinghouse
1 AMS Circle Bethesda, MD 20892-3675 USA
Tel: (301)495-4484 Fax: (301)718-6366 Tel: (877)226-4267
TDD: (301)565-2966
Email: NIAMSinfo@mail.nih.gov
Internet: http://www.niams.nih.gov/Health_Info

Ehlers-Danlos Support Group UK
PO Box 337 Aldershot Surrey, Intl GU12 6WZ United Kingdom
Tel: +44 01252 690 940
Email: director@ehlers-danlos.org
Internet: http://www.ehlers-danlos.org

MUMS National Parent-to-Parent Network
150 Custer Court Green Bay, WI 54301-1243 USA
Tel: (920)336-5333 Fax: (920)339-0995 Tel: (877)336-5333

Email: mums@netnet.net
Internet: http://www.netnet.net/mums/

Sjældne Diagnoser / Rare Disorders Denmark
Frederiksholms Kanal 2, 3rd Floor Copenhagen K, 1220
Denmark
Tel: 45 33 14 00 10 Fax: 45 33 14 55 09
Email: mail@sjaeldnediagnoser
Internet: http://www.raredisorders.dk

Ehlers Danlos Foundation of New Zealand
368 Butler Road, RD 3 Waipawa 4273 Hawkes Bay,
New Zealand
Tel: 64-06 874-7799 Fax: 64-06 874-7799
Email: flopsy@ihug.co.nz
Internet: http://www.edfnz.org.nz

EDS Today
6545 Lake Drive Mays Landing, NJ 08330 USA
Tel: (609)625-3182
Email: info@edstoday.org
Internet: http://www.edstoday.org

Genetic and Rare Diseases (GARD) Information Center
PO Box 8126 Gaithersburg, MD 20898-8126
Tel: (301)251-4925 Fax: (301)251-4911 Tel: (888)205-2311
TDD: (888)205-3223
Email: ordr@od.nih.gov
Internet: http://rarediseases.info.nih.gov/Default.aspx

Madisons Foundation
PO Box 241956
Los Angeles, CA 90024
Tel: (310)264-0826
Fax: (310)264-4766
Email: getinfo@madisonsfoundation.org
Internet: http://www.madisonsfoundation.org

European Skeletal Dysplasia Network (ESDN) Welcome Trust Centre for Cell-Matrix Research Faculty of Life Sciences University of Manchester
Michael Smith Building, Oxford Road Manchester, M13 9PTUK
Tel: 44 161 275 5642 Fax: 44 161 275 5082

Email: info@esdn.org
Internet: http://www.esdn.org

1.   A. De PaepeCenter for Medical Genetics 0K5 University Hospital Gent De Pintelaan 185, B-9000 Gent Belgium

2   Tinkle, Brad. Issues and Management of Joint Hypermobility: A guide for the Ehlers-Danlos Syndrome Hypermobility Type and the Hypermobility Syndrome. Ohio, 2008

Chapter 11 Physical Therapy in Children Presenting with Ehlers-Danlos Syndrome and Postural Orthostatic Tachycardia Syndrome -*Ashley Summers, PT, DPT*

Reviewed By Dr. Brad Tinkle, Geneticist

As a pediatric physical therapist working alongside of Dr. Brad Tinkle at Advocate Children's Hospital in Park Ridge, Illinois, I have had the opportunity of working with children ages 5-17 years old, who have been diagnosed with Ehlers-Danlos Syndrome (EDS) and Positional Orthostatic Tachycardia Syndrome (POTS). According to research, POTS is significantly more common in patients with EDS who are under the age of 25[1]. However, many patients with POTS often see improvements in their symptoms over a period of many years[2].

In our connective tissue clinic, about 75-80% of our case-load of children with EDS also have symptoms of orthostatic intolerance when changing positions. Physical therapy in general can help with increasing strength to help support the joints as well as providing training in appropriate joint protection techniques to prevent subluxations and dislocations in activities of daily living. Physical therapy also helps provide a means of which to bridge inactivity to full participation in school/gym/sports by providing physical activity suggestions that are safe and effective for patients with EDS and POTS. The most important recommendation to children and adults with EDS and POTS is to find a physical therapist that is familiar with or is willing to learn about connective tissue disorders. A physical therapist receives a generalized degree in school where they are fully equipped to treat basic pediatric, inpatient, outpatient, and post-surgical diagnoses. This does not make a physical therapist an expert in everything. Many physical therapists will take continuing education or specialize in an area of expertise in order to more fully understand their area of practice. From this principle, many physical therapists are unfamiliar with EDS and POTS; however they are fully equipped to treat patients with these diagnoses if given proper instructions on precautions in this patient population.

As physical therapy is one of the mainstays of treatment, a physical therapist can assist in relieving joint pain and preventing joint pain through exercise and treatment. Some of the major components of physical therapy visits will focus on joint stability and control, proprioceptive training, posture training, strength training, range of motion, and the instruction and development of a home exercise program. Research has not yet identified the optimal physical therapy program for patients with EDS/POTS[3]. Much of this confusion can be attributed to the difference in presentation of each patient with EDS/POTS.   A physical therapist needs to assess each individual's pain, fatigue, range of motion, strength, posture, proprioception, etc. prior to initiating a program in order to make an effective individualized treatment plan. Part of the treatment plan is also identifying the need for a multidisciplinary approach such as occupational therapy, pain specialist, neurologist, orthopedist, rheumatologist, and other specialists that may be beneficial in managing and coordinating care[4].

Although there are no specific exercises or treatments that will improve pain or decrease symptoms for every patient with EDS/POTS, there are standard recommendations[3]. The standard recommendations include promoting regular aerobic exercise (walking, biking, dancing, skating, and hiking). If the child is too sick to perform this type of exercise, it is always best to start in a horizontal position, slowly working up to recumbent exercises, like a rower or a recumbent bike.   One should also strive to promote postural and ergonomic hygiene especially at work or in school, avoid high impact sports/activities, avoiding sudden postural changes, promoting increased water and salt intake (except in cases of hypertension), avoiding prolonged sitting or prolonged recumbent positions, promoting sleep hygiene, and avoiding over-activity[4]. The most important factor in beginning a new exercise program is remembering pacing. Try to have your child focus on gradually reaching his/her goals. For instance, if he/she would like to be able to walk one mile, but are only able to walk 3 minutes today, it's okay. Tell them to listen to their body and take breaks. As their body adjusts to a new exercise program, in a few days he/she will be able to add one or two minutes to their walking time. Gradually he/she will reach their goal of walking one mile. Increasing fluid intake is especially important as it can increase blood flow, which improves circulation and decreases symptoms of dizziness. Salt intake is important as well as this helps retain fluid. Some children with POTS have noted an improvement in symptoms by pre-planning transitions/position changes prior to completing them. The brain is able to complete "motor planning" and thereby prepares the body for movement, decreasing the symptoms of dizziness. This does require the individual to slow down, think about changing positions, and think about what is involved in changing positions before completing the actual change.

Having a support system is very important in seeing and maintaining improvements in symptoms. Getting an entire family involved is key in seeing success. According to Birt et al, parents and children with hypermobility saw an improvement in symptoms with good adherence to an exercise program[5]. They especially saw improvement when an exercise program was adapted into their family routines. Seeing a benefit in exercise also increased adherence to an exercise program[5]. Parents of children with EDS/POTS can help their child by promoting family exercise time or giving rewards for completing daily home exercise programs. Parents can also help their children by highlighting improvements. Although initially these improvements may be small, gradual but steady improvements should be rewarded with positive reinforcement to continue seeing benefits. Some of these techniques may be difficult in families with teens with EDS/POTS, but they may be just as important if not more important in these cases. Your physical therapist can work with you to develop a home exercise program that promotes the greatest amount of family engagement as well as utilizes the equipment that is found at home. Ask your physical therapist how each exercise will help your child achieve his/her goals. If you have the understanding on how an exercise will help your child and you see a benefit, you will be more likely to assist them in completing it.

Keys to Success in Physical Therapy

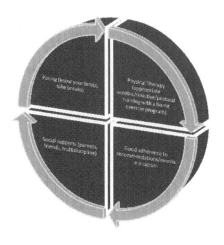

Chapter 12. Familial Dysautonomia - *President of FD Now, Ann Slaw*

Familial Dysautonomia (FD) is a genetic form of Dysautonomia and it is almost always fatal. Like those with POTS, kids with FD live in very unstable bodies. Many symptoms of FD overlap with POTS including wide swings in blood pressure and heart rate. However, unlike POTS, FD is usually only seen in the Ashkenazi Jewish population. The inability to cry tears or feel pain are two of the hallmark signs of FD. Taking a simple blood test will confirm or exclude a diagnosis of FD and can also identify carriers during a prenatal screen.

Overview of FD

FD is a rare, genetic, neurologic disease present at birth; it is almost always fatal. Approximately half of the children born with it will not make it to age 20. To best describe this disorder, consider the clues in its name. Familial means the condition is inherited. Dysautonomia (pronounced "dis – aw – tuh – noh – mee - uh") means a dysfunction of the autonomic nervous system. The autonomic nervous system controls automatic body functions, such as circulation, digestion and breathing. These functions occur involuntarily. People with FD have an impaired autonomic nervous system, rendering each breath, swallow and heartbeat undependable and erratic.

In addition to the detrimental effects of FD on the organs that function automatically (e.g., lungs, stomach and heart), FD also impairs a part of the sensory nervous system that controls pain and temperature. Thus, broken bones, burns and frostbite often go undetected.

Symptoms of FD

A newborn with FD is typically "floppy," "skinny," and may have difficulty sucking. A newborn may experience frequent aspiration pneumonia (pneumonia caused by misdirecting liquid into the lungs) and may require a nasogastric tube (a tube threaded down the baby's nostril into the stomach) for nutrition. Eventually, the baby's formula may need substantial thickening in order for the baby to coordinate a safe swallow.

The toddler with FD has difficulty gaining weight and growing. Toddlers with FD tend to wobble and stumble, falling frequently. Their eyes are often dry which may lead to numerous corneal abrasions. They don't produce overflow tears. Often, they drool and may need to wear a terrycloth sweatband to wipe their chins dry. Most toddlers receive physical, occupational and speech therapy for developmental delays. The toddler may pass out if belly-laughing or crying, especially following a startle. Many parents find themselves dialing for emergency care only to watch their child regain consciousness and then go about playing as if nothing occurred.

Children and adults with FD have difficulty regulating their blood pressure so they will often feel dizzy and will simply collapse when rising from bed or sitting in a chair. Due to the decrease in pain sensitivity, those with FD are unaware that they are hurt so, for example, cuts, bruises, insect bites, broken bones, cracked teeth, and other forms of physical distress often go unnoticed. Most alarming is when individuals with FD enter a state of *"autonomic crisis,"* usually triggered by illness, intense stress or certain chemicals found in food or medication. During the autonomic crisis, they will experience skyrocketing blood pressure and heart rate and will endure uncontrollable and violent retching.

Additional indicators of FD include a smooth tongue which may decrease taste sensations, slow digestion, swings in body temperature, cold hands and feet, scoliosis (curved spine) and kyphosis (head thrusting forward and hanging low).

Diagnosing FD

Because FD is rare, it's often undiagnosed at birth. Instead, a baby born with FD is often medically labeled with "failure to thrive," "congenital benign hypotonia," "colicky," and "failure to suck."

As the baby develops and FD symptoms emerge, a definitive diagnosis is available from a simple genetic blood test. If positive for FD, the blood test will reveal mutations in the IKBKAP gene. This genetic blood test for FD has been available since 2001.

Note that prior to 2001, parents and doctors depended on observation to detect FD. Still reliable, these indicators are:

- Both parents are from an Ashkenazi Jewish background.
- The baby's tongue is smooth, signifying an absence of fungiform papillae (large bumps that contain taste buds).
- The baby does not produce overflow tears when upset.
- The baby does not involuntarily respond when tapped with a reflex hammer.

Treating FD

Since the discovery of the FD gene mutation in 2000, researchers have made rapid progress in understanding and countering its effects. Five revolutionary treatments have helped many children and adults with FD. The benchmark of these five treatments is that they treat the underlying cause of the disease, rather than treat the individual symptoms.

These five comprehensive treatment approaches have been developed by a dedicated group of researchers led by Dr. Berish Rubin and Sylvia Anderson at the Laboratory for Familial Dysautonomia Research at Fordham University and they are:

Tocotrienol (2003) - Tocotrienol, a form of vitamin E, helps raise a lacking protein level. Those taking tocotrienol reported more stability in autonomic function, including increased energy and stamina. Some even reported the ability to spill overflow tears, a significant reversal of a telltale FD symptom. Additional research concluded that those taking tocotrienol improved their cardiac function and lowered the frequency of autonomic crisis. [1]

EGCG (2003) – EGCG (epigallocatechin gallate), a component of green tea, further helped raise a lacking protein level. Again, those taking EGCG reported additional autonomic stability. [2]

Tyramine-Free Diet (2005) - Those with FD lack a key enzyme needed to sweep tyramine from the bloodstream. Too much tyramine in the blood causes autonomic crises. By avoiding tyramine-laden foods, such as aged, fermented and smoked products, those with FD reduce the frequency of autonomic crises. [3]

Vitamin A and Beta-Carotene (2010) – Preliminary studies conducted by Drs. Berish Rubin and Sylvia Anderson demonstrate that both Vitamin A and Beta-Carotene further elevate a lacking protein level. Again, those taking Vitamin A and Beta-Carotene reported additional autonomic stability. [4]

Limiting Protein Intake (2010) – Preliminary studies conducted by Drs. Rubin and Anderson demonstrate that limiting protein intake helps reduce the number of autonomic crises. Rubin Berish.[5]

Prior to these systemic treatments, the medical community relied on a variety of individual treatments for various symptoms. In addition to the tocotrienol, EGCG, tyramine-free diet, Vitamin A and Beta-Carotene, and protein-limited diet, those with FD may still benefit from individual symptom treatments depending on the number and severity of symptoms. Typically, those with FD receive treatment options from a team of health care specialists including speech, occupational, physical and respiratory therapists, pulmonologists, cardiologists, urologists, orthopedic surgeons, ophthalmologists, and psychologists.

Planning on Having Kids? Get Tested!

A number of ethnic groups have a higher risk for inheriting specific genetic conditions than the general population. In the Ashkenazi (Eastern European) Jewish population, there are approximately nine well-known inherited conditions. The American College of Obstetricians and Gynecologists recommends that those of Ashkenazi descent and their partners be tested for genetic carrier status for four of these: Familial Dysautonomia (FD), Tay-Sachs, Canavan Disease, and Cystic Fibrosis. Carrier testing is also available for other Ashkenazi genetic disorders such as Fanconi Anemia, Gaucher Disease, Niemann-Pick, Mucolipidosis, and Bloom Syndrome. The test panel for these conditions is sometimes kiddingly referred to as *"the kosher kit."*

If you or a loved one are of Ashkenazi descent and are planning on having children, a simple blood test will determine if you are a carrier for any of these conditions. Be sure to ask if the lab tests for both of the two known FD mutations; one is more common than the other but not all labs test for both. Many insurance plans cover the cost of testing. In addition, local testing centers offer free or reduced rates. Visit www.jewishgeneticscenter.org for a list of nationwide genetic counseling and screening services to locate one near you.

For FD, you have an approximately 1/27 chance of carrying the FD mutation. If your partner also has the genetic mutation, your chance of having a baby with FD is 25% with each pregnancy. The good news is that FD is preventable. Even if both parents are carriers, your obstetrician can help you to avoid having a child with FD. Getting tested, and working with your obstetrician, are the best ways to prevent FD.

Genetic testing has had a dramatic effect on the number of FD births. Prior to 2001, the total number of reported FD births averaged 15 per year. Once testing became available for FD in 2001, the number of reported FD births steadily declined to 2 births in 2006 and 1 birth in 2007. [6]

On a personal note:

As a mom of a young adult with FD, both my husband Ken and I have been extremely active in the FD community. We founded FD NOW to support the critical work of Dr. Berish Rubin and Dr. Sylvia Anderson at the Laboratory for Familial Dysautonomia Research at Fordham University. These two researchers discovered the FD mutation in record time followed by four treatment breakthroughs with more on the horizon.

Our son, Andrew, was diagnosed with FD at age 4. He was our first child, and despite feeding difficulties, frequent hospitalizations and inability to cry tears, Andrew's pediatrician assured us that our fears were unfounded. It wasn't until Andrew smashed his finger in a door and registered no pain that he was ultimately diagnosed by a pediatric neurologist.

Andrew's FD diagnosis was both comforting and petrifying. On the one hand, we had an answer; the laundry list of FD symptoms described Andrew to a tee. On the other hand, we faced a terrifying reality; the prognosis was not good. The literature described FD as "life-threatening" or "fatal." Most sources said that Andrew would be lucky to live until early adulthood.

Immediately, Ken and I began a crusade to raise public awareness about FD and to raise money for FD research. We've been campaigning for nearly two decades, and thanks to Drs. Rubin and Anderson, we continue to gain momentum.

Andrew is a walking example of this momentum. Though he comes in a small 5' 1", 100-pound package, his personality is larger than life.

FD NOW was so named to underscore our founding principle - urgency. Children with FD, like Andrew, do not have the luxury of time. Urgency drives our researchers to test and then deliver safe substances that have an immediate positive impact in our children's daily lives; they are dedicated to "lab to life," "project to patient" research. Urgency drives our commitment to promptly forward your dollars to Drs. Rubin and Anderson, to ensure swift results. These two researchers are dedicated to improving the daily lives of our kids by making the effects of FD disappear. We eagerly await their next amazing discovery.

Need more information about FD?
Feel free to contact:
Ann Slaw, J.D., President FD NOW
   1170 Green Knolls Drive, Buffalo Grove, IL   60089
   Phone: (847) 913-0455 Fax: (847) 913-8589
   E-mail: fdnow@comcast.net Web: www.fdnow.org

1. Anderson, S.L., Qiu, J. and Rubin, B.Y. (2003) Tocotrienols induce IKBKAP expression: a possible therapy for familial Dysautonomia. Biochem. Biophys. Res. Comm. 306:303-309 and Rubin B.Y., Anderson S.L. and Kapás L. (2008) Can the therapeutic efficacy of tocotrienols in neurodegenerative familial Dysautonomia patients be measured clinically? Antioxid. Redox. Signal 10:837-41).
2. (Anderson, S.L., Qiu, J. and Rubin, B.Y. (2003) EGCG corrects aberrant splicing of IKAP mRNA in cells from patients with Familial Dysautonomia. Biochem. Biophys. Res. Comm. 310:627-633).
3. (Anderson S.L. and Rubin B.Y. (2005) Tocotrienols reverse IKAP and monoamine oxidase deficiencies in familial Dysautonomia. Biochem. Biophys. Res. Commun. 336:150-6).
4. (Rubin Berish. "Vitamin A and Beta-carotene" Familial Dysautonomia Now Foundation (FD NOW) Ed. Ann Slaw. 2010. 1 January).
5. "Protein Intake and Crisis." Familial Dysautonomia Now Foundation (FD NOW) Ed. Ann Slaw. 2010. 1 May 2010).
    <http://www.fdnow.org/RecentFind05-10.html>
6. (Lerner, Barron H (2009). When diseases disappear- the case of Familial Dysautonomia. N Engl J Med. 361:1622-1625).

Section 5. Surviving the Educational System

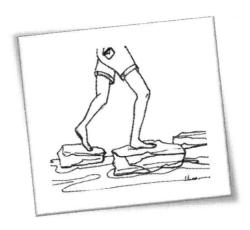

Chapter 13. Dealing with Dysautonomia in the Classroom - Tips for Teachers

"They may forget what you said, but they will Remember how you made them Feel" - Anonymous

A Brief Overview of POTS: (For teachers)

POTS, postural orthostatic tachycardia syndrome, is an illness that affects the autonomic nervous system. The autonomic nervous system or ANS, controls all of the body's involuntary actions such as: heart rate, blood pressure, breathing, digestion, etc. This illness once was believed to be rare but now new research is questioning this. Mayo Clinic estimates that 1 in 100 people may have some form of this illness. Symptoms may range from mild to life threatening. POTS is a form of Dysautonomia. Dysautonomia means a deregulation of the autonomic nervous system. There are many forms of Dysautonomia. One form, a genetic disorder, called Familial Dysautonomia, is often diagnosed at birth and is only seen in people of Eastern European Jewish descent. Children who are born with this form have a considerably low survival rate. POTS is a different format Dysautonomia and while not fatal it can be life altering.

POTS is recognized as a physical, usually neurological based disorder by every major medical university in America. It is quantifiable and verifiable.

POTS is defined as a heart rate increase of 30 beats per minute or more from the supine position (laying down) to the standing position within 20 minutes or less of standing. This is called postural tachycardia. Many people who have POTS will also have a severe drop in systolic blood pressure (20bpm or more) upon standing. This condition is called orthostatic intolerance. After the person with POTS stands, the blood pressure usually drops quickly and severely. This will cause the heart to beat faster in order to compensate in an attempt to stabilize the blood pressure. This is extremely taxing on the body and causes a myriad of unusual and complex symptoms ranging from chest pains to syncope (fainting) to shortening of breath.

There are many theories as to the causes of POTS. Most doctors agree that POTS is analogous to a fever in that the fever is a symptom of something else going on in the body. There are many reasons why one may get a fever. Like POTS, there are many underlying causes for why one may develop this syndrome. It is usually secondary to some other issue that is taking place in the body. Scientifically recognized triggers of POTS are: viral infections, autoimmune disorders, diabetes and physical trauma (such as surgeries and car accidents). A large growth spurt can often trigger POTS, which is why many people are diagnosed with POTS during their middle school or high school years.

POTS was not taught in most medical schools until recently and therefore many people who have POTS go for years searching to find the root of their illness before being diagnosed. Patients are misdiagnosed with other disease due to lack of sufficient knowledge about this disorder in the medical community. As awareness comes to the forefront more and more individuals are being properly diagnosed. POTS is believed to be one of the fastest growing syndromes in America. Researchers believe that more people have

POTS than autism. Like chicken pox, POTS symptoms can range from mild to life threatening.

Children with Dysautonomia are children first. No child wishes to be sick and no parent wishes their child to be sick. Teachers need to keep this in mind when dealing with their student who has Dysautonomia. The child is going through emotional and physical pain. They want to laugh, play, and just be children. Most kids who have POTS were once very active before their illness. Many are athletes, who now just struggle to get out of bed in the morning. Their bodies will no longer cooperate with them. Many children with Dysautonomia tell me that they feel like a young kid who has an 80 year old body. It is extremely difficult for these children to get out of bed in the morning due to low blood pressure, tachycardia, and/or extreme fatigue. Many children with POTS also have insomnia due to abnormally high adrenalin levels caused by orthostatic stress; simply the extra stress placed on the body when in an upright position. Most have spent all night staring at the ceiling, unable to fall asleep. Some POTS patients also suffer from sleep apnea. They get up to go to school exhausted, frustrated and wiped out from the night before. The act of just getting out of bed in the morning can be extremely taxing on the child with Dysautonomia. Dr. Blair Grubb, the leading cardiologist for autonomic dysfunctions, says that the symptoms of a child living with Dysautonomia are similar to a person who has COPD or congestive heart failure. Their heart has to work three times harder than a normal individual.

When the child wakes up in the morning for school, he or she is often too dizzy to stand. Some need assistance going to the bathroom. Many will use a shower chair to take their morning shower, as they are too unstable to stand for that amount of time. POTS patients may have a headache, chest pains, and a racing heart (tachycardia) throughout the day. Some children experience skipped or premature heartbeats. This makes the child feel like their heart has temporarily stopped and restarted. Obviously, this can cause great anxiety. Many have stomach pains that become worse after eating, due to blood pooling in the abdomen. This causes some children to not want to eat. As a result, some children lose weight and often rumors ensue that they have an eating disorder.

Many people who have Dysautonomia experience a phenomenon known as "brain fog." Concentration and memory are often impaired in the student who has POTS due to insufficient blood flow to the brain. This is a terrible source of frustration for the student as well as his or her teachers.

During a typical day, the child with Dysautonomia, may experience some or all of the following symptoms: visual disturbances, nausea, joint pains, frequent urination, lethargy, bloating, constipation, weakness, shortness of breath, chills, disequilibrium, numbness, brain fog, anxiety, heat intolerance,and light and noise sensitivity. 30% of kids that have Dysautonomia faint and many others have white outs and black outs (called presyncopal episodes) but do not experience full loss of consciousness. This adds to their anxiety, as they fear they may pass out at school.

To make matters worse, since so many people have never heard of this syndrome, many people including friends, family members and teachers question if they have an illness at all. After all, they look so healthy! They can often be seen in the hallways, with a group of friends, smiling and acting perfectly well. Many will appear almost hyper at times. This is due to excessive levels of adrenalin being produced in response to low blood pressure and/or orthostatic intolerance. They may appear to have drastic mood swings going from hyper to lethargic in a matter of minutes. They lose friends, because nobody understands them. Some parents even fail to understand POTS, often forcing their child to go to school when they are symptomatic. Teachers get frustrated with their students with POTS because they have not finished their homework from the night before.

Now they come to your classroom, feeling traumatized both emotionally and physically. Living with Dysautonomia is an everyday struggle not just for the child who has it but also for everyone who deals with the child from their family members to their teachers. It is an extremely frustrating, complex and unpredictable illness that has to be dealt with in a unique fashion. Below are some suggestions that may make life in the classroom easier for you and your student with Dysautonomia.

1.   Learn as much as you can about your student's condition. Every child with Dysautonomia is different and therefore has unique symptoms. Learn what their main symptoms are and ask for the parents help on dealing with each one. Pass this information on to others in the building including: elective teachers, social workers, principal, lunchroom helpers, aides, support staff, etc...

2.   Be sure the child has a 504 Plan or IEP Plan in place. Know what the plan is and be sure to adhere to the accommodations listed.

3.   Keep in constant communication with the parents and other staff, regarding your student's health.

4.   If necessary, shorten assignments. Example: when teaching math, instead of doing the entire worksheet, have the student do every other problem.

5.   Do not overload the student with homework. If they can make it through the whole school day, odds are, they will go home and crash.

6.   Do away with "busy" work.

7.   Educate the class on your student's health condition, with permission from the parents and the child.

Note: After my daughter was diagnosed with POTS and began missing a lot of school, I went in to each of her classrooms and spoke to the class about her symptoms and how they affected her life. I asked her peers to ask questions about her syndrome, so they would understand her issues when she was well enough to return to school. I showed video clips of her life before her illness and talked about how life would be different for her now. This helped the teachers to be more empathetic towards her plight as well as helped her friends to be more supportive. I was pleasantly surprised at their reaction and concern.

One boy in her classroom, who my daughter barely knew, even dropped off a note and package to our house, a few days after I came in to speak to her classmates. He wrote her a beautiful, heartfelt note that wished her well and told her if she needed homework taken home, someone to listen to her or needed a friend; he would be there for her. He left a journal and a gift card to Barnes and Nobles at our front door. My daughter and I were so touched by his thoughtfulness. It lifted our spirits and taught us the amazing impact of a kind random act.

8. Understand that this illness waxes and wanes. Little Jane may go to a birthday party on Sunday and be too sick to come to your class on Monday. The child still needs to have a social life and should not be punished or denied having fun, because they have a chronic illness.

9. Do not judge. Just because you may have never heard of this syndrome, does not mean it does not exist.

10. Remember this illness is invisible. (like diabetes) Your student may look great on the outside and still feel awful on the inside.

11. Try not to call on these students when their hand is not raised. It may cause them extra stress and exacerbate their symptoms.

12.   Children with Dysautonomia do much worse when they are overheated. Heat dilates blood vessels and diverts blood to the skin. This process reduces blood flow to the key arteries that feed the brain. Consider keeping a fan in your room or allowing the student to carry a portable fan.

13.   Have an emergency plan in place should your student faint in the classroom or if there is another emergency where your student has to leave the room in a hurry. Assign a buddy to assist as needed.

14.   Understand that sometimes your student may be late getting to class as it may take them longer to do the stairs, take the elevator or get from one room to another. Do not penalize them for this.

15.   Children with Dysautonomia usually have many digestion issues as well, especially after meals. Allow for extra bathroom time. You may want to consider giving them a permanent bathroom pass. Do not draw attention to this, as they are probably already embarrassed.

16.   If the student looks under the weather or says they are dizzy, allow them to go to a quiet place to rest. Be sure that a trustworthy student or adult escorts them. The school nurse should be informed of the situation.

17.   Have a picture of the student who has Dysautonomia, so that substitute teachers and teachers who may not know the student are familiar with what he or she looks like.

18.   Make sure any substitute teachers know of your student's health conditions and that he or she follows the accommodations set forth in the 504 plan.

19.   Most students who have Dysautonomia compensate for their condition. They want to be treated like any other child. Because of this, they may not tell you when they are feeling ill. Be sure to look for signs of discomfort. They may walk with an unsteady gate, look paler or seem extra spacey. Ask their parent's how to recognize these signs.

20.   Many children with Dysautonomia feel worse when there is a change in barometric pressure. Be prepared to see an increase in symptoms when the temperature drops, before a storm comes in or on very humid and hot days.

21.   People who have Dysautonomia have great difficulty regulating their body temperature, (as this is controlled by the autonomic nervous system) they may go from too hot to too cold in a matter of seconds, no matter what the actual temperature is. They may need to wear shorts and t-shirts in the winter and long sleeves in the summer. You may find them putting on more clothing and then removing them. As long as their clothing adheres to the school's policies try to be understanding of this seemingly odd behavior.

22.   Try to be patient when your student asks you to repeat directions. Brain fog may impair their ability to comprehend what you have just instructed. Allowing for another responsible student in the classroom to repeat instructions to this student may maintain your sanity and keep everyone's frustration level to a minimum.

23.   If a student faints or near faints, lay them on their back with their legs up in the air. Fan them with a book or piece of paper until they come around. Contact the nurse and parents immediately.

24.   Be sure to sit the child with Dysautonomia as close to you, in proximity, as possible. Also try to position her or him near a door, in case a quick exit becomes necessary. Placing the child by the door will also present less distraction should this child need to leave the room in a hurry.

25.   Allow the child to leave class a few minutes early to get to their next class. The hallways will be less noisy and chaotic for the child at this time. Also, they may need extra time to get to their next class promptly.

26.   Allow the child to have frequent motor breaks. They will need to get up and move around your classroom, as

needed, to prevent blood pooling.

28.   Snacks - Dysautonomia patients are advised to eat several small meals throughout the day, rather than 3 large meals. Allow the child to have small snacks two or three times a day. Snacks can include bananas, ½ a bagel, grapes, cherries or a granola bar.

29.   Drinks – Dysautonomia patients are required to drink much more fluids than a normal person to increase the blood volume and help stabilized their blood pressure. Allow the child to keep a water bottle with spill proof cap in his/her desk. This may lead to extra bathroom trips but it is essential to minimize fainting episodes.

Note: Note taking may be impossible for a child with Dysautonomia. Due to fatigue and "brain fog," it is difficult for these students to multitask effectively. Possible accommodations are assigning a buddy to take notes and make copies for the child, bringing a tape recorder to class, or having the notes given to the child by the teacher.

Note: My son came home from school with little or nothing written down from his school day, requiring hours to reconstruct the day by his mother! Once his teachers provided notes, we could concentrate on actually learning the material.

---

30.   If a child asks you if he or she can go to the nurse, always allow them to go. Make sure another student or adult walks them to the nurse's office to make sure they get there safely and without incident.

31.   Come up with a few signs between you and your student, so she or he can communicate to you their needs without distracting the rest of the class and causing a scene. Consider using signs for when your student needs to use the bathroom, go to the nurse, or is having an emergency.

32.   Assign a responsible buddy, especially in the younger grades, to help your student walk to the bathroom, carry his or her books, walk to the lunch line, etc.

33.   Be flexible and creative. As symptoms wax and wane from moment to moment, hour-to-hour and day-to-day, so too might the accommodations listed above. Keep an open mind and realize that your plans to help your student may change and need to be tweaked frequently.

34.   Remember that you may be the only positive influence in the child's day. Try to be understanding and patient without being patronizing. Teachers really can make all of the difference in the world for these children.

Tips for the Homebound

"Teachers who inspire realize there will always be rocks in the road ahead of us. They will be stumbling blocks or stepping-stones; it all depends on how we use them." - Author Unknown.

At some point during your child's education, school may become too taxing to attend on a regular basis. If your child is missing too many school days due to appointments, illness or fatigue, it may be time to request a homebound tutor. A homebound tutor is a licensed teacher who is required to come to your house for a certain amount of hours per week. The tutor is paid for by the school district and should not be an out of pocket expense to the parent. The amount of hours the tutor will come varies from district to district and will depend on whether the student is still in school part-time or is fully homebound. Generally there is no state mandated rule as to how many days your child has to miss in a row to qualify for a tutor, but each state may have its own rules. Many schools will not allow a tutor to be hired until the student has missed at least 10 consecutive school days in a row. As a parent, you can request that this be waived. Ask that your child get a least one-hour per day or more of tutoring for each day missed. If the school waits for the child to miss at least ten days in a row, your child will already be at an extreme disadvantage. Explain to the school staff that your child's unique chronic illness will require unique modifications.

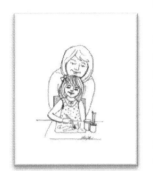

Before securing a homebound tutor, be sure that the school understands that this syndrome waxes and wanes. Be sure that the district will allow your child to return to school on a full time basis, when his/her symptoms lessen. A student who is on full homebound tutoring in the winter months should be allowed to return to school at any point, if and when they are less symptomatic. Make sure that the plan set up for your child is flexible and adaptable. My children have had many homebound tutors throughout the years. Some have worked out better than others. Below is a list of suggestions that may help the tutor to be more successful and effective with your child. You may wish to make a copy of this and give it to your child's tutor.

Suggestions for the homebound tutor

1. Familiarize yourself with the child's illness. There is a plethora of information about Dysautonomia on the Internet. You can use this book as a resource or take a look at Dynakids.org. Learn as much as you can.

2. BE FLEXIBLE- Remember the family is going through a lot. No parent wants to see their child on homebound tutoring and no child wants to be tutored. The family is under severe stress and is dealing with a chronic illness that few people understand, let alone have ever heard of. Try not to add extra stress and be understanding of the family's situation. All members of the family are going through a very emotional time. Try not to make them feel bad when sessions have to be changed due to illness, doctor appointments or lethargy. This will come with the territory.

3. The only thing predictable about this illness is that it is unpredictable.

4. Remember that your student will have good days and bad. Just because a student may have a few good sessions in a row, does not mean they are cured.

5. Listen to your student. If they tell you they are too sick to work on that particular day, reschedule. They know their body better than anyone else. If they are not feeling well, your lesson will be in vain, as they will not absorb the information any way.

6. Do not JUDGE. Just because your student looks well, it does not mean they feel well. Dysautonomia is an invisible illness.

7. Most kids who have Dysautonomia have concentration difficulties due to fatigue and low blood pressure. Lessons and concepts may have to be repeated. Do not get frustrated with your student because of this. Raising their anxiety level will only make things worse for them and you.

8. Kids with Dysautonomia tire more easily than other children. This is because their hearts work three times harder than other children due to their condition. Lessons should be short. If the student is tired allow him/her to put their head down for a couple of minutes or reschedule the lesson. If you miss a lesson, do not try to cram several lessons into one day.

9. When possible, schedule tutoring sessions in the late afternoon or early evening. Most children with Dysautonomia perform better later in the day. This is because one's blood pressure tends to go up naturally later in the day. Also, most people who have Dysautonomia have insomnia. It is better to tutor the student after they have had enough rest.

If you were to tutor them at 9:00 A.M, it is possible that they did not fall asleep until 6:00 A.M. that morning. It will not make for a very productive session.

10. Allow your student to eat salty snacks and drink fluids during sessions. Keeping them well hydrated will lessen their symptoms.

11. Students may need to elevate their feet and stretch during tutoring to prevent their blood from pooling in the legs. This will help to prevent further mental and physical fatigue.

12. If a child needs to read long novels, audio books may be a great tool.

13. On days when the child is too sick to get out of bed, be sure to know your school's policy. Some school districts do not allow the tutor to enter a student's bedroom, for legal reasons. Know your school's policy and come up with a plan, should this occur. Never force a child who is in this condition to be tutored. It is best to reschedule.

14. If the child is feeling under the weather, try placing a fan on the table or desk where you are working. Reducing the temperature of the room can make the child less symptomatic allowing for better learning.

15. If your district will allow for it, try to get the tutor to work through the summer months. This will better prepare the student for the following school year.

The Importance of the 504 Plan and IEP (Individualized Educational Program/Plan)

Accommodations for Elementary and Middle School

Establishing a 504 plan or an IEP, Individualized Education Plan/Program for your child who has a Dysautonomic condition is not only beneficial, it is imperative.

What is a 504 Plan?

A 504 plan sets out an agreement for making sure that the student with medical issues has the same access to education as any other student. It is a tool used to guarantee that all parties involved with the child's education understand and agree to their roles and responsibilities, and proactively work out potential issues. The 504 Plan provides a template for discussing, planning and implementing accommodations specific to your child. The overall goal is to ensure the child's medical needs are addressed, so that the student can learn in the best and least restrictive environment possible. The 504 Plan ideally and literally seeks to "level the playing field" for the child with Dysautonomia.

Section 504 of the Rehabilitation Act of 1973, is a Civil Rights law that prohibits discrimination against people with disabilities. This act provides reasonable accommodations within regular education settings to students who have a mental or physical disability, which limits one or more major life activities. These activities include: caring for one's self, manual tasks, walking, seeing, hearing, breathing, and learning as it pertains to education and the school setting. Section 504, as it is often referred to, applies to all schools both public and private that receive Federal funding (religious schools are often exempt from this). A 504 Plan may be requested by the parents/guardians or by the school. Your child is entitled to a 504 Plan under Federal law. If your school district is giving you trouble, you must stand up for your rights and be your child's advocate. If your needs are not being met to your satisfaction, you may need to hire an educational advocate/lawyer. The school must provide you a hard copy of the agreed upon plan. 504 Plans vary from state to state and district-to-district, so your plan may look different but essentially the accommodations would be the same for your child regardless of the school he or she attends.

In a perfect world, a 504 Plan meeting should be developed as a cooperative effort involving the family, teachers, social worker and the child's team of physicians. It is important that everyone remembers they are on the same team for the sake of the child's well being.

Who can receive a 504 Plan?

Any student who has a documented medical condition (this can include children with ADHD, hearing impairment, Dysautonomia, etc.) that interferes with his/her ability to perform in the school setting without reasonable accommodations is entitled to 504 plan. The child's doctor must then write a written report stating the diagnosis, how it impacts the child in the classroom, and a list of accommodations that have been tried in the past. A prescription from the doctor saying the child has Dysautonomia is not considered a written report and is not acceptable by itself to qualify for a 504 Plan. Simply having this diagnosis does not automatically qualify a student for accommodations. The classroom teacher/s must confer that the disability does in fact impact the child's ability to thrive in the classroom. The team of educators, social worker, counselor, psychologist, principal, etc., will then decide if a 504 is appropriate.

If there is not an agreement that your child should have a 504 (or IEP), you can take your case to higher authorities, such as the District Superintendent or School Board to push for it. If needed, the child can be tested by a neuropsychologist to validate the condition and how it affects the learning process. Again, this may be a situation in which you need to hire an educational advocate or lawyer to help you overcome bureaucratic and administrative obstacles.

It is important to note that not all children with POTS may be eligible for a 504 Plan. It depends on how significantly the syndrome is impacting one of the major life activities, and whether or not the child requires accommodations as a result of that. Accommodations must also be considered "reasonable."

Who is responsible for implementing the 504?

Your child's teachers are, by law, required to adhere to the 504 Plan accommodations, and can and should be held responsible. However, it is also the responsibility of the parents to monitor progress and communicate with the school to ensure accommodations are being met on an ongoing basis.

How do I get started on the 504 plan?

As each child with Dysautonomia is unique and has their own needs the following is just a sampling of some accommodations that may be included in the 504 Plan. There is no cookie cutter formula for children with POTS. Accommodations should be based on the individual's own needs. All accommodations should be tailored for your child, so that his/her medical needs are met.

As you are writing the 504 Plan, be sure that it is flexible and adaptable. It will need to be tweaked over time, depending on symptoms of your child. Be sure that the school has a general understanding of your child's condition. You may need to educate the staff and school district.

Have a written report with a diagnosis from your medical professional, preferably an electro physiologist or another expert in the field of autonomic disorders. Without a written report, the plan cannot be developed. Be sure that the report is written in a concise format that is easy to understand.

Below please find a sampling of possible accommodations that you may consider requesting for your child who has Dysautonomia. Remember that not all of these accommodations will be appropriate for each child who has this condition. These are only suggested accommodations and should not serve as a menu for success. They must be agreed upon by your child's Team of teachers. Simply having a doctor's note suggesting an accommodation does not by itself make it materialize.

Possible Accommodations to Request:

• A calculator should be allowed for math computation. Math that involves sequencing or steps in a process is often problematic for the child with Dysautonomia. Consider allowing the student to use a sample (or model) math problem as a reference.

• Some kids with Dysautonomia are hypersensitive to smells. They should be allowed to leave the classroom or laboratory if their symptoms are exacerbated by odors.

• Allow the student to have fluids throughout the day. Kids with Dysautonomia do much better when they are well hydrated. Allow them to have a water bottle with them or Gatorade at all times. If they forget to bring their water bottle, allow them trips to the drinking fountain as often as needed.

• Allow the child to have salty snacks throughout the day. Salt helps to retain fluids and helps keep up blood volume, helping to increase blood pressure.

• Frequent urination and stomach issues often come with this syndrome. Allow the child to have a permanent bathroom pass to prevent embarrassment.

• Taking the stairs may not always be safe due to dizziness and fatigue. Issue the student an elevator pass. Assign a friend, if the student experiences syncope, to accompany them in case of an emergency.

• Preferential seating should be allowed. The child should be placed as close to the teacher and an exit, as possible.

• Warm temperatures in the school may impact the child considerably, as children with autonomic dysfunctions have problems controlling their body temperature. Heat will exacerbate their symptoms. Consider allowing them to carry a portable fan from class to class or scheduling their classes in rooms that have air conditioning.

• Remaining upright is a problem for kids with Dysautonomia due to blood pooling in the lower extremities taking away blood flow and oxygen from the heart and brain. This results in worsening of dizziness, fatigue, nausea, chest pain and other symptoms. Accommodations may be needed for the lunch line, fire drills, etc. Assign the child a friend to assist as needed.

• Allow the student to carry a cell phone for emergencies.

• Allow the student to position themselves as needed to prevent pooling. This includes elevating feet, sitting on knees, placing knees to chest, or sitting cross-legged. These are compensatory positions to help regulate better blood flow to the heart as well as prevent pooling in the legs. This should not be viewed as disrespectful and should be permitted.

• Exercise intolerance may require elimination or modification of P.E. classes.

Note: If your child who has a chronic medical condition wants to be on an after school team sport, you must speak with the school's athletic advisor. They can guide you as to how to approach this. Most likely they will need a release from your doctor stating that your child is not a safety risk, and they can participate in the sport.

• Students must avoid germs when possible. When a child with Dysautonomia gets a cold, flu or infection, it can turn into a more serious illness than if they did not have Dysautonomia. Thus, it sets them back academically, socially and physically. A separate room, other than the nurse's office, should be set-aside for the child to rest, when the student is symptomatic. This can be the library, a teacher's office or an empty classroom, for example.

• Note taking may be impossible for a child with Dysautonomia. Possible accommodations are assigning a friend to take notes, getting a copy of the teacher's notes or bringing a tape recorder to class to record the lesson.

• Test taking may need to be modified. Children with Dysautonomia may need extended time. It may be necessary to have frequent breaks, the directions read and explained, and a scribe. Longer tests may need to be shortened, or broken into segments and taken over several periods of time. Large print format should be provided as needed. Tests should be administered in a quiet room (or in the hallway) where the student can better concentrate.

• Laptops should be allowed in class, as it makes note taking easier.

• A Kindle, an electric reading device, or books on tape may be necessary to help with reading comprehension.

• Frequent motor breaks should be allowed to improve circulation and prevent blood pooling.

• Allow the student to have extra time in between classes or allow them to leave a bit early from each class to beat the wave of students in the hall. This is especially helpful if the child is experiencing syncope.

• Allow for extended time on homework assignments when the student is symptomatic and cannot finish their work due to illness.

• If the school is large, try to arrange that all classes are close by or at least in the same building. If this is not possible, allow the child extra time to get from one side of the building to the other.

What are some other helpful accommodations for students who have Dysautonomia?

• Prioritize core academics. If a child does not have the energy for a full day, consider scheduling required classes later in the day. Elective classes may have to be added once the student can tolerate a longer school day.

• Consider half days beginning in the early afternoon. Kids with POTS do not function well in the morning because that is when blood pressure is the lowest and symptoms are usually the worst.

- Concentration may suffer due to lack of blood flow to the brain. This phenomenon is known as "brain fog". It is a common occurrence among people with Dysautonomia. Comprehension, deduction, memory storage and retrieval are often impacted. Curriculum should be adjusted accordingly.

Tip: Students who have severe brain fog may not be able to remember their locker combination. If possible allow the student to have a name combination lock instead of a number combination. Choosing a word like "dog" will be far easier for them to remember than a number combination.

- Frequent absences are to be expected with this condition. The student should not be penalized for this.
- If the student is homebound or partially homebound, teachers should coordinate how much homework is given. Avoid overloading the student.
- A student who is homebound should still be allowed to participate in all school activities, if their health allows it on any given day. These children should be apprised of all school functions and after school activities. A liaison should be appointed to collect all handouts and keep the child informed. These children are already feeling isolated and this will help them to stay connected, making the transition back to school easier. It is also critical to their emotional and social development.

Note: When my daughter was partially homebound, the teachers had a meeting and decided it would be best for her to try to come to school from 11:00AM - 12:30PM They said this way she could be at her two most important classes - math and lunch. They all agreed that the socialization of coming to lunch would help her through this rough time. I was lucky that they were so compassionate. Not all schools will respond this way.

- Noise and light sensitivity may cause an issue for kids with POTS. At times, wearing sunglasses or having earplugs on hand may be appropriate.
- Fire drills and evacuations may be very problematic. An emergency plan should be worked out for children with Dysautonomia. Keep in mind that the noise of the alarm may cause their symptoms to get worse. A plan that keeps the child safe must be put into place. Assigning a buddy to assist the child during evacuation or other emergencies may be necessary.
- An extra set of books should be provided, so that the child can have a set at home. Lugging heavy books back and forth can be physically taxing on a child with Dysautonomia.

How do I prepare for my 504 meeting?

- Bring the written report from the doctor stating the disability and how it impacts the student in the classroom. Also, if applicable, bring a list of all the accommodations that have been attempted in the past. If the child sees multiple physicians, bring the diagnosis from all the medical professionals the child deals with. Be sure that the note states the exact medical impairment.
- Have any additional pertinent information from the doctor available for review.
- Ask the doctor/doctors to make a list of suggested recommendations that should be added to the 504 to insure

for the child's success. Have this list at the meeting.

• Bring pamphlets or handouts that explain Dysautonomia and how this illness may impact school performance.

• You might consider putting together a video that explains Dysautonomia. You can find many videos on the Internet. There is one from Mayo clinic that I found on You Tube that I really like. You can run a search engine - You Tube POTS Mayo Clinic to find it. Dynakids.org also has a wonderful video called, "Goofy Slippers Lecture" on Dysautonomia. This video can also be purchased.

• Bring this book to the meeting.

• Bring some pictures of your child to the meeting. You can show pictures of before your child became sick and after. Talk about things they could do before the illness and how they have now become limited. You can even bring samples of accomplishments pre-POTS.

Note: One of my friends whose child has severe A.D.D. placed a framed picture of her son in the center of the table and played a sampling of him playing the violin. It served as a positive reminder that we were dealing with a human being who despite his learning issues has so much to offer the world.

• If you decide to do this, be sure you are not being condescending to the professionals sitting around the table. Keep in mind they hold hundreds of these meetings a year.

• Because many people are still unaware of this illness, some people will assume that your child is depressed, anxious, or has an eating disorder. Having an evaluation from a psychiatrist to dispel these rumors will help support your credibility.

• Always remember that the 504 Plan was not meant to be a power struggle but a collaborative meeting of the minds, to help your child through these difficult days. Approach the meeting with a positive attitude. Let the teachers know that you want to work with them, not against them.

• Keep all lines of communication open and remember that everyone should have one goal in mind, helping your child to achieve a successful and safe school year.

What is an IEP and how does it differ from the 504 Plan?

Your child may also qualify for an IEP. An IEP, known as an Individualized Educational Plan/Program, is different from the 504 Plan in that it is usually more specific than the 504 Plan and it deals more with the academic needs of the student. The IEP typically is directed at the child who has learning disabilities (for example an auditory processing issue). The 504 Plan addresses the medical needs and provides for necessary accommodations that need to be made to ensure your child's success and safety in school. For example, if your child has both a learning disability and Dysautonomia, you will want an IEP, which will now cover all of the accommodations set forth in the 504 Plan as well academic goals and modifications to the curriculum.

Note: Some districts do not have a 504 Plan and an IEP; you may have to have one or the other. Be sure to investigate this, so you can go into this meeting knowing your rights and your school district's policy.

In some districts it may be advantageous to have an IEP over a 504 Plan. This holds true especially during the child's secondary schooling. Some districts will allow a student with an IEP to get one hour of tutoring for every day of school missed. With the 504 Plan many schools will only allow the student to receive tutoring after ten consecutive days of an absence. Be sure to know your school's policy. If your child has only a 504 Plan in place and has been absent for a week or more, you might consider keeping them home for the remainder of the ten days, so they can get the tutoring they need.

> Note: My daughter had a 504 Plan in eighth grade. At the end of
> eighth grade I decided to try to also get her an IEP Plan to carry over
> to the High School. I made the mistake of telling the staff that I
> wanted the IEP for High School, just in case she needed it. Luckily,
> she did qualify and was given the IEP. I learned at the IEP meeting
> that an IEP will be denied if the parent's request is on a "just in case
> basis." The child's education must be currently impacted by their
> illness and if an IEP is written it must take affect for the present
> school year.

If your child has a 504 Plan but the teachers need to further
modify their expectations in order for your child to achieve success
in regular education classes, then an IEP may be a good alternative.

IEP - How to protect your child by securing an IEP

Special education allows a child to have an individual education plan (IEP) when the child's disability interferes with the student's education and performance. Special Education is available for
all children that qualify from age 3 through age 21 or upon gradua-
tion from high school, whichever comes first.

If a parent feels their child requires special education, the
first step is to contact the school the child is attending and explain
how you feel your child's disability will affect his or her education.
Most often a formal letter written by the parent requesting an IEP
Evaluation will have to be submitted by the principal or head master.

The next step is the evaluation, which will include:
- A letter or form from the physician explaining the
child's specific medical concern
- Interview with parents
- Interview with teachers

- Information from parents
- Specific testing, including all areas related to suspected disability

If the child is qualified as OHI or "Other Health Impaired" it does not require that testing be performed to show a learning disability. However, this does require proof, from your physician, of a medical disability that affects the child's education.

After the evaluation is completed, the team will meet. The team consists of the parent, regular education teacher, a school representative, which is usually the principal, and a representative from any area that the child was tested in (i.e. speech pathologist, occupational therapist, psychologist). The parent may bring an advocate, such as a more experienced parent, to this and all team meetings. At the team meeting, all findings will be reviewed, including the teacher's observations, the physician's information, and any testing that has been completed. The parent may share any literature they have on the child's disability and how it will affect him or her in school at this time.

After discussing the findings, the team will make a decision on eligibility. The student will meet the criteria for qualification for special education under one of the eligible categories.

Some of the eligible categories for special education are included below:

OHI = Other Health Impaired
D-B = Deaf Blindness
VI = Visual Impairment
HI = Hearing Impairment
ED = Emotional Disturbance
MR = Mental Retardation
MD = Multiple Disabilities
OI = Orthopedic Impairment
PI = Preschool Impairment

SM = Social Maladjustment
SP = Speech Impairment
LI = Language and Speech Impairment
TBI = Traumatic Brain Injury
SLD = Specific Learning Disability

(1) Basic reading skills
(2) Reading comprehension
(3) Oral expression
(4) Listening comprehension
(5) Mathematical computation
(6) Mathematical reasoning
(7) Written expression

There are many reasons a child may qualify for special education including a health impairment that interferes with the child's education. This can include brain fog, chronic fatigue, absences, etc. If the impairment is making it difficult for the student to master the educational material, the student may be eligible for special education services. If the child is found to be eligible, the next step will be putting together an IEP.

Developing an IEP
The team will meet and provide input on assistance the student needs to advance successfully in their education. The parent will usually be asked what they feel the child's strengths are, as well as their concerns regarding the child's education. The team will then decide on placement for the student. Students are always placed in the regular classroom whenever possible.

Some types of placement:
- Regular class (with supplementary aids and services, as needed)
- Special class (where every student in the class is receiv-

ing special education services for some or all of the day)
- Special school
- At home
- A hospital
- Institution
- Another setting as deemed fit by the team

The student's placement can be changed as needed by writing an addendum to the IEP. For example, if the child is to be in the hospital for an extended period, the team could amend the IEP to have the student receive services while in the hospital. Hospital or homebound services can also be provided as part of the services the child receives.

Some classroom modifications/accommodations:
- Preferential seating
- Provide copies of material to be copied from book or board
- Provide copies of notes (from another student)
- Peer tutoring
- Behavior contract
- Performance contract
- Highlighted textbook
- Second set of textbooks for at home
- Taped materials
- Unlimited bathroom breaks

Some assignment accommodations/modifications:
- Assignment book
- Abbreviated assignments
- Additional time
- Study guide
- Extra Grade Opportunity

Some testing accommodations/modifications:
- Extended time
- Reading instructions out loud
- Reading out loud for test items
- Repeating directions verbatim
- Use of calculator
- Modified grading scale
- Modified test format
- Abbreviated concepts
- Retesting

The final modifications and accommodations will need to be assessed for the individual, and adjusted according to specific state regulations. The team will decide on any allowable accommodations for state/district mandated assessments. The allowable accommodations will differ from state to state.

Direct services are specialized instructional services provided directly to the student. This can be done in a number of settings such as:

- Inclusion with a special education teacher or aide in general education classroom
- The special education classroom with or without a group of students
- Other appropriate settings

What are a parent's rights if you are told the child does not qualify for special education?

If the school determines that the child does not qualify for special education, the parent can request an independent evaluation (performed and paid for by the school). The second evaluation is completed by an independent, outside source that the school and parent agree upon. The school system is required to pay the cost for the independent evaluation, but only after they have conducted the original evaluation and the parent has disagreed with the results.

If after the independent evaluation, the child is still denied special services, and the parent does not agree with the decision, a due process hearing can be requested. This process varies from state to state.

Which will better protect my child, the IEP or 504 Plan?

This is an interesting question. Most schools will try to talk you into a 504 Plan. This is a much less time consuming way to go than is the IEP.

IEP or 504 Plan: What difference does it make?

Sometimes a parent is told that their child can receive all the services, specialized instruction, modifications and accommodations they need on a 504 Plan; and that there is no need to develop an IEP. The first part of this statement is true, the second is not.

It is true that any service you can get on an IEP can also be delivered via a 504 Plan. But that is where the similarities between the two end. The differences between these two documents are critical, and are based upon the laws that govern each. [1]

The 504 Plan

Section 504 is a Civil Rights Law, not an education law. Its purpose is to protect individuals with disabilities from discrimination for reasons related to their disability. The services and accommodations on a 504 Plan are meant to 'level the playing field' so that the child has an equal chance to learn. The goal of a Section 504 Plan is only to ensure that the educational needs of the student with disabilities are met as adequately as the educational needs of the student without disabilities are met.

With a 504 Plan there is no guarantee that the child will actually benefit from the services given, only that they will have the same opportunity to benefit. That is why there are no goals in a 504

Plan. The focus is on equal access, not on reducing or eliminating a student's deficits. [2]

The IEP – Goals and Modifications

The child on an IEP receives services and supports that are governed by the Individuals with Disabilities Education Act (IDEA,) a federal law. The purpose of IDEA is to ensure that eligible students with disabilities receive an education that prepares them for further education, employment and independent living. They must be given services from which they will actually benefit. This is why an IEP. contains goals and includes progress reporting for parents - so that the Team will know whether or not the child is actually benefiting (i.e., making progress) from their educational program.

Legal Protections

The other critical difference here is that the two laws have very different levels of procedural protections, with the IEP offering far more protections than Section 504. For example a child on a 504 Plan can be expelled from school, and the school has no further obligation to educate that child. While a child with an IEP may also be expelled from school under certain circumstances, the school is obligated to continue that child's education including all services on the IEP.

Section 504 does not give parents a right to an independent evaluation at public expense, as does IDEA. Section 504 does not provide a set of goals towards which the student works, does not require progress reporting to parents, and does not guarantee transitional services to older students - all things available to students under IDEA.

While other differences exist, these are some of the more important ones to be aware of.

An individual who is eligible for services under IDEA also qualifies for protection under Section 504, but the reverse is not true. In any case, the school district must comply with both laws. The school district is not free to choose which law it prefers to follow. Students who qualify for an IEP must be given an IEP [2]

The School Nurse - Creating an Individual Health Plan and and Emergency Plan Template

The school nurse is a liaison between school personnel, family, health care professionals, and the community. The school nurse participates as the health expert on the IEP and 504 teams. As the case manager for students with health problems, the school nurse ensures that there is adequate communication and collaboration among all parties. The school nurse also ensures that the student's individualized health care plan is part of the Individualized Education Plan (IEP), when appropriate, and that both plans are developed and implemented with full team participation. This team should include the student, family, and pediatrician.

Parents, especially those who have children with chronic illnesses, fully understand how critical the school nurse is to their child's well-being during the school day. The school nurse plays an integral role in making sure that each child with a chronic health condition is safe and that their medical needs are being addressed.

TIPS for Working Collaboratively with the School Nurse

- Introduce yourself to the school nurse.
- Ask the school nurse if she has any questions regarding the condition of your child.
- Tell the school nurse that she has your support and to feel free to ask you questions or clarifications about your child's condition at any time.
- Ask the school nurse if she or he would like you to provide any additional information - pamphlets, articles, videos, etc. about this syndrome.
- Never be demanding or condescending to the school nurse.

- Remind the nurse that you wish to be part of the team and to work collaboratively with him or her.
- Ask the nurse if she has any questions about your child's medications.
- Keep the nurse abreast of any medical changes that your child is experiencing.
- Ask if the school your child attends has Individual Health Care Plans for students with chronic health conditions. If so, ask to have input on this plan.
- Ask the school nurse if an Emergency Care Plan (ECP) will be created for your child.

THE INDIVIDUALIZED HEALTH CARE PLAN (IHCP)

Most schools have a certified building or district nurse. The certified nurse is often responsible for putting together an IHCP for each student that has a health related issue.

Most but not all students who qualify for 504 Plans and or IEP Plans will also have an IHCP. The IHCP Plan is set up by the school or district nurse with the parent's input. The IHCP can often be incorporated or added to the IEP or section 504 Plan. The IHCP is developed when a student has on going health issues that demand continuous nursing management. An IHCP documents the diagnosis, addresses goals and outcomes to be achieved, documents nursing interventions and explains how the plan's effectiveness will be measured, (see sample IHCP) The IHCP will vary from state to state and district to district. IHCPs should be tweaked as necessary and should be updated annually. Your child's school may also require that the child's doctor approve the IHCP and sign off on it.

Reference (1-3):
Chambers, Ellen
IEP or 504 Plan: What Difference does it make? Available at:
www.Spedwatch.org Accessed June 2008

INDIVIDUAL HEALTHCARE PLAN (IHCP)

Name: _____   Birthdate: 10/2/95   School: _____   Gr. 7

Medical Diagnosis: Postural Orthostatic Tachycardia Syndrome , March, 2008

Definition: POTS is a form of Dysautonomia, which is a malfunction of the autonomic nervous system's control of the unconscious functions of the body. POTS is characterized by a rapid heart rate (tachycardia) when a person changes positions, ie.sitting to standing, (postural). Symptoms may include chronic dizziness, lightheadedness, severe fatigue, palpitations, weakness, shortness of breath, loss of concentration and joint pain.

Assessment Date/Nurse	Functional Health Concern	Student Objective	Interventions	Outcome
2/11/2009 J.Tweten, RN	Activity intolerance related to posture changes as evidenced by dizziness, lightheadedness and decreased attention.	Student will be able to participate in school activities to her fullest potential.	Allow use of elevator when feeling dizzy or fatigued. Allow to bring salty snack and water bottle to class Allow for bathroom breaks as needed Allow for Health Office visits when symptomatic Health Office: - If becomes dizzy in halls, to sit down and cares to be called to evaluate/treat - Allow for private rest period lying down until symptoms subside. - Monitor vital sign- take pulse, resp. and blood pressure & oxygen saturations - Encourage fluids	
	Potential for injury related to general orthostatic weakness & lightheadedness.	Student will remain free from injury while in attendance.	Encourage slow changes in position Be aware of triggers in POTS, ie, dehydration, ambient temperature, stress and adjust. IMMEDIATELY assume supine (lying down) position when experiences symptoms and notify an adult.	
	Potential for impaired social interaction in school setting due to attendance limitations	Student will participate in as many school activities as able to	Encourage peer assistance with school activities as appropriate. Provide for individual counseling as necessary. Modified class schedules.	

Student Individual Health Plan

Student Name: -. .   Birth Date (Age): 10/02/1995 (14)

Gender: F   Home Rooom: Grade: 8

Medical Condition: Dysautonomia

IHP Plan:

Effective Date: 01/25/2010

Created Age: 14

Created Grade: 8

Created School:

Plan:

DEFINITION: Dysautonomia is a malfunction of the autonomic nervous system's control of the unconscious functions of the body. Postural Orthostatic Tachycardia Syndrome (POTS) is a form of dysautonomia which is characterized by a rapid heart rate (tachycardia) when a person changes positions, ie., sitting to standing, (postural). Symptoms may include chronic dizziness, lightheadedness, severe fatigue, palpitations, weakness, shortness of breath, loss of concentration and joint pain.

NURSING DIAGNOSIS #1: Potential for activity intolerance related to weakness/fatigue

GOAL: Able to function within student's capacity in the school setting

INTERVENTIONS:

1. Assess and document level of tolerance to activity. Observe for pallor, fatigue, shortness of breath, headache, dizziness
2. Monitor vital signs.
3. Allow for school facility accomodations such as use of elevator when fatigued or symptomatic.
4. May have bathroom breaks as needed.
5. Provide for private rest breaks when symptomatic.
6. Promote dietary needs such as increased fluids and salty snacks as necessary.
7. Modify class schedules, prioritizing core academics, due to periods of extreme fatigue.
8. Allow for extra time in class transitioning when symptomatic.
9. When exhibiting focusing difficulty ("brain fog")facilitate note taking in class as necessary, ie., tape recorder, sharing with friend's notes, etc.
10. If having concentration problems, offer test taking modifications, i.e., extended time, verbal directions, segmenting, use of calculator, etc.

EXPECTED OUTCOME:

1. Ability to participate in school activities to her fullest potential.
2. Increasing tolerance for daily activity
3. Maintain a well-balanced diet
4. Student able to verbalize understanding of health condition.

EVALUATION:

Ongoing assessment of attendance and level of participation in school activities.

NURSING DIAGNOSIS #2: Potential for injury related to general orthostatic weakness and lightheadedness.

GOAL: Student will remain free from injury while in attendance.

INTERVENTIONS:

1. Encourage slow changes in position and allow for compensatory self-positioning in class, ie. elevate

Student Individual Health Plan

    legs, knee to chest, cross-legged.

2. Avoid activities that involve extended periods of upright positions, accomodating for lunch lines, fire drill lines, etc.
3. Be aware of triggers to POTS, ie., dehydration, ambient temperature, stress, and make adjustments.
4. IMMEDIATELY, assume supine position (lying down) when experiences symptoms and notify an adult.

EVALUATION:

    Monitor incidences of symptoms and treatments.

NURSING DIAGNOSIS #3: Potential for impaired social interaction in school setting due to attendance limitations

GOAL: Student will participate in as many school activities as is capable

INTERVENTIONS:

1. Encourage peer assistance with school activities as appropriate
2. Provide for individual counseling s necessary

EVALUATION: Observe level of school activities integration

Individualized Health Care Plan

Demographics

Student Name _____   Birth Date _____

Home Address _____

_____

Mother/Guardian _____   Phone _____

Father/Guardian _____   Phone _____

Caregiver _____   Phone _____

Language spoken at home _____

Emergency Contact:

_____ _____ _____
Name   Relationship   Phone

Medical Care

Primary Physician _____   Phone _____

Specialty Physician _____   Phone _____

Specialty Physician _____   Phone _____

Health History

Brief health history _____

_____

_____

_____

Special health care needs _____

_____

_____

Other considerations _____

_____

Student's Ability to Participate in Care _____

Allergies _____

_____

Chapter 14. Surviving High School - Helpful Hints to Make it Through Secondary School

Surviving High School

"Every Path has its Puddle"

The transition from Middle School to High School is often filled with great trepidation as well as excitement. It can be an overwhelming experience, especially for the child who has a chronic illness. The child who has Dysautonomia may or may not be coming into high school with an existing 504 Plan or IEP. If the child does not already have one of these plans in place, you as the parent will need to research the benefits of both of these and decide which plan will offer your child more support. In order to qualify for a 504 Plan or an IEP your child's academic performance must be adversely affected by his or her medical condition. Simply having a diagnosis will not be sufficient in and of itself to be eligible for either of these plans.

Listed below are the main differences between the IEP Plan and the 504. However, it should be noted that before consideration of an IEP, districts are required to follow a three tiered intervention program called Response to Intervention. The data obtained from this tiered progression is utilized to determine eligibility for many students that may require an IEP. All three plans are discussed below. You and a team of Academic Professionals can help you determine eligibility and which plan would best benefit your child.

504 Plan
- Section 504 of the Rehabilitation Act of 1973, is a Civil Rights Law that prohibits discrimination against people with disabilities.
- The 504 Plan provides a template for discussing, planning and implementing accommodations specific to your

child.

- The overall goal is to ensure the child's medical needs are addressed, so that the student can learn in the best and least restrictive environment possible.
- Section 504 provides reasonable accommodations within regular education settings to students who have a mental or physical disability, which limits one or more major life activities. These activities include: caring for one's self, manual tasks, walking, seeing, hearing, breathing, and learning as it pertains to education and the school setting.
- Section 504 applies to all schools both public and private that receive Federal funding (religious schools are often exempt from this).
- Simply having Dysautonomia does not automatically qualify a student for accommodations. The classroom teacher(s) must confer that the disability does in fact impact the child's ability to thrive in the classroom. The team of educators, social worker, counselor, psychologist, principal, etc., will then decide if a 504 is appropriate.
- A note from the medical doctor or team of doctors stating the diagnosis is required before a 504 Plan can be established.
- The 504 Plan does not provide for modification of the curriculum.
- The 504 Plan must provide students with disabilities equal opportunity to gain the same benefit, result or to achieve the same level of academic success as students without a disability but that does not guarantee equal success. (Sedol)
- In most cases, the 504 Plan will carry over to post-secondary school; however, the 504 Plan must be current and up to date (three years or less) before transitioning to a post-secondary school.
- Each public school should have a person (usually an as-

sistant principal or a guidance counselor) who serves as the school's "504 coordinator." This person should coordinate the development, maintenance, and implementation of 504 plans.

- 504 plans should be developed by a committee, consisting of the student with a disability (if appropriate), the student's parent(s)/guardian(s), the student's teacher(s), the student's counselor, and the 504 coordinator.
- Additionally, special educators often serve as advisors to 504 committees.
- The student's disability and corresponding need for reasonable accommodation are identified and documented in the plan. Likewise, the plan delineates the specific accommodations, which will be implemented by the school. All school staff involved in the provision of accommodations should be contacted by the 504 coordinator and made aware of their duties and responsibilities.
- The 504 Plan should be updated at least annually.
- The 504 Plan is often a first course of action for students who have health impairment.

Note: If warranted, a teacher or a parent can ask that the entire process of securing a 504 Plan be bypassed. In many cases, securing an IEP, as a first course of action may be appropriate, depending on the severity of the needed intervention.

Response to Intervention

Schools throughout the United States are required to move toward a three-tiered Response to Intervention Program. The RTI will serve to more formally implement interventions within the regular classroom environment. The RTI represents a flexible delivery model that is similar to curriculum-based assessment. For example, if a student is having difficulty with reading comprehension, various scientifically based interventions would be employed to remediate this challenge. Within the context of RTI's three-tiered program, the intensity of the interventions would increase at each level until the student responded appropriately and remediation was successful. Throughout this three tier process, designated staff or teams monitor student response, data is collected, and information is formally reviewed at selected time periods. At each of these milestones, the decision to move to the next level of intervention, or tier, is considered. Once the student reaches the third tier, the most intensified interventions are implemented. If the student still does not respond to intervention at this stage, the data is compiled and utilized to determine eligibility for special education. Once found eligible, an Individualized Education Program/Plan (IEP) is developed.

If the student's concerns are the result of a significant change in medical status, (i.e. brain tumor, seizures, etc.) social emotional conditions, and/or any other areas of serious concern, the parent still reserves the right to request an evaluation to bypass the RTI process and request that the school consider an evaluation for special education services. However, it should be noted that the final decision is ultimately based on the data provided to the school (evaluations both external and internal, medical reports, anecdotal data, etc.) Within this context, the district is required to review and consider outside data and reports, and has the right to initiate its own evaluations. Upon submission of this information, parents should be notified of a meeting date to discuss these findings, within 14 school days of the request.

Individualized Education Plan/Program (IEP)

- The Individuals with Disabilities Education Act, or IDEA, is much more involved than the 504 Plan.
- A student's IEP is a legal document, which drives the

placement recommendation and support systems that will ensure that the student receives a free and appropriate public education.

- The IEP must be individualized according to the student's specific disability and medical needs.
- Most often the student who has Dysautonomia will fall under the category of OHI, Other Health Impaired.

The process

Once an educator identifies a concern regarding the performance of a particular student, with a health impairment, a period of intervention begins. The educator will try and implement standard or tier 1 interventions that would be utilized for any student with difficulties in the mainstream environment. For example, if the child is having a difficult time processing information in class due to cognitive impairment (brain fog), the teacher may first try to move the student's desk closer to the teacher. Often times proximity may be used as a tool to help the child to focus better. The educator should document the concerns and subsequent interventions. The key issue is whether the strategies enable the student to benefit from the regular education curriculum. If the intervention strategies do not work, the student is often referred to the 504 Coordinator considered for a Tier II intervention.

When a case is referred for 504 considerations, the 504 coordinator should call a meeting of the 504 team. The team should review the documentation provided regarding the concerns about the student and the interventions that have been attempted. The team should decide upon what additional intervention and evaluation is appropriate.

Over a period of several weeks, the team should closely monitor the information it obtains regarding the student's performance and the effectiveness of the methods implemented to assist the student.

Finally, the 504 team will determine three things:

1. Whether the student's performance remains problematic and whether such difficulty is the result of a disability;

2. If the problem is a result of a disability, whether reasonable accommodation is sufficient to enable the student to benefit from the regular education curriculum; and

3. If the student's needs are a result of a disability and cannot be met by reasonable accommodation alone, the 504 team should refer the matter to the special education department in the school.

As soon as a case is referred to special education either through the Response to Intervention Team, the 504 Coordinator, or a request by the parent for an evaluation, the matter comes under the control of the IDEA (Individuals with Disabilities Education Act). The IEP Team compiles a domain sheet in order to determine additional data that may be required, assessments if necessary, and existing data that may need to be required for consideration. Once the parent and the IEP team agree upon the components of the domain, the parent must sign a request for the evaluation to go forward. The IEP Team then has 60 school days between when the time consent is received and the evaluation completed to hold an IEP meeting.

All members of the multidisciplinary IEP Team should be present for the IEP meeting. The members should include:

- The student (if appropriate);
- The parent(s) or guardian(s);
- The special educator (i.e., the case manager);
- The regular education teacher or teachers;
- A "district representative" (this can be a special educator or an administrator so long as it is someone familiar with

special education services in the district); and

• Anyone else whose presence is deemed necessary or appropriate by the student, the parent(s), guardian(s), or the district.

If the parent feels intimidated by the system or does not feel knowledgeable enough about the IEP process, they may want to ask the district if they can bring a family friend, neighbor, former educator, etc. who may be able to help them interpret the details of the meeting. If the parent does bring an outside participant, it would be appropriate to inform the district ahead of time. An educational advocate can also come to the meeting if the parent feels this to be absolutely necessary; however, bare in mind that bringing in an advocate, if the parent is concerned about his/her ability to self-advocate during the meeting, may put staff members on the defensive. It is best practice to try and let the system work for you, before bringing in an advocate. If you feel the system has failed your child and that you are not being listened to or taken seriously, you could always reschedule an IEP meeting and bring an educational advocate at that time. If you decide to hire an advocate, be sure that he/she is truly out for your child's benefit. Be sure that the advocate is cooperative with the staff, because having an argumentative advocate may make your situation worse. Be sure that the advocate will work proactively and not reactively with all staff members. Remember you are all on the same team.

• During the first IEP meeting, all existing information, assessment results and other pertinent data is reviewed and discussed.

• The meeting culminates when consensus of the team determines whether or not the data support that there is an identified disability having a significant adverse impact on school performance. If a disability is identified, the student then becomes eligible for special education services.

• Once eligibility for special education is determined, an In-

dividualized Educational Plan/Program is developed.
- Before the IEP begins; the parent must provide initial consent.

The structure of the IEP begins with documentation of the student's present performance levels. Performance levels are utilized as baselines for goal development. Each performance should be linked to a goal. The goals that are written should be achievable by the child by the completion of the year. The goals are then broken down into short-term objectives or benchmarks. Goals may be academic, address social or behavioral needs, relate to physical needs, or address other school related needs. The annual goals must also be measurable. This process is often a stumbling block for the child who has Dysautonomia. It is often a challenge to find measurable goals that relate to the challenges associated with this medical issue. An example of a possible goal for a child who has Dysautonomia might include self-advocacy for their medical needs. Goals that teach independence may be fruitful. Here is where you and your team of teachers need to put your heads together and be creative.

Once goals are established other components of the IEP are addressed. This would include a transition plan that is supported by the goals, related services if necessary (Occupational therapy, speech therapy, physical therapy), accommodations if substantiated by the data provided. (See list of possible accommodations for the child who has Dysautonomia)

Finally, based on the goals, related services, and general need for support, the IEP team will review placement options and associated harmful effects. Placement is based on a continuum of options that range from the least restrictive to the most restrictive of support systems.

Once consent for initial placement is obtained, the school can go forward and implement the individualized education plan. From this time forward, the IEP Team, which includes the parents, makes all decisions regarding the student's educational program. School personnel are specifically prohibited from making such decisions without feedback from the IEP Team. As such, there are often multiple IEP meetings throughout a school year.

Once the IEP has been written, parents must receive a copy at no cost to themselves. The IDEA also stresses that everyone who will be involved in implementing the IEP must have access to the document. This includes the child's:

- Regular education teacher(s);
- Special education teacher(s);
- Related service provider(s) (for example, speech therapist); or
- Any other service provider (such as a paraprofessional) who will be responsible for a part of the child's education.

Each of these individuals needs to know what his or her specific responsibilities are for carrying out the child's IEP. This includes the specific accommodations, modifications, and supports that the child must receive, according to the IEP.

As stated above, the IEP is a legal document. The professional educators and other service providers who deal with the student must be informed of its contents of the IEP as such accommodations relate to student performance and needs.

Before the school can provide a child with special education and related services for the first time, the child's parents must give their written permission.

Regular educators must be sure to remain familiar with the contents of their students' IEP's and must also be sure to implement the required instruction and accommodations/modifications contained therein. Failure to do so can result in the educator being personally liable.

IEP implementation and the student's progress should be monitored continuously throughout the year. Reporting on student progress towards IEP goals and objectives is required to be completed on the same schedule as such reporting for non-disabled students. In other words, if report cards come out four times per year, then reports of student progress towards IEP goals and objectives should be provided at the same times.

The IEP must be reviewed annually. However, a parent has the right to have an IEP meeting at any time during the year and as often as they deem necessary. The IEP Team must meet prior to the expiration date (which is one year from the IEP's implementation) and develop a new IEP in accord with the student's progress and needs as exhibited over the year. Likewise, the formal evaluation process must be reviewed to determine whether the student remains eligible for special education and, if so, to identify the student's educational needs. The review of the evaluation is done every three years. The IEP team has the option to forgo a new formal evaluation if it feels that there has been no change in the student's eligibility.

The IDEA requires that beginning at age 14, IEP's incorporate the various goals and objectives applicable to student needs regarding transition from high school to post-high school life. Regular educators in middle school and high school should therefore be aware that IEP's will contain such goals and that the education of students with IEP's on these grade levels will involve requirements, curricula, and activities which go beyond the regular education curriculum.

Remember that whether or not, you decide to go with the Response to Intervention, process, a 504 Plan or an IEP for your child's high school years, you need to trust and work with your school's professional staff to ensure the best quality of education for your child. It is imperative to create a positive working relationship and work collaboratively with your child's teachers. It is easy to lose sight of this especially when you are dealing with a chronically ill child. Emotions are often running rampant with so many emotional, physical and educational concerns that overwhelm you, as the parent. Keep in mind that everyone wants the best for your child. It will be more advantageous to your child if you work with the system and not against it.

> *"Team means Together Everyone Achieves More!"*
> *- Author Unknown*

Thanks to Jay Miller, director of Special Education, at Stevenson High School for contributing to and reviewing this chapter.

Note: All Students should attend all 504 plan meetings or IEP meetings throughout their high school career. It will help better prepare your child for his or her post-secondary education. It is extremely important to understand what takes place at these meetings, what his/hers accommodations are and how to ensure that your needs are being met. This will teach your child to become his or her own best advocate.

Both the 504 Plan and the IEP Plan will enable your child to have accommodations that will *"Level the Playing Field"* during their secondary education career. The accommodations will be individualized according to your child's individual learning and medical needs. There is no cookie cutter recipe for establishing these accommodations. Each 504 Plan and IEP will look different. Not only will they vary according to the unique needs of the student, they will also vary from state to state and district to district. Not every accommodation that is requested will be established. Accommodations must be reasonable and realistic. They should be flexible and adaptable. Accommodations may need to be amended and revised as your child's condition changes.

Note: If the student does not use an accommodation that is set forth on their IEP Plan or 504, they may eventually lose that accommodation.

There are many other differences between Middle School (junior high) and the High School experience. Some of the main ways in which high school differs are:

- Higher academic expectations.
- New friendships
- More home work
- More stress (academic as well as social)
- More freedom
- Less hand holding
- More accountability
- Larger class sizes
- Larger assortment of extra curricular activities
- More walking from class to class
- More self-advocacy
- Classes cover more material and move at a faster pace

As you already know as a parent of a child who has Dysautonomia, stress will exacerbate symptoms. It is important to understand that the new pressures of secondary school may present a challenge to your child who has a chronic illness. High school is overwhelming for most healthy children but probably even more challenging for the child who is battling a health issue. It is imperative to closely monitor your child's academic and social well-being. Seeking the advice of a third party (social worker, psychologist, etc.) may be advisable if life becomes too overwhelming. Remember to take baby steps, lower stress levels at home when possible and take it one day at a time.

AP (Advanced Placement) Classes

Many schools offer and recommend taking AP classes during the high school years. Advanced Placement classes allow students to participate in a college level course and possibly earn college credit while still in high school. AP classes are more challenging and stimulating, but they are more time consuming, often move at a faster pace and involve more work. Most high schools give extra grade point weight on the GPA for taking an AP course and exam.

Many parents and students alike are under the assumption that taking AP courses are a MUST. It is said that about 90% of kids who have Dysautonomia are very motivated, bright and high achievers. It makes sense that many of these children would qualify for AP classes.

However, you still have a choice, not to accept this placement and put them in "at level" classes. There is no shame in this. Having a child with a chronic illness often means changing but not lowering the expectations. If putting a child in an AP class causes too much extra stress for him or her, it is not worth it. A child who is in AP classes must keep up with his or her daily work. If the child who has Dysautonomia has a history of missed school days, AP classes may cause unsolicited stress. If a child starts out in regular education classes and finds them too easy, their placement can be reevaluated. However, if your child starts out in AP classes and finds he or she cannot handle the course load, it is more damaging to their self-esteem to be moved down to a regular class. Of course, you and your Team of teachers needs to weigh the pros and cons and make the final decision that makes sense for your child's unique situation.

Helpful Hints:

- Ask to hold a meeting with your child's team of teachers, to explain your child's health condition. Do not assume that the people attending these meetings know what Dysautonomia is. Handing them a pamphlet that explains the syndrome is not the same as personally explaining it. This will also provide you an opportunity to answer questions about the syndrome that they may not understand. After explaining the syndrome, in person, you can then give the teachers a pamphlet and or direct them to this book and or the Internet to learn more.

• When requesting accommodations, never be argumentative. As I tell my son, *"arguing will get you nowhere twice as quickly."*

• Keep in mind that the teachers are trying to do the best they can to assist your child in having a positive high school experience.

• Remember that you and the teachers are on the same team.

• Try to be proactive rather than reactive.

• Keep the team updated on your child's medical status.

• Keep all lines of communication open.

• Never be condescending to the teachers. They are professionals and should be treated as such.

• Try not to let your emotions get the best of you. It is hard not to do this when your child's education is at stake. Establishing a positive working relationship with the team of teachers will get you and your child further in the long run.

• Try to keep a positive attitude for the sake of your child. This syndrome is not easy on anyone.

• Involve your child in their educational Plan. Make sure they understand their accommodations. They should attend all IEP and 504 Plan meetings, if the school will allow it.

• Teach your child to advocate for himself or herself. Be sure to guide him or her to do this appropriately. He or she should try not to come across as demanding or pushy. Advocating for oneself is a skill that does not come naturally to most children.

If you feel your child's needs are not being met to your satisfaction, you can seek the counsel of an educational advocate or an attorney. You may also contact the US Department of Education Office of Civil Rights. To file a complaint you do not need an attor-

ney. Their website is:
http://www2.ed.gov/about/offices/list/ocr/complaintprocess.html

For more information on the law, visit:
http://www2.ed.gov/policy/rights/guid/ocr/disability.html

Note: I started preparing for my daughter's high school years while she was still in eighth grade. I contacted the school she would attend for high school and explained my daughter's medical condition. I had some inside information and knew that there were at least ten other students who had POTS at this school. I also knew that at least three more from the junior high would be coming in the next year. There was also one case of FD at this school. Luckily, the social worker that I contacted listened with great empathy. I asked her if I could educate the staff on this illness so that they would have a better understanding of this complex syndrome. She made some phone calls, and they happily obliged.

I presented an hour and a half Power Point slide show for the special education staff, counselors and nurses in which I explained the syndrome and showed a video from Mayo Clinic. The school even arranged for a former Stevenson student who got POTS in college to come back and talk about the syndrome. This really was powerful. The teachers then met after the meeting to discuss how these children could be better serviced. The whole process was a huge success, and I walked away feeling like they really understood POTS and were on board with trying to make any adjustments they could to get these chronically ill children successfully through their high school days.

Interview – Counselor from a Prestigious High School in Illinois Answers Questions about Educating Students with Chronic Illnesses

JANET SUSHINSKI. Janet is a Social Worker at Stevenson High School in Illinois. Newsweek and U.S. News and World Report regularly have included Stevenson in their lists of America's best public high schools. Newsweek, which publishes its list more frequently, has included SHS seven times in the past 11 years, including the last three.

Stevenson is known for its excellent accommodations plan for students with disabilities. Stevenson has 4,500 students. The resources that are available are tremendous and atypical.

Is it more advantageous for a student entering high school to have an IEP or a 504 Plan?

This answer is dependent upon whether or not the child needs to have the curriculum modified or just needs accommodations. If the child needs to have modified coursework than the child should have an IEP. If the child is keeping up with the regular education curriculum, despite their illness, but needs certain accommodations, than a 504 Plan would be sufficient. Each case will be different depending on the student's unique needs and should be tailored to meet these needs in the least restrictive manner.

If a chronically ill child misses high school, how many days do they need to be absent in order to qualify for the district to pay for tutoring?

In some schools, the rule is that a tutor cannot be secured until after the child has missed ten consecutive days. We all know that missing just a few days of high school can put the child, who is probably already struggling because of their illness, at an extreme disadvantage. Trying to make up this amount of work could be overwhelming, even for a child who is healthy. It is important to understand the school's policy on absences upfront, especially if you know that your child has a history of missing days due to their condition. There is no State mandated rule for this (in Illinois). It is up to each individual school district to decide how absences will be handled. It is therefore critical to work with the school proactively to iron out this issue before it becomes problematic.

How do clubs and after school sport's teams handle children who are chronically ill? Is there a rule, if you are not in school that you cannot attend after school programs and sports?

Again, there is no steadfast rule that is set in stone. Each school may handle this a bit differently. More often than not, it will be the school's athletic director or club advisor that will have the final say. Having a note from the physician stating that the child has permission to participate in the sport/club may be helpful. Also, speaking to the club or athletic supervisor and explaining the illness and the extreme benefits that exercise and socialization have on this condition, may prove to be very fruitful. Most schools will follow the rule that if the child missed school for any given day, they cannot participate in any after school activities until the following school day.

Can school days be altered to accommodate for P.M. Classes?

This varies from school to school and state to state. Some schools may not have the financial support or staff to be able to make this possible. We have scheduled a later start time for several of our students that have POTS. It is also a good idea for parents to ask that the first several periods of the day be non-academic classes such as Physical Education, resource or an elective. This way if the child is not feeling well and needs to miss the first part of the day, it will not affect their core classes.

How can we ensure that the child graduates on time without having to repeat a grade?

Unfortunately, there is no way to guarantee that the child will graduate in four years. More and more students take five or more years to graduate college and there should be no shame in the child who is chronically ill to take their time to complete their high school career. Each school requires a certain amount of credits to graduate and if the credits are not met, they will need to continue their high school education until they are. Every accommodation should be made to help them achieve success along the way.

Can a child who has POTS be given extra time to get from one class to another without being penalized?

Absolutely. This can be an accommodation on their IEP or 504 Plan. If the school administration is giving you problems over this, a note from your child's doctor explaining the need for this accommodation would be advantageous.

What is the best way to approach a teacher so that the parents' concerns can be heard?

Parents and their kids need to learn to advocate for themselves and for their needs. It is vital that you learn your child's teachers and support teams. It is critical to establish the most effective means of communication. In some cases this may be through email, phone conversations, personal meetings, etc. It is best not to do this within the first several weeks of the school year as most teachers are inundated. It is best to let the dust settle. When communicating with Staff always work in a collaborative fashion. Remember that you and the teachers are on the same team. You will get much further by educating the teachers rather than making demands. Never be condescending and always treat the teachers with respect. It is far more productive to work with the team of teachers proactively rather than reactively.

What is the best way to get the school nurse on board?

Educating the nurse on this illness while also respecting her medical expertise would be the most effective way to accomplish this. Again, it is important to qualify to the nurse that most people have never heard of this syndrome, because it was not taught in most medical schools. Inform the nurse(s) that she can speak with any medical professionals that are working with your child. Let her know that your files are open. Signing a release information form may be required and is prudent. Denying this may look suspicious. Signing the form will demonstrate that you have nothing to hide and will solidify that you want to work collaboratively and openly with the school. Also, tell the nurse that you wish to keep all lines of communication open and that you will inform her of any changes that occur in your child's condition. Provide her with a list of physicians' numbers that she can contact should she have any further questions. Working collaboratively, with mutual respect, will be to everyone's benefit.

Can classes be done from home on days when the child with a chronic illness is too sick to attend?

At present, our school is investigating various options for the provision of electronic instruction to see if some coursework can be done via the computer to help the student with POTS get their required coursework complete without having to come to school every day. This program could have many advantages. It could allow the child, who has a chronic illness, to study from the convenience of their own home when they are not feeling well enough to go to school. They could also work on assignments later in the day when they are feeling better. Completing coursework on the computer eliminates distractions and will allow students to walk around the room, as necessary, in between flexible and shortened instruction time. This could certainly help with "brain fog" as well as aid in improved circulation. Children in a regular classroom setting may not be able to walk around the classroom freely as this would be a distraction for the other students.

Chapter 15. When It's Time for the Dizzy Bird to Leave the Nest- Going off to College.

"However painful the process of leaving home, for parents and for children, the really frightening thing for both would be the prospect of the child never leaving home."
- Robert Neelly Bellah.

When a child leaves his or her home for the first time, whether it is to live on their own or go off to college, it is filled with emotional complexity. Even under the best of circumstances, leaving the nest comes with a potpourri of conflicting emotions. This is especially true for the child who has a chronic illness. Both the parent and child alike are filled with emotional strife. Leaving the nest can be a perplexing time. It is often a mixed blessing filled with fear, anxiety and elation. For parents our biggest worry is the unknown. Can our ill child survive independently away from doctors and their family? Can they lead a normal existence? These same unknowns are running through your child's head as well. The now young adult, although thrilled to leave the nest, flies away with many unrequited questions. We, as their parents, pray that their journey will be safe, thrilling and steady.

All colleges/universities that get Federal money are required to address student's needs; however, these services vary widely depending on the individual school.

Notes for the College Bound:
- Try to choose a school that is close to home, if possible.
- If you are going farther away, research good doctors near the school who treat Dysautonomia before you go.
- Be sure the school is willing to work with you and your medical condition.
- The school must be willing to make certain accommodations for you such as living quarters, air conditioning,

missing classes, etc. If they are unwilling to work with you and your family, you may want to choose another school that will.

• Be sure to ask the school ahead of time what should happen if you were to get sick during the semester. Also, be sure to discuss what would happen if you have to leave school before the year is over. What will happen to your credits and tuition?

• The student should let every professor/teacher know about their medical condition and any potential glitches that may arise during the year. Be sure to discuss the probability of missing classes, tests and assignments due to illness. Be sure to have a plan in place should this become an issue.

• Try to schedule classes later in the day. This will especially be helpful if you have insomnia.

• Do not overload your schedule. Take as few classes as you can handle, especially in your freshman year.

• Mentally prepare yourself (and your parents' pocket book) that it may take you longer than 4 years to graduate as your course load may need to be lighter than most.

• Pace yourself. Do not try to do too much because you are having a good day.

• Always take a water bottle with you to all of your classes.

• Invest in a recliner chair for your room. It is best to sit in this and rest during the day than to lie down in bed. It is also a great place to put up your feet and do your homework.

• Always carry an emergency card with you in your wallet or school bag.

• Move-in day can be very taxing on your body. Be sure to drink extra fluids before attempting your move. Also, bring lots of people to help you out.

Essentials to bring with you to college:
- Pulse watch
- Ankle weights
- Blood pressure machine
- Heating pad or hot water bottle
- Sunglasses
- Wide brim hat or baseball cap
- Portable exercise equipment
- Recliner chair
- Daily pill minder
- Emergency information and phone numbers (doctors)
- Insurance card, prescription card
- Compression stockings
- Water bottles
- Cell phone
- Reusable Ice-Packs
- Salt
- Healthy snacks

These are a list of common questions and concerns that arise during the process of transition from high school to college.

Should I disclose my disability when applying for college?

The law does not require you to disclose your disability to the college. However, if you want to receive academic accommodations, you must identify yourself to the Disability Support Services Office and provide documentation of disability. Accommodations do not apply retroactively and grades will not be changed for work completed before eligibility was established.

Should I have an IEP or a 504 Plan?

It is very important to understand that IEP'S (Individualized Educational Plan/Program) and 504 Plans do not suffice as adequate documentation to accompany a student to a post - secondary institution since both are required under laws that do not apply once the student attends college. Although students are covered under Section 504 once the student goes to college, it is a different Subpart. IEP's and 504 Plans are sometimes helpful to colleges but are often insufficient as a sole form of documentation.

How does College differ from High School?

The college bound student is responsible for providing current documentation about their disability. Most schools will only accept documentation that is three years old or less. Be sure to update all documents before leaving high school.

> Note: After High School: The IEP plan ceases to exist; all students then fall under Section 504.

Even after disability is documented and accommodations are identified, students must request the accommodations each time they are needed. For testing accommodations, the student must provide the appropriate office with the dates and times of his or her exams and may be required to have more participation in the arrangements for such accommodations. Colleges are not responsible for knowing a student's schedule and arranging accommodations without initiation from the student.

Colleges are not required to provide special classes or programs, and most do not. It is up to you to find a college that offers full support. (See list of colleges for those who do provide more comprehensive support)

Parents are no longer notified of services unless the student grants permission.

Students are treated as adults and must advocate for themselves.

Colleges are required to provide accommodations only after

a formal request by the student and presentation of proper documentation verifying a specific disability and rational for accommodations.[1]

Other differences between secondary school and college.

Academics:
- Instruction is mainly by lecture, often in large lecture halls with many students.
- Independent reading is key.
- Larger amounts of reading are commonplace
- Major writing assignments are often assigned
- Essay exams are more common
- There is more emphasis on theory
- Often grades may be based on two or three large assignments or tests
- Good note taking is critical –ask your professor if you can record lectures.

Potential Stressors:
- Staying on top of assignments, especially when having a "bad day."
- There is no one to make you go to class when you are not feeling well. You must be self-motivated.
- There are many more social distractions: i.e.: parties, dances, fraternal commitments, etc.
- There is an increased work-load and faster pace. An entire course is completed in 16 weeks or less.
- Students must advocate for themselves. There is no resource room. Students must seek help when necessary.

Student Responsibilities:
- Students are responsible for time management.
- Students are responsible to get up on time, even on bad days, and get to class.

- Students must establish and maintain their own goals.
- Students are responsible to manage their own health.
- Students must be responsible to pace themselves and make good choices regarding their condition.

What is the Parent's Role?

First and foremost, parents must know and understand their child's rights as a college student with a disability or chronic illness. These rights are different from secondary school and you must familiarize yourself with them.

Section 504 and Title II protect elementary, secondary and post-secondary students from discrimination. Nevertheless, several of the requirements that apply through high school are different from the requirements that apply beyond high school. For instance, Section 504 requires a school district to provide a free appropriate public education (FAPE) to each child with a disability in the district's jurisdiction. Whatever the disability, a school district must identify an individual's education needs and provide any regular or special education and related aids and services necessary to meet those needs as well as it is meeting the needs of students without disabilities.

Unlike your high school, your post-secondary school is not required to provide FAPE. Rather, your post-secondary school is required to provide appropriate academic adjustments as necessary to ensure that it does not discriminate on the basis of disability. In addition, if your post-secondary school provides housing to non-disabled students, it must provide comparable, convenient and accessible housing to students with disabilities at the same cost.

The appropriate academic adjustment must be determined based on your disability and individual needs. Academic adjustments may include auxiliary aids and modifications to academic requirements as are necessary to ensure equal educational opportunity. Examples of such adjustments are: arranging for priority registration; reducing a course load; substituting one course for another; providing note takers, recording devices, and extended time for testing.

In providing an academic adjustment, your post-secondary school is not required to lower or effect substantial modifications to essential requirements. For example, although your school may be required to provide extended testing time, it is not required to change or modify the content of the test. In addition, your post-secondary school does not have to make modifications that would fundamentally alter the nature of a service, program or activity or would result in undue financial or administrative burdens. Finally, your post-secondary school does not have to provide personal attendants, individually prescribed devices, readers for personal use or study, or other devices or services of a personal nature, such as tutoring and typing.

If I want an academic adjustment, what should I do?

You must inform the school that you have a disability and need an academic adjustment. Unlike your school district, your post-secondary school is not required to identify you as having a disability or assess your needs.

Your post-secondary school may require you to follow reasonable procedures to request an academic adjustment. You are responsible for knowing and following these procedures. Postsecondary schools usually provide information on the procedures and contacts for requesting an academic adjustment. Such publications include recruitment materials, catalogs and student handbooks, and these are often available on school websites. Many schools also have staff whose purpose is to assist students with disabilities. If you are unable to locate the procedures, ask a school official, such as an admissions officer or counselor.

What documentation should I provide?

Schools may set reasonable standards for documentation. Some schools require more documentation than others. They may require you to provide documentation prepared by an appropriate professional, such as a medical doctor, psychologist or other qualified diagnostician. The required documentation may include one or more of the following: a diagnosis of your current disability, the date of the diagnosis, how the diagnosis was reached, the credentials of the professional, how your disability affects a major life activity, and how the disability affects your academic performance. The documentation should provide enough information for you and your school to decide what is an appropriate academic adjustment.

Although an Individualized Education Program (IEP) or Section 504 plan, if you have one from high school, may help identify services that have been effective for you, it generally is not sufficient documentation. This is because post-secondary education presents different demands than high school education, and what you need to meet these new demands may be different. Also in some cases, the nature of a disability may change.

If the documentation that you have does not meet the post-secondary school's requirements, a school official should tell you in a timely manner what additional documentation you need to provide. You may need a new evaluation in order to provide the required documentation.

Once the school has received the necessary documentation from me, what should I expect?

The school will review your request in light of the essential requirements for the relevant program to help determine an appropriate academic adjustment. It is important to remember that the school is not required to lower or waive essential requirements. If you have requested a specific academic adjustment, the school may offer that academic adjustment or an alternative one if the alternative would also be effective. The school may also conduct its own evaluation of your disability and needs at its own expense.

You should expect your school to work with you in an interactive process to identify an appropriate academic adjustment.

Unlike the experience you may have had in high school, however, do not expect your postsecondary school to invite your parents to participate in the process or to develop an IEP for you.

What can I do if I believe the school is discriminating against me?

Most post-secondary schools have a person - frequently called the Section 504 Coordinator, ADA Coordinator, or Disability Services Coordinator - who coordinates the school's compliance with Section 504 or Title II or both laws. You may contact this person for information about how to address your concerns.

The school must also have grievance procedures. These procedures are not the same as the due process procedures with which you may be familiar from high school. However, the post-secondary school's grievance procedures must include steps to ensure that you may raise your concerns fully and fairly and must provide for the prompt and equitable resolution of complaints.

School publications, such as student handbooks and catalogs, usually describe the steps you must take to start the grievance process. Often, schools have both formal and informal processes. If you decide to use a grievance process, you should be prepared to present all the reasons that support your request.

If you are dissatisfied with the outcome after using the school's grievance procedures or you wish to pursue an alternative to using the grievance procedures, you may file a complaint against the school with US Dept. of Education OCR (Office of Civil Rights) or in a court. You may learn more about the OCR complaint process from the brochure How to File a Discrimination Complaint with the Office for Civil Rights, which you may obtain by contacting them at the address and phone numbers on the following page, or at http://www.ed.gov/ocr/docs/howto.html.

If you would like more information about the responsibilities of post-secondary schools to students with disabilities, read the OCR brochure Auxiliary Aids and Services for post-secondary Students with Disabilities: Higher Education's Obligations Under Section 504 and Title II of the ADA. You may obtain a copy by contacting them at the address and phone numbers below, or at http://www.ed.gov/ocr/docs/auxaids.html.

Students with disabilities who know their rights and responsibilities are much better equipped to succeed in post-secondary school. Be sure to work with the staff at your school because they, too, want you to succeed. Seek the support of family, friends and fellow students, including those with disabilities. Know your talents and capitalize on them, and believe in yourself as you embrace new challenges in your education.[3]

To receive more information about the civil rights of students with disabilities in education institutions, you may contact the OCR at:

Customer Service Team Office for Civil Rights
U.S. Department of Education
Washington, D.C. 20202-1100
Phone: 1-800-421-3481 TDD: 1- 877-521-2172
Email: ocr@ed.gov Web site: www.ed.gov/ocr/*

Note to Parents

As parents you will continue to play a crucial role in your child's success. You can help make your child's transition from high school to college a successful one by encouraging the following:

- Self-Advocacy: It is imperative that your child be able to understand their syndrome and the accommodations they need to be successful.
- Study Skills: Be sure your child enrolls in study skills classes and orientation classes.
- Awareness: Be sure that your child attends all IEP or 504 Plan meetings throughout their high school years.
- Teach independent living skills: Make sure your child knows how to do laundry, basic cooking, use a credit card, take care of their medical needs, etc.

The Campus Tour

When you visit a potential college, be sure to take a guided campus tour. Also during the visit, make sure to meet the support personnel, observe classes and speak with students who attend the school.

Questions to ask during the Campus Visit:
- What is the average class size?
- Are course textbooks available on tape?
- Can students tape record lectures?
- Is there an advisor available who understands learning issues and is willing to help plan a course of study and balanced course load each semester?
- Is there a liaison available that can help students communicate with faculty?
- Does the college have any experience dealing with students who have Dysautonomia or have other chronic illnesses?
- How does one arrange for accommodations?
- What specific accommodations are available? (For example: note takers, extended time on tests and or assignments)?
- Are there tutorial services available?   Who provides these services? How do students access this service?
- Is there a cost for tutorial support?
- Are faculty notified of students in their class that have 504 Plans?
- Is help available for study strategies, time management and stress management?
- Are there placement tests? If so, how can I receive accommodations on these exams?
- Are there a minimum number of courses or hours required each semester?
- What happens if a student becomes too ill during the semester to finish their course load?
- How can I insure that my housing accommodations are

close in proximity to my classes and also to the cafeteria?
- Can I request that my room be on the first or second floor to avoid having to climb too many stairs?
- Are rooms equipped with air-conditioning?
- Can students keep a car on campus?

Familiarize yourself with your school's office for students with disabilities. Documentation is sent to this office. Once documentation has been sent, it is advisable for students and parents to meet with the director of this office to determine accommodations that can be offered. Here is a sampling of some possible accommodations that this office can assist in securing:
- Extended time on tests
- Books on tape
- Note takers
- Reading machines
- Separate locations

It is imperative that students seek out support from this office. This office may also be able to aid students to be able to speak with professors; however, in most cases the student will have to arrange accommodations with their professors directly.

A sampling of supportive colleges:
The list below is a working list of colleges that have been particularly supportive of students with learning issues.

Colleges with specialized programs

Adelphi University (NY)
American International (MA)
American University (DC)
Arizona State University
Boston University (MA)

C.W. Post (NY)
Catholic University (DC)
Cazenovia (NY)
Centenary College (NJ)
Clark University (MA)
College Misericordia (PA)
Concordia College (NY)
Curry College (MA)
DePaul University (IL)
Dowling College (NY)
Edinboro College of PA (PA)
Fairleigh Dickinson (NJ)
Florida Golf Coast (FL)
Gannon University (PA)
Hofstra University (NY)
Iona College (NY)
Kings College (PA)
Landmark College (VT)
Lesley College (MA)
Limestone College (SC)
Lynn University (FL)
Manhattan College (NY)
Marist College (NY)
Mc Daniel College (MD)
Merchyhurst College (PA)
Mitchell College (CT)
New England College (NH)
Niagara University (NY)
Northeastern University (MA)
Southern Vermont College (VT)
St. Andrews Presbyterian (NC)
St. Thomas Aquinas (NY)
Syracuse University (NY)
University of Arizona (AZ)

University of Connecticut (CT)
University of Hartford (CT)
University of Mass, Amherst (MA)
University of New Haven (CT)
University of Tampa (FL)
University of Vermont (VT)
Vincennes University (IN)
West Virginia Wesleyan (WV)

Review of Some Important Facts

- At the college level, education is no longer a right but a matter of eligibility, as defined by the Rehabilitation Act of 1973, Section 504 and the Americans with Disability Act of 1990.
- In order to be accepted by a college, students must first meet the admissions criteria for that school.
- Students do not have to reveal their disability, but it may be to their advantage to do so, so they can be provided with information about available services.
- Colleges vary widely in the services they offer to students. All are required to address student needs at some level if they take federal money.
- In some cases, *offer services* can help the student to speak with professors, but in most cases, the student will have the primary responsibility to arrange learning accommodations with the professors. In some cases, a plan coordinator will assist in carrying out the 504 Plan.

The following is a sample of a Post-Secondary (College) 504 Plan:

Nature of the Disability

This student has a form of Dysautonomia, called POTS, postural orthostatic tachycardia syndrome. Postural orthostatic tachycardia syndrome is defined by excessive heart rate increments upon upright posture. A person with POTS will experience heart rates that increase 30 beats or more per minute upon standing and/or increase to 120 beats or more per minute upon standing (Grubb, 2000). These exaggerated heart rate increases usually occur within 10 minutes of rising.

While the hallmark of POTS is an excessive heart rate increment upon standing, patients often exhibit numerous symptoms of autonomic nervous system deregulation, and research by the Mayo Clinic suggests POTS is a limited autonomic neuropathy (Thieben, Sandroni, Sletten, Benrud-Larson, Fealey, Vernino, Lennon, Shen & Low, 2007). Many POTS symptoms seem to be caused by an imbalance of the autonomic nervous system's control over blood flow. It is the autonomic nervous system (ANS) that regulates the needed adjustments in vascular tone, heart rate and blood pressure upon standing. Some of the messages coming from the autonomic nervous system tell the blood vessels to relax or tighten. In people with POTS, the system seems to be out of balance and blood is not going to the right place at the right time to do what the body needs (Fischer, 2007).

The symptoms of POTS are life altering and debilitating at times. POTS patients use about three times more energy to stand than a healthy person (Grubb, 2002). It is as if these patients are running in place all the time. Activities such as housework, bathing, and even meals can exacerbate symptoms (Grubb, Kanjwal & Kosinski, 2006). Research shows that POTS patients' quality of life is similar to those with congestive heart failure and chronic obstructive pulmonary disease. (Benrud-Larson, Dewar, Sandroni, Rummans, Haythornthwaite & Low, 2002) Twenty-five percent of people with POTS are disabled and unable to work (Goldstein, Robertson, Esler, Straus, & Eisenhofer, 2002). Most patients will have to make some lifestyle adjustments to cope with this disorder.

POTS can cause symptoms such as: dizziness, headaches, syncope, joint pain, nausea, insomnia, visual disturbances, digestion issues, abdominal pain, unremitting fatigue and more. Symptoms wax and wane and may come in any combination. Any autonomic (involuntary) function can be impacted at any time. The emotional and physical pieces are interrelated in complex ways, and patients can experience flare-ups of symptoms during times of emotional tension and stress. Changes in cognitive function from chronic or acute pain, or side effects of strong medications, can include compromised attention and concentration, reduced capacity to process information, disruptions in memory and reduced ability to multitask.

Patients may be on a restricted diet; may need to eat several small meals per day; and most likely will need to take medication during the course of the day.

POTS patients need to stay well hydrated and must eat salty snacks throughout the day to help keep up blood volume as well as blood pressure or fainting may result.

Often, students with POTS work extremely hard to compensate for their illness and its effects on daily functioning.

POTS is a chronic illness that is unpredictable; patients can face associated symptoms in a recurrent pattern, with periods of symptom inactivity in between active flare-ups and complications.

Symptoms may worsen and conversely, may go into remission for varying lengths of time. Medications can help manage the symptoms and improve functioning, but are not cures for POTS. However at this time there is no a cure for POTS.

Sample 504 Post Secondary Plan modified from Kings Park High School.

Section 504 Plan for :(Student Name) _____
University _____
Academic Year/Term _____

_____ shall be the point person at the university for purposes of carrying out the provisions of this Plan. This person shall be known as the Plan Coordinator. The Plan Coordinator will educate him/herself about the nature of Dysautonomia, the treatments the student is receiving, the side-effects of the treatments, and the student's particular symptoms and needs. In addition, the Plan Coordinator shall be responsible for ensuring that the provisions of this Plan are carried out and he/she shall be the liaison between the student, and the relevant university personnel.

For purposes of this Plan, _____ (the student) is a person with a disability under Section 504 and the ADA. He/she is significantly impaired in performance of the major life activity of _____.

The purpose of this Plan is to maintain the student's optimal participation in his/her academic curriculum and educational goals, aid in the management of his/her illness, and reduce the student's stress.

The Student's Symptoms and Needs
_____ (the student) has the following symptoms and needs, which may change over time:
_____ Diarrhea (estimated ___ bathroom trips per day)
_____ Pain (rated a ___ out of 10, with 10 being the worst).
_____ Syncope
_____ Fatigue

_____ Nausea

_____ Vomiting (estimated ___ times per day)

_____ Student has had surgery (___ times)

_____ Headaches

_____ Student takes medication during the day

List medications and dosages here:

_____

_____

_____

_____

_____ Student has dietary restrictions

Explain here:

_____

_____

_____

_____ Student receives treatments/office visits that require absences
  from campus/courses:

Estimated Frequency: every ____ weeks

Expected duration of absence: ___ days per treatment

Student requires university personnel assistance with:

___ Medication

___ Dietary needs

___ Loss of consciousness

___ Other (specify):

_____

Side effects of student's particular medications may cause/impact:

___ Headaches

___ Difficulty focusing, concentrating, sustaining attention

___ Tremors

___ Fatigue

___ Tachycardia

___

____ *Other (specify):*

Emergency Contacts
In case of a medical emergency, university personnel will notify the
Plan Coordinator, who will call _____ at the following
Telephone number(s):
Home: _____ Work: _____
Cell: _____ Other: _____
Signed:

_____

_____
Student Plan Coordinator

_____
Dean of Students/representative.
UNS staff
Date_____

___

Potential Accommodations (select as necessary/relevant)

1. The student will be permitted free access to leave courses for use of the restroom, without asking permission, and
without penalty.

2. University Health Services provide the student with a
place to lie down if necessary during the day.

3. The student will be permitted to carry a portable fan and
use it during classes.

4. The student will be permitted to carry and drink water,
eat salty snacks (to aid in hydration) during a course.

5. The student will be permitted to administer his/her own
medications on campus.

    a. If for medical reasons the student is not permitted
    to administer his/her own medications, the medica-
    tions will be left with a University nurse, who will
    administer them to the student at times consistent

with prescribing instructions.

b. If staff requires training in administration of the student's medication, the Plan Coordinator shall ensure that staff receives such training within ten business days of the date of this Plan.

6. Student will be allowed, "Stop the clock testing." "Stop the clock testing," means that, when the student is sitting for a timed exam, if he/she needs a bathroom break or a break due to pain, the time for completing the test will be extended by the amount of time the student spends away from the testing room.

a. This accommodation shall be provided without penalty.

7. If, because of his/her POTS symptoms or medical treatments, the student is unable to take an exam or submit a major project on a given day, the exam or major project deadline will be rescheduled. Cumulative term grades will not be determined until the student has had opportunity to take the make-up exam or complete the major project. This accommodation shall be provided without penalty and apply to course exams, term papers and projects when reasonably agreed upon.

8. Consideration should be given to the number of major exams for which the student is required to sit on the same day.

9. It would be the student's responsibility to advise the Plan Coordinator of all planned exams by the professors. If an exam needs to be rescheduled, the Plan Coordinator will facilitate the student's efforts with professors.

a. Consideration should be given to the number of major projects due on the same day.

b. It would be the student's responsibility to advise the Plan Coordinator of all planned projects by the professors.

c. If a major project needs to be rescheduled, the Plan Coordinator will facilitate the student's efforts with professors.

d. "Major projects" are defined as those that are assigned more than one week before they are due. If the student is unable to meet a deadline on any project due to anything unanticipated related to his/her POTS symptoms and treatment requirements, the project deadline will be rescheduled. This accommodation shall be provided without penalty.

10. The student will be given assistance to help him/her make up any course.

a. Time/lecture halls missed due to the student's POTS, as set forth below.

b. After a student notifies professors of symptom interference with course participation, the Plan Coordinator will help ensure that, if relevant, each professor make available an updated syllabus, lesson plans, new assignments, and copies of all visual aids, and written homework assignments within 48 hours of when they were requested by the student. This would also apply to instances where the student is present, but unable to take notes due to difficulty concentrating or writing, or when the student is out of the classroom to take care of medical needs.

11. Any and all make-up work shall be designed to show the student's competence in the subject area; quality rather than quantity of the make-up work shall be emphasized. A professor shall have the right to waive, modify, substitute or amend assignments so as to facilitate the student's ability to catch up on missed work. This accommodation shall be provided without penalty.

12. The student will not be penalized for tardiness or absences required for medical appointments and/or illness. If a professor decides that a portion of a term grade for all students is awarded based on attendance, the student will remain eligible for maximum credit of that portion of the grade if his/her only absences are due to medical appointments and/or treatment.

13. Often times, it is difficult to carry heavy books back and forth, or around to all courses for the length of the day. This may be relevant if disease activity impacts tachycardia and fatigue. Where available, the student will be permitted to use an elevator to get to classes held on various levels of the school in a timely fashion.

14. The student will not be discouraged from engaging fully in all campus activities, and will not be discouraged from taking medication on time, eating snacks when medically indicated, complying with all dietary restrictions, taking bathroom breaks, or any of the other accommodations set forth above.

15. Seating will be available to the student for easy access to the classroom door to facilitate motor breaks and reduce anxiety. The student may alter location in professors-assigned classroom seating charts, as well, if a neighboring student has or appears to have a communicable illness.

16. The university shall notify the student of a known outbreak of chicken pox, flu or other infectious diseases as to which the student is at a greater risk due a compromised immune system.

17. The student shall be permitted to carry a cellular telephone, and be allowed to use it in an emergency that precludes the student from reaching a school telephone to contact medical team members.

18. Any professor or other university personnel having questions about this Plan shall raise those questions with the student first, and the Plan Coordinator, if necessary. If the Plan Coordinator believes that there are concerns that are not addressed in this Plan, the Plan Coordinator shall notify the student and schedule a meeting that shall include the student.

19. Academic accommodations necessitated by changes in cognitive functioning due to POTS symptoms/diagnosis must be addressed and considered separately on a case-by-case basis.

All of the provisions of this plan shall be provided without penalty to the student.

The Plan Coordinator and Due Process Rights

The Plan Coordinator will help make available a copy of this Plan, with the student's permission, to any relevant professors or teaching assistants.

If the Plan Coordinator is unable to obtain compliance with this Plan by any professor other university personnel, he or she shall notify the Dean of Students. The Dean shall respond to each such communication from the Plan Coordinator within two

in-session school days with a plan for reconciling the interference with the student's educational mandates.

If the Dean declines to adopt any element or portion of the recommended action plan, he or she shall put his or her reasons in writing within two [(2)] in-session school days of receipt of the recommended action plan, and this writing shall be sent to the student and Dean.

Both the student and Plan Coordinator shall have the authority to request a due process hearing if the Dean declines to accept the plan. This hearing shall be in addition to, not instead of, any due process rights the student has under the ADA, Section 504, and/or the IDEA.[2]

Reference:
(1,2) King Park High School "Student with Special Needs – A College Guide" Advocacy Consortium for College Students with Disabilities
(3) US Dept. of Education http://www.ed.gov/ocr/auxaids.html
(4) U.S. Department of Education, Office for Civil Rights, Students with Disabilities Preparing for Postsecondary Education: Know Your Rights and Responsibilities, Washington, D.C., 2007.

Section 6. More Helpful Hints

Chapter 16. Securing a Handicap Sticker- *Jesse White, Secretary of State of Illinois*

As Illinois Secretary of State, my office is responsible for the issuance of parking placards, disability license plates, and disabled veteran license plates to residents with qualifying disabilities.

The Parking Program for Persons with Disabilities is a vital program for persons with disabilities in Illinois and across the nation. Since first taking office in 1999, I have worked to implement innovative changes to reduce the fraud and abuse of disability license plates. In addition, my office is committed to ensuring that persons with disabilities have the access they need to help them maintain their independence.

In Illinois, I initiated legislation that significantly increased the fines and penalties for those who abuse the provisions of the Parking Program for Persons with Disabilities. The illegal use of an accessible parking space is a minimum $250 fine, and municipalities have the ability to increase the fine to a maximum of $350 with the adoption of a local ordinance. Unauthorized use of disability license plates or parking placards carries a minimum of a $500 fine and a 30-day administrative driver's license suspension for a first-time offense. For a subsequent offense, the fine increases to a $750, and carries a six month driver's license suspension, and a $1,000 fine and a one-year driver's license suspension for a third offense. Law enforcement officers also have the ability to enter onto private property such as a mall or grocery store to enforce the provisions of the program, and have the authority to confiscate parking placards if they witness the placard being used illegally.

To meet the needs of Illinoisans with disabilities, the Secretary of State issues three different types of parking placards: permanent disability placards are issued to persons with permanent disabilities and are renewed every four years; Temporary disability placards are issued to persons with temporary disabilities not exceeding six months; organization placards are issued to not-for-profit organizations that transport persons with disabilities free of charge. In addition to parking placards, the Secretary of State also issues disability license plates to persons with permanent disabilities who own a vehicle, and disabled veteran license plates to qualified veterans with disabilities.

In order to obtain a parking placard or disability license plates, a person must submit a Secretary of State Persons with Disabilities Certification form signed by a licensed physician certifying that the person meets one of the following six specific medical conditions that severely impairs their ability to walk:

1. Cannot walk without the assistance of another person, prosthetic device, wheelchair, or other assistive device.
2. Be restricted by lung disease to such a degree that the person's forced (respiratory) expiratory volume (FEV) in 1 second, when measured by spirometry, is less than 1 liter.
3. Must use portable oxygen.
4. Have a Class III or Class IV cardiac condition according to the standards set by the American Heart Association.
5. Be severely limited in the person's ability to walk due to an arthritic, neurological, or orthopedic condition.
6. Has permanently lost the use of or is missing a hand or arm.

Under Illinois law, parking placards are only valid until the expiration date indicated on the placard. Placards are not transferable and it is illegal to copy or duplicate a placard for any reason. The authorized holder must be present and must enter or exit the vehicle at the time the parking privileges are being used. It is the responsibility of the authorized holder to ensure that their placard is displayed properly.

To help assist physicians with a better understanding of the eligibility requirements and the general provisions of the program, my office developed the Medical Professionals Guide to the Parking Program for Persons with Disabilities. Physicians play an integral role in preventing the abuse of the Parking Program for Persons with Disabilities by ensuring that their patients meet the eligibility requirements of the program before approving them for disability license plates or a parking placard. The medical guide is accessible on my office's Web site at www.cyberdriveillinois.com.

Disability license plates and parking placards are assigned to the person with disabilities and can be used in any vehicle in which the person is driving or is a passenger. Vehicles displaying disability license plates, placards or disabled veteran license plates may park in spaces reserved for persons with disabilities, and are exempt from parking meter fees or time limitations on parking, except at parking meters with time limitations of 30 minutes or less. Disability license plates and placards do not permit vehicles to park in areas where parking is prohibited or restricted, or in any manner that creates a traffic hazard.

Illinois honors all placards and disability license plates is-sued by other states as long as the authorized holder is present at the time the parking privileges are being used.

I remain committed to improving the Parking Program for Persons with Disabilities in Illinois. As long as I am Secretary of State, my office will continue to combat the fraudulent use of plac-ards and disability license plates as well as ensuring that persons with disabilities have the access they need to disability placards and license plates to help them maintain their independence.

If you have any questions or need additional information on the provisions of the State of Illinois Parking Program for Persons with Disabilities, please contact the Secretary of State Persons with Disabilities License Plate/Placard Unit, Vehicle Services Department, 501 Second St. Room 541, Springfield, Illinois, 62756, or call (708) 210-2843. You may also visit my office's website at www.cyberdriveillinois.com to review the various publications we offer on the Parking Program for Persons with Disabilities.

Authored by: Jesse White, Secretary of the State of Illinois

Note: Other states may have different requirements. In some states, disability parking placards are given out by counties or towns

Chapter 17. Assistive Devices - *Megan Ong, Ana Collins and Katie Ziegler - POTS patients*

POTS can compromise mobility through a variety of ways such as orthostatic intolerance, fatigue, dizziness and generalized weakness. Different assistive devices may help the POTS patient achieve functional mobility.

Types of Assistive Devices that are Available:

Canes: Those who have difficulties with balance and who feel insecure when walking may benefit from the assistance of a cane. Offset canes are often easier on the joints than straight canes and may be beneficial for those with joint issues. Canes come in all sorts of fun colors and designs and have the advantage of being highly maneuverable. There are also "seat canes" which as its name implies, is a cane with a seat. The seat can be helpful with managing fatigue and orthostatic intolerance. The seat makes the cane heavier, and will probably not be the best choice for someone who feels that they have muscle weakness as well.

Walkers: Walkers can help with more severe balance issues. There are different types of walkers, some with four wheels (often called a rollator), some with two and some with none. For patients with muscle weakness, a walker without wheels could be difficult to use since the walker must be lifted up to move. POTS patients should consider a walker that comes with a seat although these might be slightly more costly. Finally, there are walkers that also double as a transport chair, a favorite of many POTS patients.

Scooters: These are cheaper than power chairs. While they can be used indoors, they are best for outdoor use. The patient must have adequate arm strength to safely operate a scooter.

Insurance companies will help pay for the cost of assistive devices. It is often best to check with your insurance company before buying a device yourself. Sometimes, insurance companies will only pay for one device. In that case, you would want them to purchase the more expensive device. For example, if you like using a cane for short distances, you can purchase it yourself, and have the insurance company cover the cost of a power wheelchair. When purchasing out of pocket, online sites often have good prices. Make sure you are purchasing from credible companies. When purchasing through an insurance company, they will often require you to work with specific durable medical suppliers. Certain criteria must be met in order for insurance to pay for your wheelchair, via insurance.

What to look for when choosing a Wheelchair

Wheelchairs: These may be considered for patients severely limited by their POTS or for those who may need a little extra help with long distances. There are three types of wheelchairs including transport chairs, manual wheelchairs, and power chairs. Transport chairs come standard, but manual wheelchairs and power chairs can be custom fitted. It is often very useful to go to a wheelchair seating and evaluation clinic. An occupational therapist can help you decide on a chair that best meets your needs and is comfortable for you. For those planning on using their chair frequently and for longer periods of time, a proper evaluation is necessary.

Transport Chairs: These are low cost and are a good option for patients who do not need a wheelchair for long periods of time. Transport chairs have four small wheels and cannot be self-propelled. Someone else must push the chair. For those purchasing out of pocket who may need assistive transportation for "bad days" or trips to the doctor's office, a transport chair might be useful.

Manual Wheelchair: Manual wheelchairs have two large wheels and can be self-propelled or pushed. A lightweight chair is often a good choice for POTS patients since it will help reduce the amount of energy needed to propel the chair. Manual wheelchairs can be fitted with power-assist wheels. Power-assist wheels still allow the user to get exercise by pushing the wheels, but each push allows them to go a bit farther, conserving energy.

Power chairs: Power chairs are an investment. Although there are a few exceptions, most power chairs will require the purchase of a lift/ramp for the car and for the house. The lifts or ramps are not covered by insurance and patients will have to find alternate funding. An electric power chair is best for someone with muscle weakness, weak trunk support and who cannot operate a scooter. Patients with EDS may also be a candidate for a power chair over a manual since joints may dislocate using a manual chair. There are three different types of power wheelchairs: rear-wheel drive, mid-wheel drive, and front-wheel drive. Rear - wheel drive chairs generally have faster maximum speeds but have a larger turning radius than mid-wheel or front - wheel drive chairs.

Finally, add-ons like tilt, recline and elevating leg rests should be considered. These features are often very important for the POTS patient. They are designed to assist with positioning, which makes it easier to sit for longer periods of time comfortably, and helps control swelling in the extremities. For those getting a power chair, these features can also be automated. For manual chairs, keep in mind that these features add weight.

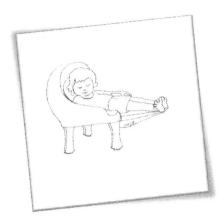

Chapter 18. 25 Necessities for a POTS friendly life

People with POTS may find it useful to take advantage of tools and equipment to make life easier. Feel free to pick and choose any or all of these ideas that may meet your own needs.

1.Ankle weights - to help improve stamina and circulation. Start with very small weights and increase the amount over time. Just walking around and wearing ankle weights may improve conditioning and muscle tone in the legs.

2.Arthritis Gloves - can help with swollen fingers and on days when your hands are too weak to function.

3.Cell phone - you should carry a cell phone at all times, in case of emergency.

4.Compression stockings - are used to improve venous return to the heart through external vasoconstriction. Manufacturers of the stockings offer graduated compression with maximum compression at the ankle and decreasing as you move up the leg. This compression, when combined with the muscle pumping effect of the calf, aids in preventing blood pooling in the legs. Compression stockings are available in a wide range of opacities, colors, styles and sizes, making them virtually indistinguishable from regular hosiery or socks. They come in various levels of compression and different lengths such as knee, thigh and waist high. You may need to be individually fitted to get the correct size, and you may need a doctor's prescription in order to purchase them. They also come with closed toes, like traditional pantyhose or open if you want to wear flip flops and show off your pedicure. A good pair can be over $100 dollars but many insurance companies can cover them if you get a prescription from your doctor.

5.Cooling vest - is a "must-have" for those planning an extended outdoor activity on a hot summer day. If medically necessary and prescribed by your physician, your health insurance company may help pay for a cooling vest. Smaller cooling neck wraps are available.

6.Disabled parking permit - You may need to apply for a disabling parking permit with the help of your doctor. The parking permit is given to people with limited mobility due to a medical, neurologic or cardiac condition and can be an invaluable asset for drivers with POTS or caretakers of individuals with POTS.

7.Emergency Information Card - always carry your medical information with you in your purse or wallet (preferably laminated). The card should explain Dysautonomia and what to do in case of an emergency. It is also a good idea to carry your doctors' numbers with you, allergies to medicines, medical conditions you may have and emergency contact phone numbers should you experience syncope.

8.Exercise equipment - A recumbent bike or a rower may be a great investment especially for those who are considering starting an exercise program. (See Chapter on Exercise and POTS, for more information).

9.Extended height rolling chair - can be very useful for a POTS-friendly household. You can use the rolling chair in the kitchen when preparing meals or when you are having a symptomatic day and need to move around the house

10. Heating pad or hot water bottle - applied to the abdomen can help relieve stomach pain. Be sure that the heating pad is not too hot in order to avoid vasodilatation and a drop in blood pressure.

11. Moldable ice packs or a bag of frozen peas – Can help with headaches and overheating.

12. Home blood pressure monitor - Your doctor or nurse may instruct you to monitor your blood pressure at home. Frequency will depend on your condition, medications and doctor preferences. Cardiologists suggest using your right arm if possible to get an accurate and consistent reading.

13. Knee, wrist foot or elbow brace - may be helpful for patients with joint disorders, such as Ehlers-Danlos Syndrome or arthritis. This may help with stability and protect the joints from injury. Be sure to check with your doctor or physical therapist to see whether you would benefit from a brace.

14. Neck pillow - Can be very helpful for long car rides since it reduces muscle tension in the neck and shoulders.

15. Pill cutter - This is great when a half dosage of a medicine is required or when you are weaning off of a medication. Most pills do not cut in half easily as they tend to crumble. Using a pill cutter makes dosage easier and more accurate. Your pharmacy may also be able to cut your pills for you.

16. Portable fan - This is a great and inexpensive way to stay cool. Some even come with misters.

17. Pulse monitor wristwatch - This is an easy way to monitor your heart rate since tachycardia is a common occurrence with this condition.

18. Recliner Chair - It is better to rest in a recliner during the day than to lay in bed in order to help improve circulation.

19. Seat Cane - may be a useful assistive walking device for those with balance difficulty or muscle weakness, in addition to orthostatic intolerance. It can be used as a cane while walking and can fold into a seat if you need to take a break. Try to find one that is lightweight and easy to open, close and transport.

20. Shower chair - This is an essential piece of equipment for those who cannot stand long enough to take a shower. Heat exacerbates symptoms. Taking a shower may be a safety concern. It is critical to avoid a syncopal episode in the shower!

21. Small snacks - you should carry small healthy snacks with you at all times in case you become hungry. Many patients with POTS experience reactive hypoglycemia or exacerbation of POTS symptoms precipitated by prolonged fasting or hungers. Eating a small healthy snack, such as raisins, banana, or a cereal bar, can quickly alleviate pre-syncope, dizziness and reactive hypoglycemia and provide a rapid energy boost.

22. Sunglasses - These may be helpful for those suffering from migraine headaches. Sunglasses can help reduce sensitivity to light and prevent migraine headaches triggered by bright lights.

23. Warm, cozy socks - Great for keeping your cold feet warm.

24. Water bottles - You should be carrying water around at all times. Stainless steel and glass water bottles may be healthier and environmentally friendlier than plastic bottles, which may contain BPA.

25. Salt packets – May help retain water thus helping to raise blood pressure.

26. Wide brim hat - prevents overheating of the head and face.

27. This book! - Use this book and other materials you collect in one place at home or office. You should have a ready reference for any problem that may arise.

Chapter 19. How to Get Job Accommodations in the work force - *Dr. Suzanne Gosden Kitchen, Senior Consultant for the Job Accommodation Network (JAN)*

Reasonable Accommodations: Employment and the ADA

"Across this country, millions of people with disabilities are working or want to work, and they should have access to the support and services they need to succeed." - President Barack Obama (USOPM, 2010)

Barriers to employment have undermined America's efforts to educate, rehabilitate, and employ people with disabilities. Breaking down these barriers through the passage of landmark Civil Rights Law, the Americans with Disabilities Act (ADA), enables employers to adequately harness the skills and talents of people with disabilities, which in turn, helps people with disabilities lead more productive lives (EEOC, 2008).

Title I, the employment provisions of the ADA, applies to private employers (which can include employment agencies and labor unions) with 15 or more employees. Title I of the ADA prohibits discrimination in all employment practices, including the job application procedures, hiring, firing, advancement, compensation, training, and other terms, conditions, and privileges of employment. It applies to recruitment, advertising, tenure, layoff, leave, fringe benefits, and all other employment-related activities (EEOC and DOJ, 2008).

Under the ADA, employment discrimination is prohibited against qualified people with disabilities, both applicants and employees. A qualified person with a disability is a person who meets legitimate skill, experience, education, or other requirements for the job, and who can perform the essential functions of the job with or without reasonable accommodation. If the person is qualified to perform essential job functions except for limitations caused by a disability, the employer must consider whether the person could perform these functions with a reasonable accommodation (EEOC and DOJ, 2008).

The ADA does not contain a list of medical conditions that constitute disabilities. Instead, the ADA has a general definition of disability that each person must meet (EEOC, 1992). Therefore, some people with Dysautonomia (because POTS is one form of it) will have a disability under the ADA and some will not. A person has a disability if he/she has a physical or mental impairment that substantially limits one or more major life activities, a record of such impairment, or is regarded as having such an impairment (EEOC, 1992). To be a disability covered by the ADA, the impairment must substantially limit one or more major life activities. These are activities that an average person can perform with little or no difficulty. Examples are: walking, seeing, speaking, hearing, breathing, learning, performing manual tasks, caring for oneself, and working. Other activities such as sitting, standing, lifting, or reading are also major life activities (EEOC, 1992).

People who do meet the definition of disability under the ADA, and who work for employers with 15 or more employees, are entitled to reasonable accommodations under the law. Examples of reasonable accommodations under the ADA include: making existing facilities used by employees readily accessible to and usable by an individual with a disability; restructuring a job; modifying work schedules; acquiring or modifying equipment; providing qualified readers or interpreters; or modifying examinations, training, or other programs. Reasonable accommodations also can include reassigning a current employee to a vacant position for which the person is qualified (EEOC and DOJ, 2008).

The ADA does not require employers to lower quality or quantity standards as an accommodation; nor is the employer obligated to provide personal use items such as glasses or hearing aids. Furthermore, an employer is only required to accommodate a "known" disability; thus, disclosure of a person's disability is a key factor in obtaining reasonable accommodations (EEOC and DOJ, 2008).

If a person with a disability requests an accommodation, the employer and the employee should work together to identify accommodations that are reasonable, effective, and not cause the employer an undue hardship. This interaction is called the "accommodation process" (EEOC and DOJ, 2008). There are many public and private resources that can help employers and employees identify job accommodations. Most provide assistance without cost, such as state Vocational Rehabilitation agencies and state Assistive Technology Projects. One such agency, the Job Accommodation Network (JAN), a service of the Office of Disability Employment Policy, can help identify accommodations for any type of disability through private, individualized consultation (Job Accommodation Network homepage, 2010).

JAN also provides information regarding the costs of job accommodations. Recent amendments to the ADA broadened the definition of disability, and once again raised public concern about the cost of providing reasonable accommodations. However, current studies show that workplace accommodations not only are low cost, but also positively affect the workplace in many ways (Job Accommodation Network, 2009). The study showed that the benefits employers receive from making workplace accommodations far outweigh the low cost. Employers reported that providing accommodations resulted in such benefits as retaining valuable employees, improving productivity and morale, reducing workers compensation and training costs, and improving company diversity. These benefits were obtained with little investment. The employers in the study reported that a high percentage (56%) of accommodations cost absolutely nothing to make, while the rest typically cost under a $1000 dollars (Job Accommodation Network, 2009).

Job accommodations may be a very useful employment strategy for people with Dysautonomia. With the right accommodations in place, people with this condition can be productive in the workplace, and fulfill their career goals as any person in the workplace would. People with Dysautonomia may develop some of the limitations discussed in this chapter, but seldom develop all of them. Also, the degree of limitation will vary from person to person. Not all people with Dysautonomia will need accommodations to perform their jobs and many others may only need a few accommodations.

The limitations specifically covered in this chapter are: migraine headaches, cognitive impairment, standing upright or walking safely, managing stress, temperature sensitivity, and dizziness or fainting. A special section on emergency evacuation from the workplace is also included in this chapter.

The following accommodations are only a sample of the possibilities available. Numerous other accommodation solutions may exist.

Accommodations for Migraines: According to the National Headache Foundation, an estimated 28 million Americans have migraine headaches, including people with Dysautonomia. (JAN Migraines, 2008). In addition to changes in blood pressure which can contribute to migraine headache conditions, migraine headaches can be triggered by light, noise, fragrance/smells, weather changes, sleep disturbance and stress.

- Add light filters to existing overhead lights to create more natural light effect
- Change the type or quantity of indoor lighting
- Provide a liquid crystal display monitor with a quick refresh rate and low-glare
- Strategically place employee's work area where lighting can be adjusted, where excessive noise exposure to fragrances/smells can be avoided
- Wear anti-glare sunglasses, wide-brimmed hat or visor
- Allow the employee to telecommute (work from home)
- Mask distracting sounds with an environmental sound machine, noise canceling headset, and/or sound absorption panels

- Keep non-work related conversation to a minimum
- Implement a fragrance-free policy or ask employees to voluntarily refrain from wearing fragrances
- Provide a modified schedule
- Provide air purification systems
- Reduce visual and auditory distractions
- Make after-hours social functions optional, particularly if an employee is affected by a disruption in sleep patterns or when the employer cannot control the environment where the function occurs (JAN Migraine Fact Sheet, 2010).

Accommodations for Cognitive Impairments: Cognitive impairment, or "brain fog" as it is commonly known, describes disturbances in brain functions such as memory loss, disorientation, distractibility, perception problems, and difficulty thinking logically. Many conditions can cause cognitive symptoms including Dysautonomia, Multiple Sclerosis, Depression, Alcoholism, Alzheimer's disease, Parkinson disease, Traumatic Brain Injury, Chronic Fatigue Syndrome and Stroke (Loy, 2010). Additionally, sometimes the treatment of a condition can cause cognitive impairment, such as treatments for cancer, or medication regimens.

- Provide written job instructions to the employee
- Prioritize job assignments for the employee
- Allow a self-pace workload
- Provide memory aids, such as schedulers or organizers
- Minimize auditory, visual and tactile distractions
- Provide space enclosures or a private office
- Reduce clutter in the employee's work environment
- Plan uninterrupted work time each day or week
- Divide large assignments into smaller tasks with specific steps
- Make daily TO-DO lists and check off tasks as each is completed
- Remind employee of important deadlines

- Allow the employee to tape record meetings, instructions, and directives
- Provide minutes from meetings or activities
- Use notebooks, calendars, or sticky notes to record information in writing
- Allow additional training time
- Post instructions for frequently-used equipment
- Provide picture diagrams of problem-solving techniques
- Assign a supervisor or mentor to be available when the employee has questions (Loy, 2010).

Accommodations for Standing and/or Walking Safely: People with Dysautonomia may have significant limitations with standing upright or walking safely, in particular after long periods of recumbency. This is likely the effect of poor circulation negatively affecting blood pressure, and can cause visual darkening or near fainting when moving from a seated (or laying) position to a standing position. Lightheadedness and dizziness can also lead to actual syncope with loss of consciousness, again related to blood circulation (Yanofsky, 1999).

- Reduce or eliminate physical exertion
- Schedule periodic rest breaks
- Allow a flexible work schedule
- Provide a scooter or other mobility aid if walking cannot be reduced
- Keep aisles clear of clutter
- Install ramps, handrails, and provide accessible parking spaces
- Assign workspace in close proximity to office machines or other frequently-visited space
- Modifying workstation design and height
- Providing lightweight doors or automatic door openers
- Use sit/stand stools in workspace
- Use standing frames to ensure a safe standing position

- Provide lumbar support stands
- Use anti-fatigue matting on hard-surface floors in the work area
- Use a cane, crutches, or rolling walkers to aid mobility
- Make workstation accessible for wheelchairs or power-scooter users (Whidden, 2010).

Accommodations for Managing Stress: Stress is a normal psychological and physical reaction to the demands of life. High levels of stress can lead to serious health problems such as high blood pressure or generalized anxiety disorder, or exacerbate existing health problems such as Dysautonomia.

- Reduce distractions in work environment
- Provide TO-DO lists and written instructions
- Remind employee of important deadlines and meetings
- Allow time off for counseling or other treatment
- Provide clear expectations of job responsibilities
- Provide sensitivity training to co-workers
- Allow breaks to use stress management techniques
- Develop strategies to deal with work problems before they arise
- Provide positive praise and reinforcement
- Provide written job instructions
- Allow for open communication to managers and supervisors
- Establish long term and short term goals
- Provide written work agreements
- Refer to employee assistance programs
- Allow telephone calls during work hours to doctors and others for needed support
- Adjust supervisory method to better manage employee
- Maintain open channels of communication between the employee and the new and old supervisor to ensure an ef-

fective transition
- Provide weekly or monthly meetings to discuss work-place issues and productions levels
- Provide for job sharing opportunities (Loy, 2010).

Accommodations for Temperature Sensitivity: Since people with Dysautonomia commonly experience significant heat intolerance due to the body's inability to regulate temperature, it is important to provide accommodations tailored to minimize the impact of temperature on the employee's ability to function in a work environment.
- Adjust work-site temperature
- Maintain the ventilation system
- Modify dress code
- Provide fan or personal air-conditioner
- Redirect vents in the workspace
- Allow flexible scheduling during extremely hot or cold weather
- Offer telecommuting (working from home)
- Provide cooling clothing such as the Cool-Vest
- Allow employee to consume hot or cold liquids at workstation
- Provide warming devices such as heated gloves
- Provide an office with separate temperature control (JAN Chronic Fatigue Accommodations, 2010).

Accommodations for Dizziness or Fainting: Employees with Dysautonomia or POTS might experience dizziness, fainting, or Syncope, as mentioned in the accommodation section for standing or walking safely, most likely caused by sharp changes in blood pressure. Employees with this limitation might have difficulty performing everyday activities such as getting out of bed; rising from a sitting to a standing position; walking; traveling; working around moving objects, under bright or fluorescent lights, or at heights; climbing ladders; viewing a computer monitor; or working in an environment that has many colors or patterns (e.g., a patterned carpet) (JAN Vertigo Fact Sheet, 2010).

- Develop a "plan of action" respond appropriately if/when employee faints
- Cushion a fall by using rubber matting on floor, and by adding padded edging to corners and edges
- Install machine guarding
- Use rolling safety ladders with handrails and locking casters
- Provide head protection and/or eye protection
- Use fall protection
- Provide parking close to the work-site
- Provide a work environment that has solid colored carpeting and walls instead of patterns and multiple colors
- Move workstation close to other work areas, office equipment, and break rooms
- Allow a flexible schedule to use public transportation to and from work
- Reduce or eliminate travel on the job when not essential to the position (Kitchen, 2008).

Emergency Evacuation Procedures: Employees with disabilities should be included in an employer's emergency evacuation plans. Identifying accommodation needs for employees with Dysautonomia will help employers with a safe emergency evacuation (Batiste and Loy, 2008).

In general, employers may implement a "buddy system" for all employees. A buddy system involves employees working in teams so they can locate and assist each other in emergencies.

Employers may also designate areas of rescue assistance. Section 4.3.11 of the Americans with Disabilities Act Accessibility Guidelines (ADAAG) specifically addresses areas of rescue assistance. If these areas do not have escape routes, they should have 1) an operating phone, cell-phone, TTY, and two-way radio so that emergency services can be contacted; 2) a closing door; 3) supplies that enable individuals to block smoke from entering the room from under the door; 4) a window and something to write with (lipstick, marker) or a "help" sign to alert rescuers that people are in this location; and respirator masks.

To evacuate employees with fainting, dizziness, syncope, or difficulty standing or walking safely, use evacuation devices such as the Evac-Chair. These devices help move people with motor impairments down the stairs or across rough terrain. If evacuation devices are used, personnel should be trained to operate and maintain them.

To evacuate employees who might experience cognitive limitations, consider communicating in alternative ways during drills or during real emergencies. For example, some individuals may benefit from pictures of buddies or color-coding exit doors or areas of rescue assistance.

Employers should consider the effects of training for emergency evacuation. Some individuals with motor impairments or cognitive impairments benefit from frequent emergency drills, but for others, practice drills may trigger anxiety or cause fatigue. Notifying employees of upcoming practice drills, and allowing them to opt out of participation, may be a reasonable accommodation. Offering another form of training for emergency evacuation procedures may be needed, such as providing detailed written instructions or watching a video of a drill in action (Batiste and Loy, 2008).

In conclusion, job accommodations are reasonable adjustments to a job or work environment that makes it possible for an individual with any type of disability to perform their job duties. Determining what types of job accommodations are needed involves close consideration of the required job tasks and knowledge of the specific limitations of the person performing the job. Job accommodations may include specialized equipment, facility modifications, adjustment to work schedules or job duties, as well as a whole range of other creative solutions (USDOL, 2010). And remember that America works best, when everybody works (Campaign for Disability Employment, 2009).

References

1. Batiste, L. and Loy, B. (2008). *Employer's Guide to Including Employees with Disabilities in Emergency Evacuation Plans.* Retrieved September 7, 2010 from http://askjan.org/media/emergency.html

2. Campaign for Disability Employment (2009). *News Room.* Retrieved September 1, 2010 from http://www.whatcanyoudocampaign.org/blog/index.php/news-room/

3. Equal Employment Opportunity Commission. (1992). *A technical assistance manual on the employment provisions (title I) of the Americans with Disabilities Act.* Retrieved August 31, 2010, from http://askjan.org/links/ADAtam1.html

4. Equal Employment Opportunity Commission and Department of Justice. (2008). *Americans with Disabilities Act Questions and Answers.* Retrieved September 1, 2010 from http://www.ada.gov/qandaeng.htm

5. Job Accommodation Network. (2009). *Workplace Accommodations: Low Cost, High Impact. Annually Updated Research Findings Address the Costs and Benefits of Job Accommodations.* Retrieved September 7, 2010 from http://askjan.org/media/LowCostHighImpact.doc

6. Job Accommodation Network. (2008). *Accommodation and Compliance Series: Employees with Migraines.* Retrieved August 31, 2010 from http://askjan.org/media/Migraine.html

7. Job Accommodation Network (2010). *Job Accommodations for People with Vertigo.* Retrieved September 1, 2010 from http://askjan.org/media/employmentvertigofact.doc

8. Kitchen, S.G. (2008). *Accommodation and Compliance Series: Employees with Epilepsy.* Retrieved August 13, 2010 from http://askjan.org/media/epilepsy.html

9. Loy, B.A. (2008). *Accommodation and Compliance Series: Employees with Chronic Fatigue Syndrome (CFS).* Retrieved August 22, 2010 from http://askjan.org/media/cfs.html

10. Loy, B.A.. (2010). *Job Accommodations for People with Cognitive Impairments.* Retrieved September 1, 2010 from http://askjan.org/media/employmentcogfact.doc

11. Mayo Clinic. (2010). *Stress Management; Stress Basics.* Retrieved September 4, 2010 from http://www.mayoclinic.com/health/stress-management/MY00435

12. United States Department of Labor. (2010). *Disability Resources: Job Accommodations.* Retrieved September 4, 2010, from http://www.dol.gov/dol/topic/disability/jobaccommodations.htm

13. United States Office of Personnel Management. (2010). *Welcome: Job Seekers with Disabilities.* Retrieved September 5, 2010 from http://www.usajobs.gov/individualswithdisabilities.asp

14. Whidden, D.E. (2008). *Accommodation and Compliance Series: Employees with Cerebral Palsy.* Retrieved August 12, 2010 from http://askjan.org/media/CP.html

15. Whidden, D.E. (2008). *Accommodation and Compliance Series: Employees with Dystonia.* Retrieved August 13, 2010 from http://askjan.org/media/dystonia.html

16. Yanofsky, Charles. (1999). *Dizziness Explained.* Retrieved September 1, 2010 from http://www.pneuro.com/publications/dizzy

Chapter 20. Dysautonomia and Disability Benefits - *Amy Michelle Krakower, Esq*

1. Introduction

Disclaimer: This chapter is intended to inform patients with Dysautonomia who have worked for a certain amount of time, about the path to receiving Social Security Disability benefits. This chapter should not be construed as legal advice. If you believe you are entitled to receive disability benefits, please contact your local Social Security Administration office and an attorney who specializes in disability benefits.

Choosing to apply for disability can be an extremely difficult decision for those with Dysautonomia. There is undoubtedly a social stigma associated with receiving disability from the government. I have talked to countless patients, mainly with POTS, who feel as though they have failed somehow because they are too sick to work. Even worse, the process of applying for disability is difficult when many patients who apply don't "look" sick.

Adding insult to injury, Dysautonomia lacks recognition in both the medical community and the general community. The Social Security Administration deals with recognizable illnesses every day: degenerative disc disease, rheumatoid arthritis, bipolar disorder, depression, cancer, heart failure, etc. Add in "Postural Orthostatic Tachycardia Syndrome," "Neurocardiogenic Syncope," "Orthostatic Intolerance," "Pure Autonomic Failure" and "Autoimmune Autonomic Gangliopathy" and rest assured, very few in the business of government benefits have heard of these disorders, including attorneys hired to help people entitled to benefits.

First, if you can work in some capacity, I recommend trying. Work gives most a sense of purpose and a sense of accomplishment. Even if you have to modify the type of job or career you intended, many with Dysautonomia are able to work in some capacity. I have seen many people with Dysautonomia enter career paths not suited for people with this disorder. For example, if your job requires you to be on your feet for several hours at a time, and you have severe orthostatic intolerance, nursing may not be the right profession for you. However, if you are passionate about nursing, there are other capacities in which you can work in a hospital or healthcare setting. For example, you could work in an administrative role within the nursing field so that you may be able to sit, instead of remain on your feet for hours at a time.

2. General Framework

If you are too ill to continue working, then applying for disability benefits would be the next step. In short, you must be very ill to qualify. A mild or moderate case of POTS would not likely be sufficient grounds for receipt of these benefits. A severe case may qualify. If you pass out every now and then, you are likely not severely ill enough to qualify. If you pass out several times a week, you are more likely to receive benefits.

In order to qualify for disability benefits, a worker must be under the age of 65, have a qualifying disability and be disabled for a full five months (Social Security Act, 1965). The "five months" portion of the regulation means "the Social Security Administration will withhold five months of an approved claimant's benefits before starting monthly payments (or, more likely, before calculating back payments owed to the claimant, since it takes so long to get a disability approval)" (Laurence, 2012). You also must have worked for a certain amount of time prior to your disability depending on your age. For example, if you are a 27 year-old patient with severe POTS, you would need to have worked three years (12 credits) out of the past six years (between ages 21 and 27) to qualify for benefits (Social Security Administration, 2012).

Note: while many of us may think that an employer must make a "reasonable accommodation" for those with Dysautonomia to be successful in the workplace, do not confuse receiving a disability-related accommodation with receiving disability benefits. An applicant does not need to refer to "reasonable accommodations" when applying for Social Security Disability Insurance (Cleveland v. Policy Management Systems Corporation, 1999).

3. Your Doctor and Your Medical Records

Most patients with Dysautonomia have amassed volumes of binders of medical records throughout the years, mostly because it takes a while to find a competent doctor who can diagnose the disorder. Keep all of your records. Make copies of those records and organize them by date. You may even want to color-code them. Even more important: Find a competent specialist who treats patients with Dysautonomias. Make and keep appointments with this doctor consistently to discuss symptoms and medications. Document your reactions to medications. Make sure your progress is accurately recorded in the doctor's notes.

Undergo as many autonomic tests as you can afford so that there are objective scientific tests that confirm your autonomic dysfunction: tilt table tests, skin biopsies, echocardiograms, abnormal EKGs, abnormal 24 hour Holter monitors, abnormal 30 day Holter monitors, abnormal findings from loop recorders, emergency room visits, urgent care visits, ambulance rides, dates and names of people who saw you have an autonomic crisis, hospitalizations, sleep studies, brain wave studies, abnormal MRIs, abnormal blood work, abnormal sweat tests, abnormal catecholamine tests, abnormal responses to Valsalva maneuver testing, genetic testing, etc. If you have completed any of these tests, be sure to include them. You do not have to complete every test, but the above tests can help indicate a severe disability. Be as thorough as possible in the documentation of the progression of your Dysautonomia and here's why:

The Social Security Administration evaluates medical evidence including records provided by your treating doctor or doctors (Wooster, 2012). In 1991, the Social Security Administration added a provision to the original Act that if the treating physician's opinion on the nature and severity of the disability is well supported with acceptable diagnostic tests and is consistent with other evidence in the case history, then that doctor's opinion will be given controlling weight (Code of Federal Regulations, 1991). In laymen's terms, this means that while your medical records and the opinions of your doctor are not the ultimate deciding factors in determining your case, both taken together are very, very important. If you have only seen a doctor for Dysautonomia once, the weight given to his or her opinion is small. If the doctor you saw was not a Dysautonomia specialist (or at least a cardiologist or neurologist), again, this will likely hurt your case. If the tests you received were not thorough, or the doctor analyzed the results incorrectly, this may hurt your case. If your doctor's opinion of your disability is somehow inconsistent with your test results, this may hurt your case.

4. The Process

If you are ill enough to consider applying for disability because of severe Dysautonomia symptoms that impede your ability to continue to work, you can begin the process of applying without a lawyer. You will fill out a claim for benefits either via Internet, or in a Social Security branch office. This office will then transfer the claim to the cooperating state agency. A state agency evaluation team, which includes a doctor and an evaluation specialist, will evaluate your claim (Smith, 1977). While it seems unfair for a physician who does not know you and a non-physician who has likely never heard the word "Dysautonomia" to decide if you are "disabled enough to qualify," there are several levels of appeal if the decision is not favorable.

If the agency denies your initial claim, this would be the best time to find a lawyer. Do your homework and shop around. While some lawyers are trained in the area of disability benefits, this does not alone make a good lawyer. Find out how many successes the lawyer has had in winning cases. What is his or her reputation in the community? Has the lawyer ever had disciplinary action taken against him by the Bar? If you interview a lawyer, and something doesn't feel "right," then trust your instinct. Your instinct likely helped you receive a Dysautonomia diagnosis in the first place, which is a feat in itself. Use that instinct in choosing your attorney; after all, the attorney can and likely will charge you up to 25 percent of past-due benefits if you win your case on one of the many appeal levels (42 U.S.C. § 406). If your initial claim was denied and you cannot afford a lawyer, or do not want an attorney taking 25 percent of your benefits, you may go it alone. I have heard several stories of Dysautonomia patients winning on their own. Whether or not you choose a lawyer to represent you, or you decide to navigate the waters alone, after initial claim denial, there are several appeals stages as outlined below.

"reconsideration" is a review of the claim by someone who was not part of the first decision. The representative will look at all the original evidence presented, plus any new evidence. If the reconsideration decision is unfavorable, you may ask for a hearing. An Administrative Law Judge, who was not part of the original decision or the reconsideration stage, will conduct the hearing. At the hearing, the Administrative Law Judge will question you and any witnesses you bring. It will be to your advantage to attend this hearing and explain how Dysautonomia has rendered you unable to work. The judge will make a decision based on all the information in the case, including any new information or evidence you present. If you disagree with the hearing decision, you may ask for a review by Social Security's Appeals Council.

The Appeals Council looks at all requests for review, but it may deny a request if it believes the hearing decision was correct. If the Appeals Council decides to review your case, it will either decide your case itself or return it to an Administrative Law Judge for further review. If you disagree with the Appeals Council's decision, or if the Appeals Council decides not to review your case, then you can file a lawsuit in a Federal District Court (Social Security Administration, 2008).

1. *Social Security Act. 42 U.S.C. § 423 (1965).*

2. *Laurence, B. (2012). What Is the Five-Month Waiting Period for Social Security Disability? Retrieved October 7, 2012 from*
http://www.disabilitysecrets.com/five-month-waiting-period.html

3. *Social Security Administration (2012). Benefits Planner: Number Of Credits Needed For Disability Benefits [Official Website]. Retrieved October 7, 2012 from*
http://www.ssa.gov/retire2/credits3.htm

4. *Cleveland v. Pol'y Mgmt. Systems Corp., 526 U.S. 795. (1999).*

5. *Wooster, A.K. (1998). Determination and Application of Correct Legal Standard in Weighing Medical Opinion of Treating Source in Social Security Disability. In American Law Reports: Federal (Vol. 149). Eagan, Minnesota: Thomson Reuters.*

6. *20 C.F.R. § 404.1527 (1991)*

7. *Smith, J. (1977). Social Security Hearings and Appeals in Disability Cases. In American Jurisprudence: Trials (Vol. 24). Eagan, Minnesota: Thomson Reuters.*

8. *42 U.S.C. § 406*

9. *Social Security Administration. (2008). The Appeals Process (SSA Publication No. 05-10041). Washington, D.C: Government Printing Office. Retrieved October 7, 2012 from*
http://www.ssa.gov/pubs/10041.pdf

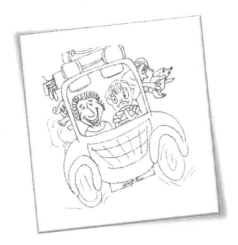

Chapter 21. Tips for Vacationing with someone who has Dysautonomia.

Family Vacation!

Written by: Sharon Cini, MD and Jodi Rhum

A vacation trip is one-third pleasure, fondly remembered, and two-thirds aggravation, entirely forgotten. - Robert Brault

Vacationing with someone who suffers from POTS can be challenging, yet fun and rewarding. The family does not need to miss out on a deserved holiday because one member has a chronic illness. Traveling with people who have a chronic illness often requires extra time and planning. The more you retain your normal schedule, the more your family will enjoy their vacation. Since every case of POTS is unique, each person's capability is different. These tips and suggestions have been assembled by trial and error. They may not help all POTS patients. Hopefully by adhering to some of these suggestions, you will have a more enjoyable, safe and relaxing trip. It is important for long lasting health that all families take a vacation.

Two of my four children have problems when a plane descends. The pain in their ears is so excruciating, that they actually scream out loud. This is unpleasant for everyone around us on the plane. We are not popular to sit near. Several years ago, when we were flying to Virginia, my daughter had a severe pain in her neck that extended into her head and ear. I was so frightened; I thought we might have to make an emergency landing. I was not looking forward to ever flying again. Forty-eight hours on a train sounded like paradise.

One year after this disastrous flight, we were offered an opportunity to go to Beijing for the Olympics. I wondered if we could take a boat, bus, rocket ship, anything but a plane. The thought of fourteen hours on a plane with screaming children did not excite me. We almost opted not to go. Before completely abandoning the China trip, we decided to speak with my daughter's cardiologist. He told us to give each POTS child one Sudafed and 2 Motrin one hour before landing. (Sudafed can make the heart race faster. When using Sudafed, be careful not to mix with caffeine and make sure you have your doctor's permission.) We decided to go ahead with the trip, and I am so happy we did. The suggestion miraculously worked, and we had an uneventful and wonderful flight and a phenomenal and memorable family vacation. - Jodi Rhum

Note: One of my daughter's doctors suggested that Afrin be used before the door of the airplane cabin is shut. He believes that once the door to the airplane is closed and the cabin is pressurized, it may be too late to achieve an optimal effect. Other doctors have recommended using Afrin instead of Sudafed, since there is no systemic absorption; it's generally safer and just as effective. The same cannot be said for other nasal decongestant sprays since they will not open the Eustachian tubes.

Listed in this chapter are suggestions that have worked for us or other POTS patients. Remember, these are only suggestions. They may not work for everyone all the time but can still be useful.

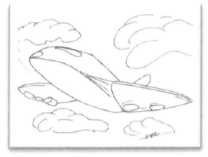

Air Travel

1. Before going on a trip, call the airlines and inform them about the person's medical condition. It may be your child, spouse, friend or traveling companion. I usually tell them that POTS is a cardiac condition. There is some disagreement among experts whether or not it is a cardiac condition, however, since most POTS patients see a cardiologist, and have cardiac symptoms, I do not feel I am stretching the truth. What you say or how you say it is completely your judgment call. Everyone seems to understand that a cardiac condition is serious and may require extra assistance. I use this term because it is simple for the airport staff to understand, it takes less time to explain and provides faster service. Ask the representative to reserve seats in the bulkhead for you. Note that some bulkhead seats are located in the exit row with the age restriction of at least 18 years old. If this is the case, ask them to upgrade you to economy plus.

Also, should the POTS or NCS patient become very dizzy, the bulkhead gives you more room to lay them on the floor in front of you with their legs up in the air. This will help return the blood flow back to the brain. In case of syncope you will not have to lay them in the aisle, which can be dangerous for everyone. The bulkhead provides space to stretch your legs, stand up or lay on the floor if needed. This is important for circulation. If the representative will not do this for you, ask to speak to their supervisor.

Prior to traveling, it may be useful to obtain a letter from your cardiologist requesting special seating but also starting that is safe to fly so long as accommodations are made. Once you get to the ticket counter, explain that you have pre-arranged seats and present the letter to the gate agent. It also helps if you have an article explaining the illness. I often show them my emergency card. I carry it with me at all times. If they still do not accommodate you, once you are on board the plane, ask to speak with the senior steward or stewardess. We have never been denied. Persist until you get what your patient needs.

2. Traveling is often exhausting for the person with Dysautonomia, especially since most airports are so large and spread out. When making your reservation or checking in at the gate, request a wheelchair for your POTS traveler; it will be waiting for you when you get off the plane. All airlines and airports should offer assistance to disabled passengers. Using a wheelchair can be a great way to conserve their energy. Flying can also be particularly difficult for POTS patients and may make them prone to vertigo because of the changes in altitude and diminished oxygen due to cabin pressure changes.

3. Request pre-boarding for all flights to ensure your POTS traveler can get on the plane safely without being rushed. POTS patients require extra time and assistance to board. As soon as you arrive at the gate, walk up to the podium. Find out which gate agent will be in charge of boarding passengers. Inform that gate agent you are traveling with a disabled person and that they require pre-boarding. Explain that your traveler may look completely normal but they are not and that they require extra time and assistance.

4. It is important to plan your flight times carefully. Schedule your departure according to when your POTS patient has the most energy. Some do better after a good night sleep and are exhausted by the evening. Most, however, function better if their return flights are scheduled in the early to late afternoon or evening hours. This is because their blood pressure is lowest in the morning and naturally goes up later in the day. Also, many POTS patients have insomnia and are up all night. Leaving later in the day allows the majority to rest before their trip.

5. Pack as little as possible. Agree on what's essential to bring and stick to that. It is easier to travel with light luggage.

6. Barometric pressure can affect those with POTS. They tend to do better in places like San Diego, Honolulu, Hawaii, and Arizona where the barometric pressure is high and stable. When possible, choose a vacation location at sea level or with stable barometric pressure. Mountainous areas have low barometric pressure and less oxygen at higher altitudes. This can be problematic for POTS patients. Also, you do not want to choose a place that is too warm. As we all know, heat, especially accompanied by humidity, is not ideal for people with POTS. We mistakenly took a trip to Disneyworld in Florida a few summers ago. Standing in lines in the 100-degree heat was not a good idea for my POTS clan. Big Mistake!

7. Do not pack your medications in a checked bag! All medications should be accompanied by a letter from your doctor and packed in your carry-on bag. If you pack your medications in your checked bag, the airlines can lose it and you will be stranded without your medications. This could ruin your vacation. Getting them replaced is difficult when you travel domestic and even worse when you travel international. Pack liquid medications in a plastic bag to comply with airline regulations. Always carry extra medication and plastic bags in case you have to stay somewhere longer than expected.

8. Drink plenty of water and eat salt before and during the flight. Avoid drinking soda, caffeine or alcoholic beverages on the plane. Bring salty foods and protein snacks. It's often cheaper to buy them at your local grocery store rather than at the airport. Some travelers always take a large empty bottle. They fill it with water once they are past security, so they don't have to ask the stewardess for constant refills. If you forget, once you are on the

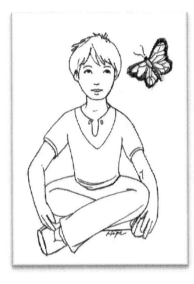

plane, you can inform the flight attendant that you have a medical condition that requires you to drink excessively and they will often provide you with your own bottle of water.

9. To prevent ear pain: Chew gum, suck on candy, and drink water or V-8 Juice upon departures and arrivals (the sport bottle is effective). Earplugs, a warm washcloth or compress for the ears can help lessen some ear pain. Afrin Nasal spray, used thirty minutes to one hour prior to take off and landing, can eradicate sinus and ear pain. Speak with your doctor first. Alternatively some doctors recommend starting a steroid nasal spray a couple of days before, twice a day, and to use it an hour before the flight departure and landing. These suggestions have helped anyone with a Eustachian tube dysfunction; that is what causes sinus and ear pain. This is not unique to POTS patients. Be cautious taking Sudafed if you have POTS, since it can lead to tachycardia, vertigo, near syncope and headaches.

10. Walk around the plane as often as permitted to prevent blood clots and venous pooling in the legs. Wearing compression stockings, sitting with legs crossed or squeezing thigh muscles together also helps prevent pooling in the lower legs. The latter also improves circulation.

11. Dress in layers on the plane. Controlling body temperature is often a problem for people with POTS. They should not become overheated or too cold.

12. Standing for long periods can also be difficult. After landing, get up slowly and wait until most people have exited the plane.

Car Travel

1. Make sure the group you are traveling with is aware of your illness.

2. You will need to make frequent stops for bathroom breaks, fresh air, and just to get up and walk around to prevent venous pooling in the legs caused by sitting still in the car for long periods.

3. Hydration is crucial when traveling. At all times, carry water, fluids that contain electrolytes, and salty snacks. Allow for frequent bathroom breaks.

4. As with all travel, be sure to have medical information, emergency card and doctors' phone numbers with you.

5. Wear loose fitting clothes to avoid restricting blood flow. Sit comfortably with legs elevated or crossed.

6. Have medications readily available, not packed away in luggage. Make sure you have an ample supply of food with you as some of your medications may require you to take them on a full stomach. Eating may also prevent queasiness or upset stomach.

7. Be sure to keep cool in the car. It is not advisable to take a trip in a car that does not have air conditioning in hot weather. If you don't have air conditioning, then consider riding with the windows open or taking a battery-operated fan.

8. When traveling long distance, break the trip up into small segments to prevent sitting in the car for prolonged periods. Also, allow for adequate sleep at night.

9. Use a stress ball or weights to retain muscle tone and circulation. It also lessens boredom and preoccupies children.

10. People with Dysautonomia have difficulty keeping a stable body temperature. Blankets can be used to cover and uncover as needed.

11. Bring pillows for comfort and to prop up the legs from time to time. Larger vehicles, which allow you to lie down, may be helpful to POTS patients.

12. Distractions are great for the chronically ill person. Watching movies on a portable DVD player, listening to audio books on CD, playing with a Gameboy, listening to music on an MP3 player, using your laptop, playing with a deck of cards, reading magazines, working on puzzles, playing with toys or similar items are excellent diversions and can provide hours of fun for the whole family.

13. Car and airplane rides can often be noisy. Using earplugs will decrease the sensory overload. Noise canceling earphones are also a fabulous investment.

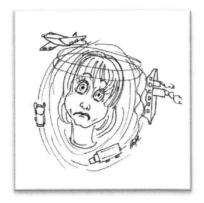

Motion Sickness – Car, Plane, Cruise

Motion sickness is the result of your body sensing a discrepancy between you and what you see outside a moving vehicle. Even though you are sitting still, the vestibular system (inner ear) tells the brain you are actually moving. The conflict between what you feel and see causes a neurotransmitter to be produced. Your brain interprets this as a hallucinogenic poison and responds by trying to rid the cause. Motion sickness occurs more often and suddenly in children with Dysautonomia. Here are some helpful tips:

1. Always keep tissues and a plastic bag nearby.

2. Look out the window. Focus on a non-moving object in the distance, such as the horizon. Don't do anything that involves focusing on a fixed spot, such as reading, watching a video, playing a card game. Don't turn around or look from side to side.

3. Sit in the front. Drive, if possible. Drivers rarely get car sick as they are always focused on the road. Sitting in the passenger's seat is the next best thing. The front of the car is less bumpy so there is less motion sickness.

4. Take a nap or close your eyes.

5. Ride with the windows open. Many people find that smelling fresh, cool air helps make them feel better. If it is not possible to open the window, lean towards the bottom of the window and breathe.

6. Avoid odors in the car such as perfume, air fresheners, and cigarette and cigar smoke. Sometimes spraying a bit of lavender in the car may help to eliminate other foul odors.

7. Take frequent breaks. Go outside. Stretch your legs. Relax using deep breathing techniques, however, be careful with too much deep breathing, since it lowers your blood pressure and can make you dizzy. Take some deep breaths in through your mouth and exhale out your nose, breathing deeply from your stomach.

8. Eating a few ginger biscuits (cookies) before or during your car ride may help with nausea. Other foods that may relieve some of your nausea: hot ginger tea, ginger candy, lemon drops, peppermint candy or peppermint tea, fresh mint, and pickled ginger.

9. Acupressure may relieve some of your symptoms. Apply gentle pressure between the two tendons about an inch back from the wrist joint. This should temporarily alleviate nausea. You can also buy Sea Bands or acupressure wristbands at a local pharmacy. Some people use a rubber band fitted snugly around the wrist.

10. There are many over-the-counter and prescription medications that prevent motion sickness. Some popular brands are Dramamine and Bonine (Antivert). They come in tablets or patches. Look into the side effects and drug interactions before using these medications. Check with your doctor or pharmacist to be sure it is safe for you. Any sedating antihistamine like Benadryl will also work if these are not available.

11. Some people swear the smell of newspaper makes them feel better.

12. Eating a dill pickle, saltine crackers, salty snack, or chewing gum helps some with these symptoms.

13. Don't eat a heavy meal or consume alcohol right before or during your trip. If you stop to eat, wait at least 20 minutes before getting back in the car.

14. It has been reported that eating chocolate can exacerbate motion sickness.

15. Don't talk about motion sickness, or even look at someone else who's experiencing it.

16. Taking a B-complex supplement for several weeks before the trip can make a difference in motion sickness. Many people, who get nauseous easily, actually have a Vitamin B6 Deficiency.

17. Chewing herbs, like parsley may also help relieve nausea.

Once At Your Destination

1. Rest or do something very low key on your first day. It is worth the sacrifice to enjoy the remainder of your vacation.

2. Beware of amusement parks. The rides often make you dizzier. If you decide to go to an amusement park, Disneyland in California is a better choice than Disneyworld in Florida. The weather in California is more moderate. It is best to go to amusement parks in the winter, not in the summer, when the temperature is cooler. The summer is too hot for most POTS patients. If you go to an amusement park, once inside, first, take your doctor's note to customer relations. They can rent you a wheelchair if needed and issue a permit to bypass the lines. Some of the newer parks, like Animal Kingdom and California Adventure, do not issue special passes; you will have to wait in the regular lines.(check this out before going). For these parks, you may need to rent a wheelchair before going to the park.

3. Even though you may not normally need a wheelchair you might be able to obtain one for trips that require long distance walking, with a prescription from your doctor, you may be able to get your health insurance to pay for this. Alternatively, you may consider buying or renting a walker that has a built in seat. This way, if you get tired, you can sit down wherever you are. Your physician can also write a prescription for a walker. Prior to your vacation, check with your insurance company to see if you have coverage for a walker and wheelchair.

4. Always carry bottled water, Smart Water, electrolyte drinks or V-8 Juice. Smart Water has no calories and provides electrolytes.

5. Always carry a cell phone, or make sure someone in the family or group has one. Don't forget the charger!

6. Be sure to pack sunglasses and a wide brimmed hat or baseball cap to keep cool in the sun.

7. You might consider purchasing a portable fan that has an attachment to squirt water. This saved our lives when we were at Disney!

8. Keep extra water bottles in your hotel room so you can drink in the middle of the night, if needed. Some people take an extra suitcase filled with bottled water and snacks to last a couple of days, in case they cannot get to a store early on.

9. Carry salty snacks with you at all times to maintain hydration and blood pressure.

10. Always carry your emergency medical information card that explains Dysautonomia. You can also wear a medical alert bracelet.

11. Do not plan too many activities. Include periods of downtime to prevent extreme fatigue. You can always add more activities if you feel well.

12. If your family is staying in a hotel, be sure to choose a floor that is on the ground level or 2nd floor. Going up the elevator is not easy for some people with POTS, as it often makes them dizzier. Also, if an emergency arises or a false alarm goes off, lots of stairs, flashing lights and loud noises are a bad combination for people with POTS.

13. If you have to use an elevator, such as for site seeing or in a hotel, there are techniques you can use to minimize dizziness.

For example, my daughter crouches and squeezes her buttocks muscles. It looks peculiar, but she swears by it! A cardiologist who works with kids with POTS recommends jumping into the air while the elevator is moving. You should experiment to see what works best for you.

14. Choose a room that is located away from most of the action. You do not want a room near the lobby, elevators, game room, exercise room or swimming pool. Noises and distractions in the middle of the night for the POTS insomniac could make for more symptoms the next day.

15. Plan time for naps in the day whenever possible.

16. Bring a hot water bottle to reduce stomach discomfort.

17. Allow enough time to recuperate, at least a day or two after your vacation, before you return to work or school.

Finally, just understand that traveling with a person who has POTS will be different. You will need to adjust your expectations for the vacation and be sure the whole family is accepting of this fact. Your vacation can still be wonderful! Your family probably is not going to be able to do as much as your pre-POTS vacations. Instead, plan a more relaxing laid-back trip. Isn't that the real purpose of a vacation anyway? Vacations should not be measured in how many sites you see or how many rides you can go on but by how many precious family memories are made. You may actually be surprised to find this way of vacationing more relaxing and more enjoyable.

Everyone in the family not only needs a vacation every so often, but deserves one as well. Though traveling with POTS is never easy, it can be a wonderful, bonding experience for the entire family.

Bon Voyage!

Checklist for Vacations:

✓ Medications (Take extras)

- ✓ Emergency medical information: Emergency card, doctors phone numbers, and insurance information
- ✓ Sunglasses
- ✓ Cell phone and charger
- ✓ Brimmed hat or baseball cap
- ✓ Sun tan lotion
- ✓ Portable fan with attachment to squirt water
- ✓ Walker or wheel chair, if necessary
- ✓ Compression stockings
- ✓ Hot water bottle or heating pad
- ✓ Doctor's note: Explain condition, limitations, if any, Bulk head seating for planes, and allowing liquids to go through security
- ✓ Salty snacks
- ✓ Water bottles
- ✓ Earplugs
- ✓ Warm compress or washcloth
- ✓ Chewing gum
- ✓ Quart sized Ziploc bags for liquid medications
- ✓ Neck pillow
- ✓ Motrin and Afrin for descent on flight
- ✓ Blankets and pillows for the car
- ✓ Squeeze ball, weights or other exercise equipment
- ✓ Blood pressure monitor
- ✓ DVD player, DVD's, toys, books, games, puzzles, and any other forms of entertainment.

Added items for motion sickness

- ✓ Vitamin B Complex
- ✓ Ginger or peppermint products, Ginger Ale
- ✓ Saltine crackers, dill pickles, chewing gum
- ✓ Wrist-bands, Sea Bands, or rubber-bands
- ✓ Motion sickness medication: Bonine, Dramamine, Benadryl

✓ Battery-operated fan
✓ Newspaper
✓ Lavender, Eucalyptus, and Arnica oils

Chapter 22. Finding a Physician that is right for you

Finding a good physician to treat your illness can be very challenging, to say the least. It is extremely important to find not only a qualified physician but also one who is also compassionate, supportive, approachable, and has good bedside manners.

Tips for Doctors' Visits (and or hospitalizations)

During our journey to find a diagnosis for my oldest daughter, I was told by a very prominent physician to produce a medical history form paraphrasing my daughter's medical history. He said that most physicians do not have the time to search through files upon files of medical history (as most patients with Dysautonomia have). He said that coming up with an abbreviated sampling of symptoms, tests administered; types of physicians seen as well as a family history of illness would be a far more effective way of helping the doctors to find the correct diagnosis. This would also prevent duplicate tests and lab work from being unnecessarily repeated. I took his word for gospel and produced a sample medical form that I brought religiously with me to every doctor's appointment (see the following example of a complete medical history). Not only were the doctors appreciative of this background history, but also it helped us to find a quick and accurate diagnosis.

Putting together the background history for me was also very enlightening. I felt like a scientist putting together a complex laboratory experiment. The more symptoms I wrote down, the more the puzzle pieces began to fit together. Things I never thought were connected before suddenly began to come together like an impressionistic painting.

Note: As soon as the doctor would walk into the room to examine my child, I would hand them the medical history form that I had produced. This way, I could witness first hand that they read it and considered it in their diagnosis. Using bullet points seemed to help the doctors to read through the form more thoroughly and with greater ease. I felt I was better able to accentuate my points, by using them.

Example of a Complete Medical History of Emma Anderson

- Pregnancy achieved through IVF.
- Mother had mild gestational diabetes, controlled by diet.
- At 26 weeks, in utero, mother had Campylobacter (food poisoning) and was hospitalized for four days. IV fluids stopped pre-term labor.
- October 10, 1996, Emma was born by C-section, weighing 5 pounds, 5 ounces. She was three weeks early. No medical issues noted.
- As an infant Emma was fussy. She would projectile vomit and had reflux. She was put on a special baby formula, Nutramigen. This seemed to help.
- Emma reached all milestones on time.
- At age 3, a sofa table fell on Emma. She sustained a concussion.
- At age 4, Emma started doing competitive dance.
- At age 6, Emma first started complaining of headaches and dizziness. She had a CT scan and was diagnosed with a sinus infection.
- At age 8, she injured her lower back during a dance competition. The next day, she was taken for an x-ray and although the x-ray was clear, the doctor treated her for pneumonia (she had been coughing before the injury). No bones were broken. From that day on, she has had lower back and neck pain.

- At age 9, Emma complains on and off of stabbing chest pains. She says she is often out of breath, but does not appear to be in distress.
- At age 9, Emma is diagnosed with Sever's Disease in her heels, after months of complaining of intermittent feet pain.
- At age 9, Emma complains on an airplane ride, on descent only, that her ears burn worse than any other pain she has ever had.
- At age 9, Emma breaks navicular bone in foot. She is put in a hard cast. Dr. Simonis, her Orthopedic Doctor, tells us he has never seen anyone fracture this bone in other than a car accident.
- At age 10, Emma begins to have wrist pain in both wrists.
- Emma has a hard time falling asleep and it is difficult to wake her in the mornings.
- At age 11, after continued chest pains, Emma has an EKG that says she has borderline prolonged QT. Dr. Deal, Cardiologist at Children's Memorial Hospital in Chicago, says that when it is read by hand, she does not have this condition. She finds that she is Orthostatic and tells her to drink more fluids and continue with heavy exercise.
- At age 11, Emma has headaches, dizziness and a stomachache that last three weeks. Her eyes started to blink, uncontrollably. She says she sometimes sees squiggly lines. The blinking disappears after a month. The Neurologist diagnoses her with migraines and abdominal migraines. Her MRI is normal. She is put on Periactin for the headaches.
- The Periactin causes her to gain 15 pounds in 3 months. Emma then breaks her 5th metatarsal on her right foot. Not knowing it is broken; she tapes it up and continues dance competitively. A month and a half later, she breaks the other foot (1st metatarsal). After the casts come off, she is diagnosed with RSD (Reflex Sympathetic Dystrophy) and anx-

iety. She is sent to a pain clinic.

• Emma has a large growth spurt.

• At age 12, one day after her birthday, she wakes up with terrible abdominal pains. The next day, she wakes up with a migraine and dizziness. These symptoms do not go away. She is put on Topamax and Lyrica but the pain in her feet, headache and dizziness still remain.

• Emma complains that elevators make her dizzier. Exercise hurts her head more. She complains of body twitches and some weakness in her hands. She says her hands sometimes feel numb and she feels like she sometimes slurs her words. She complains of gas and severe stomach pains. She says that when she is making a bowel movement, she gets dizzier.

• Hot showers and baths; seem to make Emma lightheaded.

• Emma sees Dr. Hain. He finds that she has tachycardia and orthostatic blood pressure. He wants to give her meds for migraines.

• Emma sometimes has red blood in her stool.

• Emma complains of off and on ear pain.

• Emma's feet are always cold and she seems to have difficulty controlling her body temperature.

• In February of 2008, her symptoms worsen. She now complains of shooting pains all over her body. These pains are mainly in her neck, head and chest. They are sharp and usually short lived (60 seconds or less)

• She complains that she is always dizzy. She is having many visual disturbances. She says that the walls feel like they are closing in on her, objects that are far away appear closer and the floor appears to be coming up at her. She says she feels like she has just gotten off of an elevator.

• Emma says she has strange, warm feelings in her stomach that feel like they shoot up into her throat. She says sometimes she feels like butterflies are in her stomach.

- Emma now begins to lose weight. She says her stomach always feels full. Eating makes her stomach hurt worse and makes her symptoms more pronounced.
- October 2008 - Dr. Blair Grubb in Toledo, Ohio, diagnoses Emma with Postural Orthostatic Tachycardia Syndrome. She is put on Proamatine and Florinef.
- November 2008 - Emma's feet still give her pain where they were broken. She complains of popping in her feet and grinding in her knees, the pain is so intense that it stops her in her tracks and she has to sit down immediately. Stairs are becoming a tremendous effort for her.
- February of 2008 - Emma is now being home tutored. Going to school is too strenuous.
- July 2008 - Emma's #1 complaint as of July 2008 is extreme dizziness.
- March of 2010 - Emma is diagnosed with Ehlers-Danlos Syndrome. It is postulated that Ehlers-Danlos Syndrome is causing her POTS symptoms.

Family History

- Parental grandfather has Mitral Valve Prolapse. He passes away at age 57 from rectal cancer.
- Grandmother, brothers, mother and several first cousins have history of migraines.
- Younger sister has chest pains. She has an innocent heart murmur.
- Younger brother has low tone, postural orthostatic tachycardia syndrome and a minor heart anomaly.
- Strong history of ADHD and anxiety in the immediate family.
- Maternal grandfather has a rare neurological disorder, PPA, Primary Progressive Aphasia. This has left him mute

and in a wheelchair.
- Maternal grandmother, brother and uncle have had blood clots.
- Maternal grandmother has a thyroid imbalance.
- High blood pressure runs on father's side.
- First cousin and maternal uncle have diabetes.
- Maternal grandfather has IBS (Irritable bowel syndrome).
- Both brothers have speech issues and allergies
- Mother has had one episode of unexplained fainting.
- Father has had two episodes of fainting.
- Emma's Known Allergies - Ragweed, cucumbers and bananas.

Doctors seen:
- Orthopedic Specialist- diagnosed with foot fractures (3) and Reflex Sympathetic Dystrophy
- Rheumatologist - Diagnosed with hyper mobile joints
- Endocrinologist - Diagnosed with borderline low blood sugar
- Neurologist - Diagnosed with migraine headache and abdominal migraines
- Cardiologist- Diagnosed with orthostatic blood pressure and POTS
- ENT - Normal findings
- Ophthalmologist - Normal findings
- Psychiatrist - Normal findings
- Urologist - Normal Findings

Medicines Tried:
- Topamax
- Lyrica
- Florinef
- Periactin
- Midodrine

- Proamatine
- Lexapro
- Zyrtec

Medicines presently taking:
- Lexapro
- Proamatine
- Vitamin B complex
- Motrin
- Omega 3 fish oil
- Calcium Magnesium
- Motrin for EDS
- Glucosamine, Chondroitin & MSM Complex for EDS
- Vitamin D supplement
- Multiple vitamins

Tests Administered:
- MRI
- CT Scan of brain
- Echo
- EKG
- X-Ray (feet and wrists)
- Ultra Sound - back and heart
- Spinal tap

More Tips:

Always bring a list of all medications and dosages to all doctor appointments. Sometimes bringing the actual bottles themselves may help avoid confusion and may be prudent.

Always ask for copies of all MRI's, CT scans, X-rays and related radiologist reports as soon as they are taken. Trying to get a hold of these at a later date is often time consuming and can be a lengthy process. All imaging and reports should be placed in a file and ready to go should you need to bring them to any given appointment.

Always have a list of questions ready to ask the doctor. Do not assume that you will remember all of your questions in the short amount of time you get to see the doctor.

Always be prepared and organized for all doctors' appointments. Have a file containing blood work-ups, imaging studies and reports, medical history bullet points, (see example) questions to ask the doctor, all other pertinent medical records and history, and phone numbers or business cards of all other doctors and therapists seen (in order to enhance communication).

What you need:

You will need to get a Pediatrician or Primary Care Physician who is knowledgeable about Dysautonomia. Make sure the physician supports the fact that Dysautonomia is a real illness. If you cannot find a physician in your area who is familiar with this syndrome, make sure that they are willing to research it and educate their nursing staff. If they are not willing to do so, find another doctor.

You will also need to find a local cardiologist or another specialist who specializes in autonomic disorders. This doctor may be an electro physiologist, pediatric cardiologist, neurologist or endocrinologist.

Questions to ask when choosing a Pediatrician or Primary Care Physician:

- How many patients in your practice have autonomic disorders?
- How long have you been treating people who have Dysautonomia?
- Is your staff educated on Dysautonomia? If not, are you willing to familiarize them with the illness?
- What is the protocol for follow-ups?
- What are your plans to communicate with the other specialists involved in my care?

- Do you have a special home care coordinator that will be overseeing my health plan?

For a current list of physicians who specialize in autonomic dysfunctions around the globe, please refer to *DysautonomiaInternational.org*

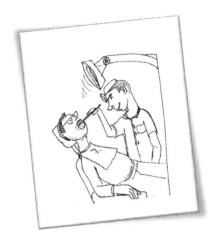

Chapter 23. Going to the Dentist, Orthodontist or Oral Surgeon - *Jodi Rhum and Dr. Mark Cannon, DDS*

It is imperative that people, who suffer from POTS, let all medical professionals who deal directly with them, know of their diagnosis. Do not just assume that all doctors understand this condition. Many health care providers have unfortunately never heard of this syndrome. If this is the case, take time to explain the illness. if necessary or bring a medical emergency card with you that they can read. It is especially important that you make your dentist, oral surgeon and orthodontist aware of your condition, as certain modifications in your treatment should be documented.

When treating a patient with a history of POTS, the dentist should assess his or her blood pressure and heart rate before administering local anesthetic, particularly one containing the vasoconstrictor epinephrine or levonordefrin. [1]

Surgical procedures require several precautions. Dentists and or oral surgeons must vigilantly check vital signs during all procedures. "Clinicians can maintain the patient's blood pressure and heart rate with isoflurane titration and improve vascular tone by administrating low doses of phenylephrine. Blood expanders, such as crystalloid, also should be on hand during procedures." (JADA) Dr. Abdallah recommends not getting wisdom teeth pulled when symptomatic. This could really set the patient back.

About one half of patients who have Dysautonomia also have MVP (mitral valve prolapse) or another minor heart anomaly. Be sure to inform your dentist and oral surgeon of this so it can be added to your chart. You then must follow the antibiotic regimen prescribed by the American Heart Association before any dental work is done. In most cases, the antibiotic has to be given one hour before treatment. Check with your doctor for the correct dosage.

Postoperative care may also need to be modified for the POTS patients. Approximately 15% of people with POTS have drug allergies. Clinicians must therefore be prudent before prescribing postoperative medications and should do a pharmacological review.

Many people who have POTS have a heightened level of anxiety. If this is the case, the dentist may want to prescribe pre-medication with oral anxiolytics. Photosensitivity is another symptom of people who have POTS. If this is an issue, you may want to consider wearing sunglasses to your appointment to alleviate the discomfort of the overhead lighting that is used during the visit.

Syncope is another risk factor that needs to be addressed with your clinician. If you have ever experienced syncope it is important to let the doctor know this and make sure he/she is prepared should this happen. Be sure to sign all insurance forms while sitting down. At the completion of any procedure, make sure someone assists you to an upright position slowly. If the clinician notices the onset of a syncope episode, he or she should be instructed to raise your legs slightly above your heart and place a cool towel on your head. The clinician should then contact your primary doctor and get further instructions. Any adult patient who loses consciousness during a visit, should never leave the office unescorted and should not drive themselves home.

The orthodontist needs to adhere to these same guidelines. If the patient with POTS also has Ehlers - Danlos Syndrome, or EDS, the capillary fragility can increase the risk of bleeding, during procedures. In this case, hemostatic agents, like desmoropressin can be used. Delayed wound healing can also be an issue with patients who have EDS. Placing braces on a person who has both POTS and EDS may lead to rapid tooth movement and increased mobility, often times requiring more than usual time to achieve the desired effect.

Before performing any orthodontic procedure, the POTS patient may want to take Motrin or Tylenol in anticipation of discomfort. It is also very important that fluids are pushed. Many times after a procedure, it is difficult to eat. This can make all of the POTS symptoms worse. It is then doubly important, to keep up with fluid and salt intake. Having homemade smoothies (you can add vitamins and protein powder), applesauce, soup, and yogurt are all good choices that can provide some of the necessary nourishment that the POTS patient requires. Making your own popsicles can also be a healthy treat. Making Gatorade popsicles or any other beverage of your choice that contains electrolytes can help make fluid intake possible.

Going to the dentist, orthodontist or oral surgeon to have a procedure done is anxiety provoking in and of itself, even for the healthiest of people. It is important that your clinician recognize your unique situation and that he or she is empathetic to your needs.

Preventive care is essential, as with all patients, but every effort should be made to insure that the dental professional is using all techniques currently available to alleviate oral pathology. The preventive measures available are commonly used by Pediatric Dentists, specialists in the dental care of children. Pediatric Dentists are dental specialists with extensive additional training in care of the young. In addition, many are hospital trained and have treated patients with almost every type of disability or medical condition. After the additional hospital training, most remain on staff at large hospitals and in constant contact with medical colleagues.

The preventive measures that a dental professional treating patients with POTS are as follows: fluoride analysis of the drinking water, as believe it or not, many people still do not have fluoridated water, fluoride varnish treatments, daily MI Paste home application and appropriate diagnostic testing. Minimally Invasive Dentistry (conservative dentistry) should include many of the following regimens; therapeutic sealant application, soft tissue laser treatment, Single Tooth Anesthesia, and Ultrasonic Cavity preparation.

MI Paste or minimum intervention paste is a cream that is applied to the teeth every night. The cream contains high levels of amorphous calcium phosphate (calcium and phosphate that is bioavailable, actively benefiting the patient) and casein phosphopeptide (a pre-protein from dairy sources that inhibits cavities as effectively as fluoride). MI Paste is safe if accidentally swallowed, unlike many high fluoride products, so it is ideal for little children. Fluoride varnishes replace many of the old ways of topically applying fluoride. It adheres well to the teeth and the dose to the patient is no more than what happens when brushing with fluoride toothpaste. Older methods of fluoride application often required the use of a foam tray that could irritate the inside of the mouth. Fluoride varnish helps the enamel to become more acid resistant and is well tolerated by almost all patients.

Therapeutic sealants are sealants that release fluoride or calcium phosphate into the surrounding teeth. Also, therapeutic sealants are easier to apply than the older types of sealants because they do not require a perfectly dry tooth surface prior to placement. The ease of application is important because that potentially reduces oral structure manipulation and should minimize the anxiety during sealant application.

There are many wonderful xylitol products that help prevent decay. Xylitol is a naturally occurring sweetener that is found in birch trees, plums and many berries. Xylitol is not digested by pathogenic bacteria so it inhibits their growth. Xylitol is used in lollipops, candy, sprays, varnishes and other dental applications to help prevent decay. The lollipops also may contain Chinese licorice root (use licorice root with caution especially if you are on Florinef), another natural inhibitor of cavity producing bacteria.

Probiotics - the use of probiotic supplements is also important. Whenever there are any changes to the oral environment the type of bacteria found in the oral microflora is also changed. Many medications have also been associated with saliva reduction that not only decrease the saliva's buffering and antibody capability but may increase the growth of unhealthy (pathogenic) bacteria. Probiotics are defined by the World Health Organization as "live microorganisms which when administered in adequate amounts confer a health benefit on the host." Probiotics have created a great amount of interest and has resulted with a "surge" in published research. In 2006 there were 528 hits in the Pub Med data base for the key word "probiotic" and 47 human studies reported. Articles on Probiotics Therapy have been published in numerous refereed medical journals, including the Archives of Disease of the Child, Pediatrics, Journal of Pediatrics, Journal of Clinical Immunology and Allergy, Lancet and many others too numerous to mention. The preponderance of the publications reported positive results for Probiotic Therapy as an important adjunct in the treatment of a host of pathologic processes.

Beneficial bacteria work by preventing the growth of pathogens; with competitive displacement of pathogens, by regulating gut microbial ecosystems, with improving gut function/nutritional uptake and by modulating immune responses to improve health. By augmenting the natural L. reuteri colonization in humans positive health effects have been reported. A Swedish company, BioGaia, has produced probiotic supplements for Dental applications. The Probiotic Lactobacilli reuteri is available in the following formats; chewing gum, drops, chewables, straws and lozenges. These convenient application formats allows for the Probiotic Therapy of all types of patients; infants, disabled persons, teen or adults. These applications contain Lactobacillus reuteri strain ATCC 55730, an extensively studied strain that colonizes the stomach and intestine after ingesting the tablets. The colonization results in a significant boost to the immune system and has been reported as significantly reducing the level of pathogenic (bad) bacteria and significantly decreasing the effects of periodontal (gum) disease. Many patients utilize probiotic supplements to reduce the risk of dental disease.

What happens if the patient starts to get cavities? Small cavities may be treated with ART, atraumatic restorative technique, whereas the patient does not require an anesthetic. The surface of the cavity is gently removed and a re-mineralizing filling material is bonded into the cavity. The remaining decay is hardened and the decay process stopped or reversed with this technique. This technique is very useful with small children and patients with a history of previous negative medical experiences. Another very useful way to "prepare the teeth" for restoration (fillings) is the use of Ultrasonic Dentistry. Ultrasonic dentistry uses ultrasonic wavelengths to remove un-salvageable tooth structure and does not require anesthesia. Although available in many foreign countries, it is not readily found here in the USA. AquaCut, air/water abrasion is also a gentle conservative method for preparing teeth for restoration. Both methods are less expensive and even kinder to tooth structure than the hard tissue lasers. Soft tissue (gum and tongue) Lasers are extremely useful in dentistry and have improved significantly just the last few years. Many soft tissue procedures are done with minimal anesthesia and yet with great comfort during and after the treatment.

If a cavity has grown too large for ART to be performed or if the tooth structure itself is not suitable then a rubber dam should be used for the filling procedure. A rubber dam is a sheet of rubber that holds the cheek and lips away from the area the dentist is working on. The rubber dam also protects the airway, which is vitally important! Restoration of the child's dentition (teeth) may be accomplished with either local anesthesia (Single Tooth Anesthesia or block), nitrous oxide analgesia, sedation or general anesthesia.

Treatment under either sedation or general anesthesia should be performed in a Pediatric Medical Facility by experienced Pediatric Dentists working with Pediatric Anesthesiologists. This will insure the safest treatment method possible. Local anesthesia is the most prevalent way to insure comfort during tooth restoration. Single Tooth Anesthesia (STA) is a computer controlled method of just making the tooth being restored numb, leaving all the lips, cheeks and tongue completely un-numb. Obviously, many patients prefer STA, even without any sensory issues. Nitrous oxide analgesia combined with STA will allow the dental specialist to restore many teeth without any significant amount of local anesthesia levels in the patient's system. But as with all other events in life, the best is always provided by those who have the most experience and training! Don't hesitate to review the background of the health professionals who care for your children.

1. JADA John J. Brooks,DDS and Laurie A.P. Francis.

Chapter 24. POTS and Visual Disturbances
Doc, are these Spots from POTS? - *Dr. Dawn Kaplan, OD*

When is a visual disturbance or symptom involving your eyes something to be concerned about? Or...when is it something to chalk up to "another POTS symptom?" I have been a practicing Optometrist for almost 20 years and, although I am not a POTS specialist, I have certainly seen my share of patients suffering from POTS. Indeed, the diagnosis has become more prevalent. Common visual complaints I have heard from POTS patients include:

- Blurry vision
- Double vision
- Flashes of light
- Floaters and spots
- Tunnel vision/ reverse tunnel vision
- Pain around the eyes
- Twitching eyelids
- Frequent blinking
- Room spinning/vertigo
- Light sensitivity
- Visual perception sensitivity
- Visual "snow" (spots in the vision that actually look like snow)
- Dry Eyes

If you have never had an eye exam or it has been over one year since your last eye exam, all of the above complaints warrant a doctor visit. Many of the above symptoms may be brought on by inadequate blood flow to internal organs in the eye and to the optic nerve, a fairly common issue with POTS patients. In addition, many of these symptoms can be the result of a faulty autonomic nervous system. Conversely, some of these symptoms may be more serious and should be checked out with more urgency. **A good rule of thumb is if the symptom is temporary (lasting only minutes or a**

few hours) generally it is not something to worry about. If it is something that has lasted for a day or more and seems to not be resolving and possibly getting worse, then definitely schedule your visit - the sooner the better!

During your eye exam your doctor should get a thorough case history including any medical diagnoses and what medications you are taking (this part is very important). Be very specific with what kind of visual disturbances you are experiencing. For instance, are you seeing flashes in only one quadrant of your vision in one eye or is it all over in both eyes? Also, the medication question is very important because many medications and combinations of medications can cause any of the above visual disturbances. The doctor will then do a series of tests to determine if you need a prescription for eyeglasses or contacts. He or she will also do tests to rule out any of the more serious diagnoses like retinal detachments, glaucoma, and tumors (yes, some brain tumors can be detected during a routine eye exam). An **automated visual field test, dilation, and retinal imaging** should also be performed to further rule out the aforementioned conditions.

After the eye doctor has performed a thorough eye exam and if nothing abnormal is detected, then your visual disturbances are most likely POTS-related and should be discussed with your physician treating you for POTS. Most importantly, if something abnormal is detected, your eye care professional will take care of the problem or refer you to the appropriate specialist. Your Optometrist is like your primary care doctor, but just for your eyes.

I will now go over the above symptoms in a little more detail:

Blurry vision speaks for itself. This is the most common chief complaint of any patient coming in for an eye exam. If the blurriness is of sudden onset, this is an emergency. Otherwise it could simply mean a change in refractive error (prescription). Fluctuating vision can be due to hormones, diabetes, or other causes such as POTS.

Double vision (diplopia) is also a potential for an emergency if it is of sudden onset. There are many possible etiologies for double vision but the most common is a muscle decompensation between the two eyes. This is often treated with eyeglasses or vision therapy. More serious reasons for sudden onset of diplopia could be a stroke or diabetes.

POTS patients often suffer from **migraine headaches**. Many of the above related visual problems are related to migraines, specifically flashes of light, tunnel vision, or blurry vision in only one quadrant. These symptoms could also be indicative of any retinal disorders such as holes, tears or detachments.   That is why these specific symptoms could be serious and should not be ignored.   If your doctor determines the retina is completely healthy, then it is safe to say these are most likely POTS symptoms due to abnormal blood flow and vessel constriction. **Vertigo and light sensitivity** can also be migraine related. It would be helpful to keep a log of when you are suffering from these symptoms and see if they occur before or during a migraine headache.

Twitching eyelids and frequent blinking are also common symptoms to POTS patients and non-POTS patients alike. Twitching is caused by stress. It could be physical stress, such as not using the proper eyeglasses or working on the computer too much, or mental and emotional stress. Twitching can be very disconcerting, but it is actually harmless. It can come and go throughout the day and often alternates between the eyes.   It usually lasts about one month.   Frequent blinking is much less common but because blinking is controlled by the autonomic nervous system it therefore could be POTS related.   Sometimes people develop something called a "blepharospasm" where the muscles around the eyebrows actually spasm and cause the upper lids to appear to be twitching. These types of spasms are more constant and involve both eyebrows. Botox injections can control these types of spasms.

Pain around the eyes could be as simple as needing a new prescription for eyeglasses or contacts. It could also be sinus related or muscle tension. **Pain on *eye movement*** can be a more serious condition related to inflammation of the muscles and nerves surrounding the eye.

A whole chapter could be written about **dry eye**, as it is an extremely common disorder that mostly affects adults but sometimes affects younger people, as well. It can cause quality of life impairment comparable to migraine headaches. It is the single most common complaint among contact lens wearers. Because of this, research is abundant and ongoing regarding treatment of dry eye. POTS in and of itself does not necessarily cause dry eye but often an underlying autoimmune disorder, such as Sjogren's syndrome, can be the cause.

Treatment of dry eye is guided by symptom severity. We treat dry eye symptoms both pharmacologically and non-pharmacologically. Artificial tears are the mainstay of dry eye treatment and they often resolve the symptoms. However, often the dry eye disease is accompanied by inflammation of the ocular surface and sometimes a short-term use of a steroid drop can be helpful.

These are but a few of the myriad of symptoms involving your eyes. Although I am not a POTS eye doctor per se, in my experience I have not seen any higher incidence of eye disease in POTS patients than in any other population.

That said, remember the eyes aren't only for looking out but, like windows, the doctor can use them for looking in. Your eyes are essentially a window into your brain. We can detect diabetes, high blood pressure, multiple sclerosis, strokes, and many other conditions via a routine eye exam. So even if you aren't experiencing out of the ordinary visual disturbances, it's always a good idea to get an annual eye exam! And if you are experiencing visual disturbances of an unknown etiology, remember that when in doubt, check it out! It is always better to err on the side of caution and to be safe rather than sorry.

Section 7. Pass the Salt

"You are what you eat"

Most of us are well aware that a diet high in sodium can have negative effects on our bodies. Salt raises our blood pressure and retains fluid intake. Too much salt can lead to high blood pressure, congestive heart failure, stroke, kidney stones and a myriad of other ailments. Most doctors recommend a diet low in sodium. People with POTS on the other hand, are one of the few categories of illness, where doctors actually recommend an increase in salt intake. Most people with POTS need extra sodium in their diets for the exact opposite reason. (POTS patients may be the only people in America looking down the grocery aisle to find foods with high sodium content).

Many doctors recommend taking salt tablets to help retain water thus increasing blood volume. Many people, however, complain that the salt tablets give them an upset stomach or that they find the tablets to be ineffective. If you choose to not take salt tablets here is a list of foods that are high in salt content and that are healthy at the same time. Many other foods are high in salt content but are unhealthy choices. They include: bacon, processed meats, hot dogs, canned food, canned soups, condiments, fast foods, etc. As they are not healthy choices and can exacerbate POTS symptoms, I do not recommend them. I therefore will stick to the foods that are high in sodium as well as good food choices.

Foods high in sodium include:
- Tomato juice
- Most veggie juices
- Bullion cubes - be sure they do not contain monosodium glutamate (MSG)
- Whole grain saltine crackers
- Soy sauce - do not use one that contains MSG
- Corn flake cereal (Cornflakes contain as much sodium as a bag of chips)
- Celery

- Organic peanut butter
- Cheese
- Cheese pizza
- Salted popcorn
- Whole grain bagels
- Most breakfast cereals
- Organic salad dressing
- Organic Mac and cheese
- Organic pancake mix - try a multigrain mix
- Miso soup (Be sure it does not contain msg)
- Wheat germ
- Tuna in oil
- Artichoke hearts
- Chili
- Organic canned veggies
- Annie's Organic Snack Mix Bunnies - contains 290 grams of sodium and 3 grams of protein. It is a mixture of baked cheddar crackers, pretzels, and buttery Rich crackers. My kids love this!
- Turkey bacon
- Organic canned soup (be sure there is no MSG in it)
- Organic canned baked beans
- Wheat thins
- Corn chips
- Veggie sticks
- Veggie chips
- Organic tortilla chips
- Chinese Food (Ask them to hold the MSG)
- Most salsas
- Pickles (be careful because garlic and vinegar can lower blood pressure)
- Almost all organic canned items. One of my kids' favorites is Annie's P'Sghetti Loops with soy meatballs. It has 650

mg of sodium and 9 grams of protein. It does contain wheat, so beware if you are on a gluten free diet. I often serve this with whole grain bread and butter and an organic apple. It makes for a great POTS meal.

Healthy Snack Suggestions
- Celery or apple and peanut butter, sunflower seed butter or almond butter
- Organic tortilla chips and salsa
- Organic chips or veggies and fresh guacamole (add a pinch extra salt to the guacamole)
- Veggies and organic salad dressing
- Miso soup packet with sour cream makes for a fabulous dip. You can even add fresh dill or fresh chives. Dip veggies and chips in miso dip.
- Whole grain crackers and cheese
- Bowl of popcorn
- Hummus and chips
- Pirates' Booty
- Salty pretzels dipped in peanut or sunflower butter

A great way to get your sodium in is to try CERALYTE. CeraLyte is a rice-based version of PediaLyte. CeraLyte oral electrolytes are scientifically formulated with the right concentrations of salts and water and complex carbohydrates to maximize absorption. This quickly and effectively increases blood volume and pressure, helping people feel less tired and fatigued as nutrients are now better able to reach organs and the brain.

Note: You can also sneak table salt or sea salt into every meal or snack you eat.

Chapter 25. The Importance of proper Nutrition - *Darren Friedman, Nutritionist*

Improving the quality of life of individuals afflicted with POTS can be achieved through mindful nutritional practices and supplementation. Although there are general guidelines that most individuals with POTS can follow, each person has their own unique chemistry and therefore, specific needs.

To better understand what Biochemical Nutrition is it would be helpful to have a working knowledge of what General Nutrition is. General Nutrition, as most dietitians practice it, is concerned with the general balancing of foods with the proper intake of proteins, carbohydrates, fats, vitamins and minerals. Nutritionists use a standard set of guidelines that produce a balance for most healthy individuals. They also assume that everyone's body functions exactly alike.

How is Biochemical Nutrition different? Biochemical Nutrition is the usage of vitamins, minerals and amino acids to alter biochemical pathways in the human body to correct metabolic problems and chemical malfunctions. Biochemical nutrition does not assume that everyone's body functions the same. In fact, it assumes that each person has his or her own specific pattern of needs and sensitivities. Biochemical nutrition treats each person's body as a unique chemical system with different requirements.

How do medications compare to Biochemical Nutrition? Medications target specific organ functions, whereas Biochemical Nutrition works on a molecular level. For example, if your sinuses are dripping and you took an antihistamine, it would block the activity of the body chemical histamine and your sinuses would stop dripping. This is one way a medication works. Using Biochemical Nutrition, it would be determined what is causing the production of histamines. Then, either the chemicals used to produce histamine found in your diet would be removed, or the pathway of histamine production would be altered to lower production. The results would be the same; your sinuses would stop dripping. However, the approach of one is short-term and the other is on a more long-term basis.

Proper nutrition and supplementation can not only significantly improve the quality of healthy or otherwise disease free people's lives, but can have a greater impact on those suffering from debilitating conditions such as POTS. It can make the difference between succumbing to a sedentary and unproductive life style, to leading a very active and accomplished one. In order to establish what the special needs of individuals with POTS are, we must first understand what this condition is. POTS is basically characterized as Dysautonomia or a malfunction of the autonomic nervous system. This particular malfunction is known as Orthostatic Intolerance, that is when moving from a supine position to that of an upright one, an abnormal increase in heart rate or tachycardia occurs. In addition to the nervous system, the cardiovascular system, and other mechanisms are involved with Orthostatic Intolerance. However, for simplicity and practical reasons, the autonomic nervous system is what we will be focusing on.

The nervous system is comprised of three unique systems or chemical highways. They are the sympathetic, the parasympathetic, and the non-adrenergic/non-cholinergic system.   Each system has its own distinct neurotransmitter or chemical messenger. They are epinephrine (sometimes called adrenaline), acetylcholine and nitric oxide, respectively. Now that the fundamental chemicals used to govern the autonomic nervous system have been identified, it's time to find the necessary building blocks, from either food or supplements, needed to produce them. Phenylalanine and tyrosine are used to produce epinephrine, phosphatidyl choline is used to produce acetylcholine and arginine is used to produce nitric oxide. Foods rich in tyrosine are pork and walnuts. Eggs are plentiful in acetylcholine and chicken and almonds are loaded with arginine. Although these foods contain the building blocks needed to produce the chemicals that fuel our nervous system, the body is only so efficient in metabolizing or processing them.

In many cases, and especially if one has a health related condition such as POTS, food alone is not enough to optimally meet the demands of the human body. However, with proper supplementation these gaps can be met. Not only are the building blocks necessary to produce the chemicals used by the nervous system, but there are critical cofactors that need to be present too. For example, in order to synthesize adrenaline, vitamin C and biopterin must be available. Biopterin is also a cofactor needed by the body to produce nitric oxide. Furthermore, NADH and other vitamins and minerals play an integral part in the functioning of the nervous system. To sum it up, both the necessary building blocks and cofactors need to be present for even a normal nervous system to function properly, let alone people with POTS.

Now what role does each of the three chemical messengers (epinephrine, acetylcholine and nitric oxide) of the autonomic nervous system play and how does it relate to POTS? Well it's actually quite simple. Epinephrine is like the gas pedal in a car; it speeds things up. Acetylcholine is like the brake; it slows things down. And nitric oxide is like the oil; it reduces friction. Okay, now let's apply this to the human body. Adrenaline increases the heart rate, acetylcholine slows it down, and nitric oxide can increase the heart rate indirectly by opening up the blood vessels and reducing resistance. In healthy individuals, the nervous system is functioning properly and these neurotransmitters needed to maintain a normal heart rate and blood pressure are appropriate for any given activity level. With that said, how are individuals with POTS different? First, the nervous system itself does not function normally. Secondly, the chemicals that regulate it are often in excess or in deficient amounts needed to help keep homeostasis or equilibrium (normal heart rate, blood pressure, and well-being}. On the bright side, we don't have to have to accept it all, we can take action!

So what can people with POTS do to help themselves?

Eating the necessary foods and taking the appropriate sup-plements to support the autonomic nervous system is key. Howev-er, each individual has his or her unique chemistry or needs and even these change over time. With that said, it would be in the best interest of individuals who are afflicted with POTS to seek counsel-ing from a skilled biochemical nutritionist who has experience in this area.

Now what can people with POTS do in the meantime to help themselves? Most individuals can benefit by consuming an ample amount of water and salt. Both of these are helpful by in-creasing blood volume and pressure. Although salt is not for every-one, it can be advantageous by decreasing nitric oxide production. Nitric oxide lowers blood pressure by dilating the blood vessels. An-other chemical that not only opens up the blood vessels, but also contributes to many of the symptoms associated with POTS includ-ing chronic fatigue, muscle aches, headaches, dizziness, brain fog, irritable bowel, nervousness, sleeplessness, inflammation and aller-gies, is histamine. It's worth noting that even in healthy individuals who consume high histamine and histidine (an amino acid precursor to histamine) containing foods regularly; it can overly stress the ad-renals and wreak havoc on the body. Therefore, most people should restrict their intake of high histamine and histidine containing foods. Some of these foods include dairy, wheat, corn and tomato products, bananas, strawberries, eggplant, spinach and oatmeal. Now let's talk about methionine, a sulfur containing amino acid, one of twenty such acids that makes up proteins. What makes me-thionine unique is that many individuals have difficulty metabolizing it and it promotes the release of adrenaline. People, who have dif-ficulty processing it, respond by producing an excessive amount of histamine. This is obvious in those with peanut, orange, and fish allergies to name a few. Furthermore, sulfur metabolism varies from one individual to another in one's ability to remove sulfur from the body. If an individual's sulfur level climbs too high as a re-sult of consuming too much methionine, he or she runs the risk of having either a too high or too low adrenaline level. Until one knows what his or her sulfur level is, it would be wise to limit the amount of foods rich in methionine and also avoid anything containing sulfur, sulfur dioxide, potassium metabisulfite, sulfites and sulfates. Some foods rich in methionine include fish, oranges, celery, peppers, onions, cabbage, rice, peanuts, and soybeans. These are some dietary changes individuals with POTS can do right now, but it's only the beginning. Not only is it important to restrict certain foods, but it's just as important to choose the right foods as well.

How can dietary supplements help people with POTS?

Certain vitamins, minerals, amino acids, herbs and other nutrients can help improve a number of the symptoms associated with this syndrome. Because minerals have been reported as the number one deficiency among Americans and are needed in almost every chemical reaction that takes place in the human body, it would be wise for everyone, with or without POTS, to consider taking a high potency multimineral supplement. Another compelling reason why an individual with POTS would be interested in minerals is that the nervous system depends on them to regulate the heart rate and blood pressure. Now why not just take a multivitamin? Although it has all the vitamins and minerals too, most multivitamins simply do not have enough of everything to optimally support the needs of someone who has POTS, let alone a healthy individual. Furthermore, not everyone needs to supplement with everything that is found in a typical multivitamin. The advantage to this approach is that an individual can take only what he or she needs, in therapeutic amounts, and can take them multiple times a day. As with most water-soluble vitamins and minerals, they can be taken two or even three times a day. This helps keep the levels high throughout the entire day. A second supplement to consider taking is vitamin C as it helps boost the immune system and it's critical for the production and release of adrenaline. A third supplement to look into taking is B-complex. The B vitamins assist in the transformation of protein, carbohydrates, and fats into energy. They can also aid the body in the removal of excess histamine. The next four supplements are the remaining vitamins found in most multivitamins, Vitamins A, D, E, and K. Depending on an individual's need and food intake, it may or may not be necessary to supplement with these. The eighth supplement to consider is an omega-3 fish oil. Omega-3 fish oil can help reduce inflammation, although be aware that in some individuals it can contribute to lowering blood pressure. Other supplements that can be beneficial to individuals with POTS are the autonomic nervous system precursors discussed earlier. Individuals who have high sulfur levels can consider taking an amino acid lysine, which can be helpful in removing sulfur. However, before taking these or any other supplements, one should consult with a qualified health care practitioner.

People with POTS should be aware that their histamine and sulfur levels are not only affected by what they eat and drink, but also by the air they breathe. The air quality varies according to the weather, the seasons, the geographical location, pollution and natural disasters. Changing weather conditions can change the particles in the air. If any of these particles are perceived as an allergen, the body would respond by releasing histamine. Arthritis sufferers are often hit hard by weather changes. Just like the weather, the different seasons will change the air composition. Common seasonal allergens include pollen and ragweed. There are specific geographical locations that tend to be better tolerated by people with POTS and other health conditions. San Diego is one of these places where the weather is stable all year round. Although there are many exceptions, in general, the air quality is better in the West than in the East. The reason being is that the weather typically travels in an easterly direction, carrying all the pollution and sulfur along the way. Remember, sulfur promotes the release of adrenaline. Lastly, there are things beyond our control that can suddenly change the composition of the air. For example, the recent volcano eruption spewed out massive amounts of ash and sulfur into the air. Individuals with POTS should maintain a constant awareness of the air quality in their environment and take a proactive approach if necessary. If the air quality is poor outdoors, one can turn on his or her air conditioner or air cleaner.

Precision Nutrition opened to the public in Oceanside, NY in 2005 and has retained its original home phone number of (516) 244-1302. In addition to seeing patients in his office, Darren does phone consultations, making it possible for almost anyone to use his services. He can also be found on the web at www.precisionnutrition1.com and can be emailed at *dfriedman@precisionnutrition1.com*.

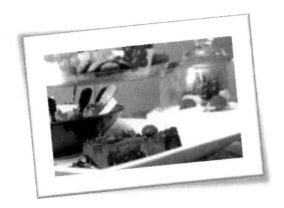

Chapter 26. Nutritional Recipes Designed for POTS patients - *Created by Chef Randy Ordonio of San Francisco*

Tips for a POTS diet...

- Water, water, water! - Hydration is the most important factor to any good POTS diet. Minerals and electrolytes in general are essential!
- Foods or drinks high in salt/sodium help in maximizing blood volume for those with POTS.
- Remember, salt is used to flavor your food and enhance the quality of your special dish.
- Foods that help to regulate the blood sugar are also helpful for most people with POTS, as blood sugar fluctuations cause palpitations, nervousness and fatigue. Don't eat too many carbohydrates, and don't eat too few. Think about how a diabetic might eat.
- Salts that are great for your everyday health are:
    - o Mediterranean Sea Salt - fine, medium, or coarse. Fine salt is great for cooking and measuring, strong flavor and loaded with natural components.
    - o Himalayan Pink Sea Salt - A little bit goes a long way, often found in large chunks or even slabs.

o   Kosher Salt - Fine granules are the most common household salt found in the pantry.

APPETIZERS

Smoked Trout Mousse - Serves 6-8 People

Ingredients
- 2 Filets of Smoked Trout / or Smoked Salmon
- 12 oz. Soft Cream Cheese
- 2 Tangerines Juiced
- 1 1/2 Tablespoons of Honey
- 1 Teaspoon of Dill Weed
- 1/2 Teaspoon Fresh Cracked Pepper

Directions
Remove the skin from the fish and gently crumble the fish into a medium size mixing bowl. With a spatula, mix in the cream cheese, tangerine juice, honey, dill weed and pepper. Place the mousse in your favorite bowl and lightly sprinkle the top of the mousse with dill.

This Smoked Trout Mousse is great with whole grain crackers, or pretzel stick.

Grilled Turkey Bacon Wrapped Shrimp - Serves 4-6 People

Ingredients
- 18-20 Shelled Large Shrimp
- 9-10 Cut Turkey Bacon Sliced in half

Sauce:
- 1/2 Cup of Mayonnaise
- 2 Teaspoons Relish
- 1 Tablespoon Capers
- 1 Tablespoon Dijon Mustard

Directions
Tightly wrap the shrimp with the 1/2 strips of bacon and grill until bacon is crispy. (You can use 1/4 strip of bacon as long as it wraps completely around the shrimp.) Approximately 3-5 minutes per side. Mix sauce ingredients altogether. Place shrimp onto an appetizer plate and set the sauce aside for generous dipping!

Roasted Asparagus and Stilton Blue Cheese - Serves 4-6 People

Ingredients
- 18-20 Pieces of Asparagus
- 1/4 Cup Stilton Blue Cheese
- Olive Oil Spray
- 1 Teaspoon Fine Salt
- 1/2 Tablespoon of Fresh Cracked Pepper

Directions
Preheat the oven at 425ºF. Wash the asparagus and dry with a paper towel. Place the asparagus onto a large rectangle baking pan. Generously season with olive oil spray, salt and black pepper. Mix the asparagus, salt and pepper. Let it marinate for about 5-10 minutes so the salt permeates the asparagus. Arrange the asparagus equally at the base as close together as possible. Sprinkle the blue cheese 1-2 inches at the base of the asparagus. Roast in

the oven for 10-12 minutes or until the asparagus is slightly crisp and the cheese is melted. With a flat spatula, carefully place onto an appetizer platter and eat them while they are still hot!

SOUPS

Carrot Ginger Soup - Serves 4-6 People

Ingredients
- 1 Medium Onion Diced
- 3 Tablespoons of Freshly Grated Ginger
- 1/2 Tablespoon of Freshly Chopped Garlic
- 1 Pound of Coarsely Chopped Carrots
- 1/2 Quarts of Vegetable Broth
- 1/2 Cup of Cream or Milk
- 1 Tablespoon of Honey
- 2 Bay Leaves
- 1-2 Sprigs of Thyme
- 1/2 Teaspoon of Cinnamon
- 1 1/2 Teaspoons of Fine Salt
- 1 Teaspoon Fresh Cracked Pepper

Directions
In a stockpot sauté onions, ginger, garlic, salt and pepper until the onions are translucent. Add the carrots to the pot and lightly brown the carrots. Add the bay leaves, thyme and cinnamon; stir for about 2-4 minutes so the flavors can melt together. Add the vegetable broth and bring the soup to a boil. Let it boil until the carrots are tender, approximately 7-10 minutes. Fish out the bay leaves and the stem of the thyme. Add the cream or milk and honey; with a hand mixer, place the mixer gently at the bottom of the soup and mix on high until the soup is nice and smooth. If you need to add a touch more salt, sprinkle and taste.

Note: If you think it may be too salty, add more cream or milk to neutralize the salt.

Mexican Chicken Cilantro - Serves 4-6 People

Ingredients

- 1 Pound of Diced Boneless Chicken Thigh
- 1 Medium Onion Diced
- 2 Cups of Chopped Carrots
- 1 Cup of Chopped Celery
- 1 Can of Roasted and Diced Tomatoes
- 1 Small Jalapeño Finely Diced
- 1 Teaspoon of Freshly Chopped Garlic
- 1 1/2 Quarts of Chicken Broth
- 2 Teaspoons of Basil
- 1 Teaspoon of Oregano
- 1/2 Teaspoon of Cumin
- 1 Small Bunch of Cilantro
- 1 Tablespoon of Olive Oil
- 1 Tablespoon of Fine Salt to taste
- 1/2 Teaspoon of Fresh Cracked Pepper

Directions

In a stockpot sauté onion, garlic, cumin, black pepper and 1 tablespoon of salt. Add the carrots, celery, jalapeño, basil, and oregano; sauté the veggies until they are slightly tender. Add the chicken and stir vigorously and pause 2 minutes in between each stir; about 3 times. Then, add the chicken broth and canned tomatoes and bring the soup to a boil for about 4-6 minutes. Lower the heat and let it simmer for about 15-20 minutes. Finally, wash the cilantro very well and remove the leaves from the stem and add them to the soup. Let it sit for a couple minutes and gently stir to have the flavors mix together. Gently add more salt to your soup, just to your taste.

Top with your favorite tortilla chips and let it soak up this hearty soup!

SIDES

Mashed Cauliflower Bake - Serves 4-6

Ingredients

- 2 Heads of Cauliflower Cleaned and Coarsely Chopped
- 1/2 Cup of Sour Cream
- 1/3 Cup of Grated Parmesan Cheese
- 1/2 Teaspoon of Garlic Powder
- 1/2 Teaspoon of Black Pepper
- 1 Tablespoon of Dill Weed
- 1 Tablespoon of Freshly Chopped Chives
- 1/2 Teaspoon of Fine Salt
- 1 Tablespoon of Butter

Directions

Preheat oven to 375ºF. Fill a stockpot with water (enough to cover the cauliflower). Add 2 tablespoons of salt to the water and cauliflower for a faster boil. Boil the cauliflower until the cauliflower is incredibly soft. Approximately 20-25 minutes on a high boil. Strain out the water and sauté the cauliflower with the garlic powder, black pepper and butter until the majority of the water is dissolved. Then, lower the heat to medium and add the sour cream and stir. With a hand mixer, mix the cauliflower on high until coarse or smooth to your liking. Stir in the Parmesan cheese, dill weed and chopped chives. Place the mashed cauliflower into a rectangle baking dish, and bake until you have a golden crust.

Brussels Sprouts and Prosciutto - Serves 4-6 People

With Prosciutto, a little goes a long way! Fantastic for getting a lot of flavor, with little "guilt."

Ingredients

- 1 Pound of Brussels Sprouts
- 8 Ounces of Chopped Prosciutto
- 2 Tablespoons of Olive Oil
- 1/2 Tablespoon of Fine Salt
- 1/2 Tablespoon of Fresh Cracked Pepper

Directions

Preheat oven to 375ºF. In a large mixing bowl, mix all ingredients well. Pour the mixture onto a baking pan and let it roast in the oven for 15-20 minutes until tender and crispy.

Green Beans Sautéed with Lemon - Serves 4-6 People

Lemons have super antioxidant components

Ingredients

- 1 Pound of Fresh Cut Green Beans
- 1 Small Meyer Lemon Juiced
- 1 Heaping Tablespoon of Sliced Sun Dried Tomatoes (in olive oil)
- 1 Teaspoon of Freshly Chopped Garlic
- 1 Teaspoon of Fine Salt
- 1 Teaspoon of Fresh Cracked Pepper

Directions

Sauté garlic and sun dried tomatoes for 2-3 minutes. Add the green beans and lemon and sauté all ingredients together. Lower the heat to medium and pour a 1/4 cup of water and let the water steam the green beans as you stir. As soon as the water is dissolved, place the green beans onto a serving platter and let the wonderful smell greet your guests!

MAIN COURSE

Poached Ginger Honey Salmon - Serves 4-6 People

Ginger is so great for nausea and dizziness
Natural antibacterial and anti-inflammatory properties

Ingredients

- 1 Pound of Salmon Filleted and Skinned
- 2 Tablespoons of Freshly Grated Ginger
- 2 Tablespoons of Honey
- 1 Cup of Apple Cider Vinegar
- 1 Medium Onion Chopped
- 1 Teaspoon of Freshly Chopped Garlic
- 3 Sprigs of Fresh Dill
- 2 Bay Leaves
- 1/4 Cup of Fine Salt
- 2 Quarts of Fish Stock
- 1 Tablespoon of Fresh Cracked Pepper

Directions

In a large pan, add the ginger, honey, vinegar, onion, garlic, dill, bay leaves, salt, fish stock and black pepper. Bring these ingredients to a boil for 10-12 minutes. Lower the heat to low medium, and gently place the salmon into the stock. Let the salmon poach and soak in the flavors for 4-7 minutes or until the salmon is fully cooked. Gently remove the salmon from the stock, and place it onto a serving platter. Ladle one scoop of the stock on top of the salmon to keep its moisture.

You may reserve the fish stock for a wonderful broth or fish chowder!

Chicken and Green Veggie Sauté - Serves 4-6 People

Ingredients

- 1 Pound of Small Diced Chicken Breast and Thighs
- 1 Medium Onion Chopped
- 1/2 Pound of Broccoli
- 1/2 Pound Brussels Sprouts Sliced in Half
- 2 Large Zucchini Sliced
- 1 Tablespoon of Freshly Grated Ginger
- 1 Teaspoon of Freshly Chopped Garlic
- 1 Tablespoon of Sesame Oil
- 1 Teaspoon of Honey
- 1 Teaspoon of Fresh Cracked Pepper
- 3 Tablespoons of Soy Sauce
- 1/4 Cup of Chicken Broth

Directions

In a large sauté pan, heat the sesame oil and sauté the onion, garlic, ginger and black pepper for 3-4 minutes. Add the chicken and sauté for 2-4 minutes. Then, add the soy sauce and honey and stir well. Add the Brussels sprouts and broccoli and sauté for 2 minutes and add the chicken broth. Let it simmer on high for 2-4 minutes, then add the zucchini and let it cook for 2-4 more minutes. This dish will be nicely accompanied with brown rice.

Slow Roasted Pork Loin - Served 4-6 People

Ingredients

- 1 - 1/2 Pounds of Pork Tenderloin
- 2 Tablespoons of Dijon Mustard
- 1 Tablespoon of Basil
- 1 Teaspoon of Paprika
- 1 Teaspoon of Olive Oil
- 1 Tablespoon of Fine Salt
- 1 Teaspoon of Fresh Cracked Pepper
- 1 Cup of Chicken Broth

Directions

Preheat oven to 425ºF. Lay the pork tenderloin onto a baking pan. Mix the Dijon mustard, basil, paprika, olive oil, salt and black pepper together in a small mixing bowl. With a spoon or brush, spread the mixture all around the pork tenderloin. Then, add the chicken broth, pouring it at the bottom of the pan. Place the pork in the oven for 15 minutes to get a good sear to seal in the juices. Then reduce the heat to 350ºF and let it continue to cook for 45-60 minutes. For every 15 minutes, spoon over the drippings to keep it moist. The internal temperature should be 155ºF. Once cooked, let it rest for 20 minutes before carving.

DESSERTS

Balsamic Parfait with Whipped Ricotta - Serves 4-6 People

Ingredients

- 1 Pound of Fresh Strawberries, sliced in half (or any other berries/fruit)
- 1/2 Cup of Balsamic Vinegar
- 1 Tablespoon of Honey
- 1 Teaspoon of Vanilla
- 1 Teaspoon of Sugar
- 1 1/2 Cups of Ricotta Cheese
- 1 Teaspoon of Fine Himalayan Pink Salt (set aside / as needed)
- 1/2 Cup of Salted Almonds

Directions

In a small saucepan, bring the balsamic vinegar to a boil and let it reduce to half. Then, reduce the heat to low and add the sugar. Let it simmer for 2-4 minutes, and set the sauce aside. In a medium mixing bowl, add the strawberries and mix in the balsamic sauce. In a small mixing bowl, add the honey, ricotta and vanilla; mixing them well.

For the fun assembling; use your favorite dessert dish and first layer the bottom of the dish with the honey-vanilla ricotta. Then, top it with the balsamic strawberries. With the Himalayan Pink Salt on reserve, use a tiny pinch of the salt to top this treat! Finally top with a few or more almonds to your liking.

Poached Pears with Oatmeal Crunch - Serves 4-6 People

Ingredients

- 4-6 Bartlett Pears (peeled)
- 1 1/2 Quarts of Water
- 1/2 Cup of Apple Cider Vinegar
- 1/4 Cup of Sugar
- 1 Tablespoon of Honey
- 1 Cinnamon Stick

Crunch:

- 1 Cup of Oatmeal
- 1 Tablespoon of Brown Sugar
- 1 Tablespoon of Honey
- 1/2 Teaspoon of Cinnamon Powder
- 1/4 Cup Chopped Salted Walnuts (optional)
- 1 Tablespoon of Melted Butter
- 1 Teaspoon of Fine Himalayan Pink Salt (as needed)

Directions

Preheat oven to 375ºF. In a medium size mixing bowl, add the oatmeal, brown sugar, honey, cinnamon, walnuts and butter. You can always subtract the sugars, or replace them with stevia or other sugar substitutes. Then spread out the mixture onto a baking pan and bake the oatmeal for 10-14 minutes or until golden in color. Set aside for the oatmeal crunch to cool.

In a stockpot, add the water, apple cider vinegar, sugar, honey and cinnamon stick. Bring the mixture to a boil until the sugar is dissolved and all ingredients are well combined. Then gently drop the pears into the syrup and let it poach for 10-12 minutes or until the pears are soft and tender.

For the fun arrangement with your favorite dessert dish; spread the oatmeal crunch evenly on the bottom of the dish. Then, lay the pears on top of the oatmeal crunch with the top of the pear standing up. Lastly, sprinkle the top of the pears with a pinch of the fine Himalayan Sea Salt.

Section 8. Alternative Therapies and Exercise

Chapter 27. Tips, Natural Supplements and Vitamins that May Help with Symptoms - *Co-written by Sharon Cini, M.D. Edited by Rosalee Jaeger*

The contents of this chapter are provided for informational purposes only and should not be used as a substitute for professional medical advice, diagnosis or treatment. Please keep in mind that new treatments are continually emerging and some of the older treatments may rarely be used. In the event that your doctor has recommended a supplement from this list, you can use this as a reference to understand why your doctor has made this recommendation. These suggestions may help and as with everything else MUST first be approved by your team of physicians.

POTS causes a myriad of complicated and strange symptoms. This is a list of vitamins, natural supplements and home remedies that have helped other people who suffer from POTS. These alternative remedies may lessen some of the more bothersome symptoms associated with Dysautonomia. Remember that what works for one person may not work for another. You should only try these with your doctor's prior approval and with medical supervision. Always consult your physician before taking any supplement.

Many physicians will not recommend the use of alternative supplements because currently there is no FDA regulation. Additionally, there is no standardization. There is no regulation that what you are buying actually contains the amount that is recommended and additionally there is no regulation that forces companies to remove impurities.

Many doctors who specialize in alternative and complementary medicine recommend that if you are going to purchase a supplement that you do so from one of their recommended compounding pharmacies or a manufacturer of pharmaceutical grade supplements. They recommend that you only purchase pharmaceutical grade supplements.

Any company that manufactures or sells supplements can say that they test their supplements for purity and standardize their supplements but there is no one regulating them to be sure that what they say is true and accurate. Supplements are not covered by most health insurances, as well, so it can be more costly to pursue this avenue. For these reasons, many traditional physicians will not use non-FDA regulated substances.

You should only take a supplement if recommended by your physician and do so with utmost care. Also note that some people who suffer from Dysautonomia have a lower tolerance for medications and supplements. They are generally more sensitive, even at low doses, to adverse effects. Our doctors recommend that when starting a new medication or supplement, to start only one at a time. If you take more than one supplement and have a bad reaction you won't know which one is the culprit. They also recommend starting at a very low dose and then gradually and slowly increase. For this reason it can take a long time before a true benefit is seen. You may not tolerate a higher dosage, but at low or homeopathic dosages, you may find them to be very helpful.

Anxiety

- *B-Complex Vitamins:* The B-vitamins are often called the "stress" vitamins. When our bodies are forced to withstand the demands of physical or emotional stress, the B-vitamins and other key nutrients are the first to be depleted. The body not only needs specific nutrients to combat stress, but it must also replace the nutrients that stress directly uses up.
- *GABA* is a chemical in the brain that creates a sense of well-being. GABA is also involved in the production of endorphins, brain chemicals that create a feeling of calm. Endorphins are produced in the brain and released during physical activity.

There are many foods that help to increase GABA production. These include: Almonds, Tree nuts, Bananas, Beef Liver, Broccoli, Brown Rice, Halibut, Lentils, Oats, Whole

Grain, Citrus Fruits (Oranges), Rice Bran, Spinach, Walnuts, Whole Wheat and Whole Grains.

- *L-Theanine*, an amino acid that boosts GABA, can be found as a supplement in most health food stores. This amino acid is known to help to reduce anxiety as well as create a sense of alertness.

- *Glutamine* when taken with B6 is also converted to GABA. It acts to calm as well as decrease heart rate. POTS patients have reported having more chest pains with Glutamine and B6 just as they would with a beta blocker. If taken, it is best used at night as it can improve sleep. Caution should be used with drinking anything containing alcohol and you should take care to drive or operate machinery as it causes sedation. Also, use caution while climbing ladders, when under the influence of glutamine or GABA.

- *Valerian* is a plant that was used for medicinal purposes dating back to ancient Greek and Roman Times. It was used as a folk remedy for a variety of conditions such as sleeping problems, digestive complaints, nervousness, trembling, tension headaches and heart palpitations. Valerian helps relax the central nervous system. It promotes feelings of calm and decreases levels of anxiety and stress. Valerian is also an effective sleep aid. Unlike many prescription sleep aids on the market, valerian is non-addictive and does not create morning grogginess. It can be harmful to mix supplements such as Valerian with Kava or benzodiazepine medicines like Valium, Xanax and Klonopin. Additionally, do not take these supplements with beverages containing alcohol.

- *Pregnenolone* is used as a mood stabilizer and improves emotional well-being.

Chest Pains
- *Ice Pack:* Placing an ice pack on your chest can help slow

down your heart rate and may help alleviate some of your chest pain.

• *Tiger's Balm* is an ancient Chinese herbal ointment that has been used for over 100 years. It can provide temporary relief from joint pain, muscle ache, chest pains and headaches. It can be purchased at most health food or vitamin stores. Visit www.Tigerbalm.com to learn more.

Dizziness

• *Cooling devices* can help POTS patients. www.CoolSport.net sells personal body cooling vests that may help patients tolerate hot environments (1).

• *Ginger* also helps to prevent dizziness and vertigo although you must take caution as it can also lead to increased heart rate and cause insomnia. Ginger is used as a caffeine substitute.

• *Manganese* has been helpful in reducing dizziness, but caution that you do not take too much as that can lead to electrolyte imbalance.

• *ResQGARD* is new product that is being used by the United States Army to raise stroke volume in injured soldiers. ResQGard is an Impedance Threshold Device (ITD) that provides a safe, simple and convenient way to treat states of low blood pressure in spontaneously breathing patients. The ResQGARD provides therapeutic benefit as soon as a patient begins to breathe through it. Animal and clinical studies have shown that the ResQGARD increases blood pressure during hypotension from a variety of causes. ResQGard may help alleviate symptoms of dizziness in some patients by helping provide increased blood flow to the brain.

• *Rinsing off with cold water* after taking a shower can relieve some dizziness.

• Try sitting in a squat position and squeeze legs and buttocks. You can also lie on your back with your legs up in the air. This helps return the blood to your brain and heart.

- *Vision Check:* Have your eyes evaluated for prisms by a qualified vertical hetorophoria specialist, like Vision Specialists of Michigan at www.VSofM.com. Vertical hetorophoria occurs when the eyes become misaligned. This is a common source of dizziness and headaches that few physicians recognize. The prisms help align the eyes and lessen the headache and dizziness.

Eye Twitching

- Eye twitching may be due to insufficient calcium. Try adding more calcium to your diet and see if this helps. For a short-term resolution, hold your eyelids down with your fingertips. This should help the twitching to cease, at least temporarily.
- Eye Twitching can occur as a result of fatigue as well. If you are not getting enough restful sleep this will occur with increased frequency. Anything that calms the central nervous system should help lessen these episodes.

Fatigue

- *Acetyl L-Carnitine* improves concentration, memory and energy.
- *Cerefolin* is a vitamin supplement that may help improve patient's symptoms of fatigue and help them feel more alert. Some possible minor side effects of this drug include upset stomach, headache or unusual or unpleasant taste in your mouth.
- *D-ribose* is a simple, five-carbon sugar that is found naturally in our bodies. When Ribose is consumed, the body recognizes that it is different from other sugars and preserves it for the vital work of actually making the energy molecule that powers our hearts, muscles, brains, and all

other tissue in the body.

Normal, healthy heart and muscle tissue has the capacity to make all the D-Ribose it needs. However, when the muscle is chronically stressed by disease or conditions that affect tissue energy metabolism, the cells and tissues simply cannot make enough Ribose quickly enough to recover.

- *Function Alternative Energy Drink*: It is all natural and has no preservatives. It contains Vitamin C, folic acid, zinc, vitamin B and sodium. It contains natural caffeine (a combination of catuaba, muira pauma, epimedium and yerba) and provides stamina support for up to eight hours. We have tried the citrus Yuzu and strawberry Guava flavors. They are both very good. Look up www.functiondrinks.com to learn more about this product.

- *Liquid Iron Supplement:* Some say this works wonders for increasing energy levels. Sometimes iron supplements can cause constipation, so beware. Too much iron can also cause liver damage and is not recommended for most men. Some forms of Iron can also cause gastritis. You should only take Iron when recommended by your doctor. Toxic levels can build up if you are not deficient in Iron.

- *Lucidal* has been marketed to improve memory, but some have found that it improves energy.

- *Max GXL and Lipoic acid* can also increase energy but caution their use since they can also lead to increased GI symptoms and exacerbate GER.

- *Fizz drink* sold at Costco can also improve energy, but it may also cause chest pains in POTS patients.

- *Ginger* can improve energy; however, caution that it may also lead to increased heart rate.

- *Siberian Ginseng* can also improve energy and sense of well-being.

- *Coq10* can also increase energy and mental alertness. Coq10 can also lower your blood pressure, so use with caution.

- *DHEA* also increases energy and mental alertness. However, use cautiously and only under medical supervision. It can also lead to insomnia.
- *N-Acetylcystein* is a precursor to glutathione, which is also a potent antioxidant, and improves memory and energy.
- *Spark Energy Drink by Adovocare* – Spark may enhance energy as well as mental focus. It is sugar free and contains more than 20 vitamins, mineral and nutrients. Spark does contain caffeine so use with caution and only the guidance of your team of doctors.

General pain

- Chronic pain is common in patients with Dysautonomia. This type of pain is usually better treated with traditional medical therapies such as the SSRI's, *NSAIDS, and Steroids such as Prednisone*. Use caution when taking SSRI's as they can exacerbate symptoms of POTS patients.
- *Homemade ice pack or heating pad-* Fill a tube sock with uncooked white rice. Tie a knot around the end of the tube sock. Place the rice filled sock in the microwave oven for approximately 70 seconds. Place the warm sock on your head or stomach to help with discomfort. If you prefer cold, you can also place the sock in the freezer instead of the microwave. Add fragrances (like lavender or chamomile) to the inside of the sock for an even more calming effect.
- *Arnica* is a homeopathic preparation that has been used since the 1500's for medicinal purposes by Europeans and Native Americans. When used topically, Arnica can help with bruises, muscle aches, rheumatic pain, wound healing and general inflammation.

Gastrointestinal Complaints

- *Chamomile* is one of the mainstays of European medicine; it is the dried flowers of a daisy family plant. The name chamomile comes from Greek words meaning, "ground apple." When brewed into tea, chamomile flowers release this same aroma and flavor along with a slightly bitter taste. Chamomile tea is an excellent home remedy for upset stomachs, heartburn, and indigestion. It has no side effects. It also has mild relaxant and sedative properties.

- *Small meals* are recommended. Eat six small meals throughout the day instead of three larger meals. Larger meals tend to increase the amount of blood needed for digestion, often depriving the brain and heart of needed oxygen. Many POTS patients feel more symptomatic after eating. Ingesting smaller meals will cut down on the amount of blood needed to digest the food, and will hopefully result in fewer symptoms.

- *Probiotics* are products containing the helpful bacteria that normally inhabit the human digestive tract. Probiotics help to maintain the healthy flora of the intestines. Most of these "friendly" bacteria occur naturally in cultured milk products, such as yogurt with active cultures or acidophilus milk. Consider taking probiotic foods or supplements whenever you are on antibiotics, which can wipe out intestinal bacteria indiscriminately, including those that help keep the digestive system functioning properly. Taking probiotics daily, even when you are not on an antibiotic, may help relieve some stomach pain often associated with Dysautonomia.

- *Ginger* is also used as a digestive aid. It is used to prevent nausea and helps to regulate gastrointestinal complaints.

Headaches

- *Butcher's Broom* is an herb that acts as a vasoconstrictor and seems to have a favorable effect on the legs. Veins constrict after consumption of the herb and swelling seems to subside. By acting directly on the blood vessels, Butcher's Broom increases blood flow and thus an increase in circulation occurs. Butcher's Broom has been shown to have benefits for those suffering from orthostatic hypotension by improving blood pressure response with movement without raising resting blood pressure. Butcher's Broom has also been used effectively in POTS patients to help ward off headaches.

Butcher's Broom has proven so effective that it is used in some European Countries as a post-surgical precaution to ward off blood clots.

> *Note: This herb should not be taken if you are pregnant, have hypertension or in combination with an MAO inhibitor (used to treat depression.) Butcher's Broom is a bitter herb and is often better tolerated in capsule form than in a tea. Butcher's Broom is also a mild laxative as well as diuretic and should be used only under the close supervision of your doctor.*

- *Feverfew*, a member of the daisy family, has been used for centuries for fevers, headaches, stomachaches, toothaches, allergies, asthma, nausea, and vomiting. Feverfew was mentioned in Greek medical literature as a remedy for inflammation and swelling. The name "feverfew" is derived from the Latin for "chase away fevers." Beginning in the 16th century, it was used by British herbalists for the treatment of fevers and rheumatic aches and pains. Recently, feverfew has been used to treat migraine headaches. Feverfew blocks platelets from releasing serotonin, which may help to explain how it works to prevent migraines. People who are allergic to Ragweed should not take this herb.

- *Magnesium supplements* can be very useful in treating Dysautonomia. Some studies suggest that taking magnesium supplements may help prevent migraine headaches. In addition, a few clinical studies suggest that magnesium supplements may shorten the duration of a migraine and reduce the amount of medication needed. People who have migraine headaches tend to have lower levels of magnesium compared to those with tension headaches or no headaches at all. Magnesium can cause diarrhea, which may be balanced by taking a calcium supplement.
- Some experts suggest the combination of magnesium, the herb feverfew, and Vitamin B2 (riboflavin) may be helpful in alleviating a headache.

Leg Cramps
- Try adding more calcium and or potassium to your diet. Often cramping occurs when your body is calcium and or potassium deficient. Bananas, orange juice and white potatoes are great food choices that are high in potassium. Almonds, tofu, yogurt and dairy products are high in calcium. However, too much potassium can cause diarrhea. *Bananas and orange juice* contain a lot of natural sugar; so if you are diabetic, beware.
- *Quinine*, an ingredient of tonic water, can reduce or eliminate leg cramps.

Orthostatic Hypotension
- *Caffeine* helps some POTS patients due to its stimulative effects; however, other patients report a worsening of symptoms with caffeine intake.
- *Compression stockings* are used to improve venous return to the heart through external vasoconstriction. This compression, when combined with the muscle pumping effect of the calf, aids in preventing blood pooling in the legs.

Compression stockings are available in a wide range of opacities, colors, styles and sizes, making them virtually in-distinguishable from regular hosiery or socks. They come in various levels of compression and different lengths such as knee, thigh and waste high. You may need to be individually fitted to get the correct size, and you may need a doctor's prescription in order to purchase them.

• *Fluids Containing Electrolytes*, such as Smart Water, Pe-dialyte, V-8 Juice or coconut water will help to raise blood pressure by retaining fluid intake. Electrolytes are lost when the body sweats; therefore replacing the body's lost fluids with electrolytes will prevent a dehydrated state and will allow for proper electrolyte balance within the body. Al-ways look at the label of a hydrating supplement. If it con-tains sugar, the sugar can cause stomach cramps.

• *Licorice root* is an herb that has been used for medicinal purposes for centuries. It has been used in ancient Greece, China, and Egypt, mostly for gastritis (inflammation of the stomach) and ailments of the upper respiratory tract. Lico-rice is the most widely used herb in Chinese medicine. It is widely recognized for its anti-inflammatory properties. Licorice root can sometimes be used as an alternative to Florinef in that it helps the kidneys to retain sodium and fluids. It might provide a good alternative to those who are sensitive to Florinef. Licorice root can throw off the electro-lyte balance, so it is imperative, if using this as an alterna-tive to Florinef that you check with your doctor first. Similar to Florinef, Licorice root can cause the body to excrete po-tassium; therefore, it is critical to check potassium levels frequently. Licorice root can be fatal if you are diabetic, have kidney or liver damage, or coronary heart disease. It must strictly be used under a physician's guidance.

Do not look for licorice root in the candy aisle. The licorice sold in America today has little to no licorice root in it and therefore, no medicinal value. You can find licorice root extract under the name of Glycyrrhizin.

• *Salt Loading* refers to adding salt to your diet. Sea Salt or Celtic Salt is best. This is a very effective way to increase blood pressure for those who have orthostatic hypotension, or a drop in blood pressure upon standing as well as anyone who suffers from near syncope or orthostatic intolerance. (Be sure the salt you add is aluminum free. Aluminum is added to table salt to give it a white appearance. Natural salt contains discolored specs.) Adding salt to your diet also helps the body to hold on to fluids as well as helps to expand blood volume. Salt tablets are available as an alternative to those who do not want to add extra salt to their diets. Some; however, feel that the tablets are hard on their stomachs and prefer to add extra salt to their food.

Caution: do not use salt if you have a history of coronary artery disease or congestive heart failure. Salt has been touted in the press as the number one cause of high blood pressure and can lead to heart attacks and death. Salt loading should only be used when recommended by your physician.

Physicians often recommend consuming anywhere from 3-15 grams of salt per day for many patients with Dysautonomia.

• *Thermotab* is a salt supplement. If you decide to get your additional salt in your diet by taking salt supplements, Thermotab may be an option. Many people feel that this is a very helpful and effective way to add salt to their diet. When taking Thermotab be sure to drink it with plenty of water and to take it on a full stomach. The capsules are often easier on the digestive tract than are the tablets. Ask your pharmacist to keep this product in stock, as some pharmacies do not carry this product unless preordered. Be sure to consult with your physician before using this product and make sure to inquire about how many grams you should be taking.

Insomnia

Please, also refer to the section, "Combating Insomnia."

• *Chamomile* Tea helps lessen insomnia. You can buy Chamomile tea bags in most supermarkets. This is a great natural product to use when your stomach is upset or when you are having sleep issues.

• *Melatonin* is a hormone that is released in the pineal gland. It helps to regulate the sleep wake cycle. Melatonin is released in total darkness and is often referred to as the "hormone of darkness." No food product is known to contain melatonin. Melatonin can be purchased over the counter or as a dietary supplement. It should be taken with an acidic drink such as orange juice or apple juice as most over the counter preparations contain other ingredients. The acidy of the drink will break down these undesirable ingredients. Take the melatonin several hours before your desired bedtime (preferably 1 to 5 hours before) and be sure your room is completely dark, as the melatonin will be more effective. Check with your doctor for dosaging. Use caution with liquid preparations of Melatonin as they could contain 7% to 13% alcohol. [2]
Possible side effects of melatonin are that it may lower blood pressure and one report showed that melatonin increased seizure activity in children with significant neurological conditions and seizures.[3]

• *Valerian Root*: See Description under Anxiety

• *Warm Milk* contains Tryptophan, an amino acid that promotes sleep naturally. Try drinking warm milk and honey before bedtime.

• *Glutamine* also causes sedation when taken at night,

however, caution-taking glutamine since it has similar properties as beta-blockers. It can also lower heart rate and lead to chest pains.

Joint Pain

Try taking a liquid fish oil (Omega) supplement. Be sure the fish oil comes from sardines and not a larger fish. Liquid fish oil will get digested faster and will be less rough on your stomach.

Miscellaneous Natural and Alternative Medicines

- *Counter maneuvers* can help to decrease symptoms by lessening the amount of blood that pools in the legs. Useful counter maneuvers include: standing with your legs crossed, sitting in a low chair, sitting in the knee to chest position, leaning forward with your hands on your knees when sitting and tightening the buttocks, thigh and leg muscles when standing (particularly when standing for any length of time). Research shows that tensing the leg muscles while standing enhances brain blood flow. [4] Squatting can also be a useful counter maneuver, although some patients report an increase in symptoms after squatting.
- *Correcting anemia* has been shown to improve orthostatic tolerance. A simple blood test can determine if you are anemic.
- *Cranio-Sacral Therapy* is an alternative therapy for many POTS patients. It is not invasive and can relieve symptoms in some patients.

Cranial manipulation has been practiced in India for centuries. The ancient Egyptians and members of the Paracus culture in Peru first developed it in 2000 B.C.

Cranio-Sacral Therapy (CST) was pioneered and developed in the United States, by osteopathic physician John E. Upledger following broad scientific studies from 1975 to 1983 at Michigan State University, where he served as a clinical researcher and Professor of Biomechanics.

CST is a gentle, hands-on method of enhancing the functioning of a physiological body system called the cranio-sacral system. The cranio-sacral system is comprised of the membranes and cerebrospinal fluid that protects the brain and spinal cord.

Using soft touch, practitioners release restrictions in the cranio-sacral system to improve the functioning of the central nervous system. By complementing the body's natural healing processes, CST is frequently used as a preventive measure to augment resistance to disease, and is effective for a wide range of medical problems associated with pain and dysfunction, including: chronic fatigue, headaches, chronic neck and back pain, central nervous system disorders, traumatic brain and spinal cord injuries, stress and tension, fibromyalgia, orthopedic problems, connective tissue disorders, neurovascular and immune disorders, sinusitis, digestive issues, insomnia, temporo-mandibular joint (TMJ) problems, motor coordination impairments, and more. [5]

When looking for a practitioner to perform cranio-sacral therapy, it is best to consult with your team of physicians for a recommendation. Cranio-sacral therapists are an unlicensed group and are not doctors. Cranial osteopaths, on the other hand, are fully licensed doctors of osteopathic medicine (medical physicians), having gone to medical school, passed medical boards and as such have a deeper and broader knowledge of the human body. The cranial osteopath will most likely have a better understanding of POTS.

• *Elevating the head* of the bed by 4 to 12 inches has helped some POTS patients become less symptomatic. It has been reported that elevating the head of the bed generates mechanisms that expand plasma volume (6). Sleeping on a wedged pillow or incline can achieve a similar affect.

- *HAWTHORN* was once used as a "living fence" in much of Europe. Besides protecting estates from trespassers, hawthorn has also been used medicinally since ancient times. Roman physicians used hawthorn as a heart drug in the first century AD.

During the Middle Ages, hawthorn was used for the treatment of dropsy, a condition we now call congestive heart failure. It was also used for treating other heart ailments as well as for sore throat.

Today hawthorn is believed to be a safe and effective treatment for congestive heart failure (CHF). Like other treatments used for CHF, hawthorn improves the heart's ability to pump more effectively and may therefore help to lessen some bothersome symptoms of POTS and other forms of Dysautonomia.

- *Glutamine and B6*: Glutamine is an amino acid that is released in small amounts by the brain and lungs. Glutamine helps to protect the lining of the gastrointestinal tract known as the mucosa. Clinical studies have found that glutamine supplements may strengthen the immune system and can reduce infections (particularly infections associated with surgery).

If you try glutamine, divide your doses throughout the day, as it can cause constipation. Large amounts of glutamine may also be hard on weak kidneys. Make sure you have adequate supplies of coenzyme B6 before using glutamine. Coenzyme B6 is needed to convert glutamic acid into GABA. GABA is the calming, or "peacemaker" chemical in the brain, GABA induces relaxation, reduces stress and anxiety, and increases alertness.

Excess glutamine can cause an imbalance that can contribute to seizures. Anyone prone to seizures should be very wary of using glutamine.

When taken properly the combination of Glutamine and B6 can reduce headaches and can help promote restful sleep in some patients who have Dysautonomia.

Glutamine and B6 also stimulate the hypothalamus and can regulate women's menstrual cycles.

- *Ice* has reportedly helped some POTS patients. Rubbing ice on the body, especially on the bottom of the feet or neck, may help some POTS patients ward off an episode. In our family we like to use bags of frozen peas as ice. This conforms nicely to the body.

- *Stay well hydrated.* Drinking plenty of fluids, preferably ionized water is critical to the well-being of patients who have Dysautonomia. This does not include soda, which has a very high positive ORP and may actually be more harmful to patients with Dysautonomia. Fluids help to increase blood pressure as well as blood volume. Drinking water or other liquids that contain added electrolytes may prove especially fruitful. Often drinking water before getting out of bed in the morning may help lessen feelings of dizziness and other symptoms. It is recommended that patients drink approximately eight, eight ounce glasses of liquid a day. [7] Warning: Drinking too many liquids can cause an electrolyte imbalance, which can potentially lead to an abnormal heart rhythm.

- *Manganese* is a supplemental nutrient that helps retain salt in the body. Manganese is an essential nutrient for enhancing low sodium levels. Often, a craving for table salt is due to a manganese deficiency. Other specific nutrients, which assist adrenal activity and sodium retention, are potassium, vitamin B-1, vitamin B-5, vitamin C and vitamin E.

- *Magnesium* is used by every organ in the body; especially the heart, muscles and kidneys need the mineral magnesium. [8] Magnesium may prove to be one of the most essential supplements for those with POTS and Orthostatic Intolerance. Studies in the late 80's and early 90's, done originally on patients with MVP (Mitral Valve Prolapse) and orthostatic intolerance, have shown that the majority of these patients were deficient in magnesium. A magnesium deficiency can cause many of the symptoms associated with POTS. Magnesium is sometimes suggested for people who have *Ehlers Danlos Syndrome.* Some patients report a decrease in heart arrhythmias after taking magnesium on a daily basis.

Many Americans do not get enough magnesium from their diets and thus may benefit from supplements. Foods rich in magnesium include whole grains, nuts, and green vegetables. Green leafy vegetables are particularly good sources of magnesium.

• *Nuun* Tablets are a sugar-free, electrolyte flavored drink that contain Vitamin C, magnesium, calcium, and riboflavin. Nuun recharges your salts without sugars or carbohydrates and is absorbed more effectively than most leading sports drinks.

• *Protein, vitamin C, and all vitamins of the B* group have been found beneficial in preventing and treating low blood pressure. Of these, pantothenic acid is of particular importance. Liberal use of this vitamin alone often helps in raising the blood pressure. A diet that contains adequate quantities of complete proteins, B vitamin and, particularly, the nutrients that stimulate adrenal production, quickly normalizes low blood pressure.

• *Treating allergies* might help one to feel better. It has been reported that people with POTS lose their ability to vasoconstrict. [9] This means that many POTS patients have problems with their blood vessels being excessively dilated. Histamine is known to dilate blood vessels, which can further lower blood pressure in POTS patients. Many people who have POTS have allergies. Finding out exactly what you are allergic to, should help to alleviate at least some of your symptoms.

Avoiding foods that are high in histamines may also help to alleviate some symptoms. Some foods that are high in histamines include: dairy products, spinach, pineapple, corn, tomatoes, cream sauces, strawberries, red wine, wheat and wheat products, eggplant, bananas, pasta, cakes made with wheat flour, oatmeal, pinto beans and black beans.

The following supplements help lower histamines and are used as alternative treatments for allergies: Quercetain, Stinging Nettles Leaf, Bromelain, and Butterbur. This list is not all-inclusive; there are many more that can be found on the web. Orthomolecular makes D-Hist Jr., which contains a combination of these.

- *Vitamin C* is the body's basic support for connective tissue. Vitamin C is required for the synthesis of collagen; it helps collagen in connective tissue. It plays a vital role in the formation of collagen, a structural protein in connective tissue, amino acid metabolism and hormone synthesis, and the utilization of many nutrients, such as folic acid and iron. It is also a key factor in the body's immune system. Vitamin C is required for the production of collagen, a protein necessary for the formation of connective tissue in muscles, skin, bones, and cartilage. Vitamin C also plays an important role in the synthesis of the neurotransmitter, Norepinephrine. Neurotransmitters are critical to brain function and are known to affect mood. It has been postulated that Vitamin C may be beneficial for those who have Ehlers-Danlos Hypermobility Syndrome.

- *Vitamin D* is found in many dietary sources such as fish, eggs, fortified milk, and cod liver oil. The sun also contributes significantly to the daily production of vitamin D, and as little as ten minutes of exposure is thought to be enough to prevent deficiencies. [10] Most people, especially in the Mid-west have low vitamin D levels. This is also true of those that have Dysautonomia. A good Vitamin D supplement may help counteract some of the symptoms of Dysautonomia. You should have your vitamin D level checked prior to starting Vitamin D. If low, there are recommended guidelines that your physician will suggest. If you have adequate vitamin D levels, they may not recommend any supplements. Most people will remain in a normal level from 1000 – 4000 IU daily. Caution though, as you can also become toxic if taking too much vitamin D. People who live further away from the equator, in northern areas, where there is less sun exposure are particularly prone to low vitamin D levels.

References:

1. Dysautonmia Information Network (Dinet.org) POTS Place: A Guide to Postural Orthostatic Tachycardia Syndrome.

2. Tan D.X., L.D. Chen, B. Poeggeler, L.C. Manchester, R.J. Reiter (1993) Melatonin: a potent, endogenous hydroxyl radical scavenger. Endocrine J. 1: 57-60

3. Lounsbury ML, Bates JE: The Cries of Infants of Differing Levels of Perceived Temperamental Difficultness: Acoustic Properties and Effects on Listeners. Child Dev. 1982; 53:677-686)

4. Niels H. Secher , Johannes J. van Lieshout, Frank Pott, Per Lav Madsen, Jeroen van Goudoever   Cerebral Artery Blood Velocity Muscle Tensing During Standing : Effect Cerebral Tissue Oxygenation 2001; 32:1546-1551.

5. Kern, Michael DO., R.C.S.T., M.I. Cr.A., N.D. Introduction to Biodynamic Craniosacral Therapy Available at: craniosacraltherapy.org. 2003

6. Low, P. A. Autonomic neuropathies. Current Opinion in Neurology, October 1994: vol. 7, 402 - 406.

7. Low, P. A., Schondorf, R., Novak, V., Sandroni, P., Opfer-Gehrking, T. L., & Novak, P. Postural Tachycardia Syndrome. In P.A. Low (Ed.), Clinical Autonomic Disorder. 681 - 697. Philadelphia: Lippincott-Raven Publishers; 1997

8. Johnson S. The multifaceted and widespread pathology of magnesium deficiency. Med Hypotheses. 2001; 56(2): 163-170. Available at: www.umm.edu/altmed/articles/magnesium

9. Grubb, B. P. Orthostatic intolerance. National Dysautonomia Research Foundation Patient Conference. Minneapolis, Minnesota. July 2000.

10. Vitamin D; Mayoclinic.com. Accessed August 1, 2011.

Chapter 28. The Basics of Going Gluten Free

Removing wheat from your diet might be one of the most beneficial, non-invasive, non-pharmaceutical things you can do to help decrease some of your POTS symptoms. While no scientific research has been done to evaluate the impact of a gluten free diet on POTS patients, anecdotally, we hear from many patients who have switched to a gluten free diet and stick with it because they have noticed an improvement in their symptoms. POTS patients have reported improvement in their gastrointestinal symptoms, rashes, hives, flushing, joint pain, headaches and migraines after switching to a strict gluten free diet. It may not work for everyone, but if you try it and it helps relieve some of your symptoms, it may be well worth the effort.

In the book Wheat Belly, author Dr. William Davis, a re-nowned cardiologist, says that wheat we find at the grocery store today is not the same wheat that our grandparents ate 50 years ago. It has been completely genetically modified and no longer even resembles the wheat that was once only in our pizzas, pastas, breads and bagels. Modern wheat consists of many components; for our purposes, we will mostly discuss gluten and how this component can wreak havoc on the human body.

Gluten is a collection of proteins that are found in wheat. Gluten is what determines the characteristics of baking properties like firmness, ability to stretch, chewiness, crust formation, etc. [1] Now, no longer just used in baked items, modern gluten is used as an additive and is found practically everywhere, from licorice to seasoning mixes. It is found in frozen foods, deli meats, granola bars, soy sauce and instant soups (many of which the average POT-Sy lives on due to quick protein and high sodium count). Why, you ask? Because it is abundant, cheap to produce and, according to Dr. Davis, acts as an opiate on the brain and produces addictive cravings for more. This all adds up to more money for the food industry, but at what cost to us as consumers, who often experience poor health due to this protein?

According to Dr. Davis, gluten is responsible for increased inflammation in our bodies, thus leading to poor health and eventual disease. He believes that gluten is the culprit in many health conditions today - ranging from acid reflux to diabetes. Davis strongly believes that no one can escape the ill effects of gluten (whether or not you have symptoms now), and he advocates that we should all remove gluten from our diets, even if we do not have a sensitivity or intolerance for the protein.

Going gluten-free can be more expensive, and this is one of the primary reasons why some patients seem unwilling to give it a try. However, add up the cost of doctor appointments, ER visits and hospital stays and this argument is not as valid. Even if going gluten-free reduces these visits by five percent, it seems like a positive trade-off. Also, preparing many gluten-free foods from scratch and not buying prepared gluten-free items, which are not as healthy anyway, will help make this transition more cost effective.

Many patients have attempted to go gluten-free at one point and have not seen many changes in symptoms, at least not enough to stay committed to this lifestyle. After all, it is not easy and can be quite inconvenient, especially when you are first learning about it. It is possible that those that have tried to go gluten-free and have not been successful may not have noticed improvements of symptoms for one of the following reasons:

1. Going gluten-free may require up to a month or more of commitment to notice any significant changes in health.

Some people will see improved symptoms after several days, while others may even experience worsened symptoms for a few days as they experience what is known as wheat withdrawal.

2.   Many people try to replace their favorite gluten-filled products, such as pastas, breads, bagels and baked items, with gluten-free alternatives. Keeping too many of these in your diet still raises your blood sugar levels and these alternatives can cause their own health issues. Instead, try eating more single-ingredient natural foods, like fresh fish, meats found in the butcher shop, and organic fruits and vegetables.

3.   A lot of people who try to go gluten-free make the mistake of not fully understanding what has gluten in it and what does not. Many foods that you think are gluten-free might actually not be and, therefore, you think you are completely gluten-free but in fact are still inadvertently digesting the protein. For that reason, it is prudent to study up on all things gluten before attempting this routine. Simply reading this chapter will not give you enough information to make this change properly. You will need to do more research, stock your cabinets and refrigerator with fresh gluten-free foods and ingredients, as well as prepare your kitchen and your family for this new lifestyle.

The following should help you have a better understanding of the foods you can and cannot eat but in no way should this serve as your only resource to making the transition to gluten-free.   The following list is just a starting point to teach you the very basics. It will be up to the reader to learn more and do his or her own research.

Basic gluten-free foods include:

- Fresh meats, fish and poultry (not breaded, batter-coated, fried or marinated)
- Fruits
- Most dairy products
- Vegetables
- Wine and most liquors

Grains and starches allowed in a gluten-free diet include:

- Amaranth
- Arrowroot
- Buckwheat
- Corn
- Cornmeal
- Gluten-free flours (rice, soy, corn, potato, bean)
- Hominy grits
- Polenta
- Potatoes
- Pure corn tortillas
- Quinoa
- Rice
- Tapioca

Always check labels to make sure your foods haven't been contaminated with gluten during processing.

Be sure to avoid the following products in your food or drinks. They always contain gluten:

- Barley
- Bulgur
- Durham (also spelled durum, durhum)
- Farina
- Graham flour
- Kamut
- Matzo meal
- Rye
- Semolina
- Spelt
- Triticale
- Wheat

Avoid these foods/drinks unless they are specifically labeled 'gluten-free' or if you can confirm with the manufacturer that the product is gluten-free.

Also, check all labels to see that the item is processed in a facility that is free of wheat:

- Bacon
- Beers
- Breads
- Bread crumbs
- Candies
- Cakes and pies
- Cereals
- Cookies
- Crackers

- Croutons
- Gravies
- Imitation meats or seafood
- Marinades
- Mayonnaise
- Oats
- Pancake and waffle mixes
- Pastas
- Processed luncheon meats and sausages
- Salad dressings
- Sauces (including soy sauce)
- Seasoning mixes
- Self-basting poultry
- Soups

Hidden sources of gluten and other products that you come in contact with on a daily basis may also contain gluten.   Some of these include:

- Chewing gum (some brands are gluten-free)
- Cottage cheeses (some brands are gluten-free)
- Dextrimaltose
- Emulsifiers
- Hydrolyzed vegetable protein
- Hydrolyzed wheat starch
- Licorice candies (natural licorice root is gluten-free)
- Lipstick and lip balms (some brands are gluten-free)
- Malt, malt flavoring and maltodextrin (malt is made from barley)

- Medications and vitamins that use gluten as a binding agent
- Modified food starch (modified food starch made in the US is made from corn)
- Natural Flavors
- Stabilizers
- Textured vegetable protein
- Toothpaste (most popular brands are gluten-free, but just double check the manufacturer's website)

Some of my personal favorite gluten-free products include:

Bacon:
- Boar's Head
- Apple Gate

Bakery Items:
- All Pamela's Products, especially the pancake mix and chocolate chip cookie mix
- Enjoy Life brand, especially the double chocolate brownie cookies
- Glutino Breakfast Bars (strawberry, cherry and blueberry)
- Udi's Muffins

Bread and Buns:
- Udi's white
- Udi's whole grain

Cereals:

- EnviroKidz organic gluten-free cereals, especially Amazon Frosted Flakes and Leapin Lemurs (peanut butter and chocolate)
- General Mills - Chex - gluten-free cereals
- Kellogg's Rice Krispies gluten-free (note, the regular Kellogg's Rice Krispies are not gluten-free because they contain malt)
- Puffins – Honey Rice Cereal

Pastas:

- DeBoles gluten-free
- Quinoa gluten-free

Sandwich Dressings and Spreads:

- Hellmann's Mayonnaise
- Veganaise

Snack Foods:

- Colby's Kettle Corn (low in calories, as well)
- Glutino's gluten-free pretzels
- Snyder's gluten-free pretzels
- Hersey's Chocolate
- Kernel Fabyan's popcorn
- Kind Bars
- Pirates Booty - corn and rice puffs
- Mr. Krispers Baked Rice Krisps (sour cream and onion)

- Snikiddy baked fries
- Trader Joe's or Tate's gluten-free chocolate chip cookies

Soups:
- Health Valley gluten-free chicken noodle soup
- Health Valley gluten-free vegetable noodle soup
- Swanson Chicken Broth, Chicken Stock or Beef Stock

Soy Sauce:

Tamari Sauce (note, regular soy sauce has wheat in it, but tamari is a higher quality soy sauce that does not contain wheat)

More and more restaurants are now offering delicious gluten-free options, making it easier than ever to be gluten-free. There is a fantastic new app called Find Me Gluten Free. It is compatible with many mobile devices. Find Me Gluten Free helps you locate gluten-free friendly restaurants in whatever area you happen to be in. It allows you to view ratings and reviews, browse gluten-free menus, get directions, and call restaurants right from the app.

Going gluten-free may be one of the most life-altering, beneficial decisions you ever make towards better health. There is little to lose and much to gain. For more information on going gluten-free, check out any of the great resources below:

- The G-Free Diet: A Gluten-Free Survival Guide [Paperback] by: **Elisabeth Hasselbeck**
- Wheat Belly: Lose the Wheat, Lose the Weight, and Find Your Path Back to Health [Hardcover] by: **William Davis, MD**

- Wheat-Free, Worry-Free: The Art of Happy, Healthy Gluten-Free Living [Paperback] by: **Danna Kornhttp**

Reference:
1. Davis, William MD. (2011). Wheat Belly: Lose the Wheat, Lose the Weight, and Find your Path Back to Health. New York, NY: Rodale Inc.

Chapter 29. Yoga, Meditation and Spirituality - *Lynda Dresher, Cantor*

Cantor Lynda Hope Dresher, Cantor.

Spirituality and Meditation for the Soul; Gaining Control of the I in sick.

It is at these times when we feel the worst, when we cannot continue, when our pains and negativity consume us that we find our deeper purpose, our greatest joy and our divine spark that keeps us going. We are struck by our amazing courage and resilience. We see that what may look like a curse is actually a blessing and sometimes the other way around. We know that we cannot blame our circumstances on others; it is always about us, what we can learn from it and how we can grow our souls.

We find ourselves surrounded by angels who give so much of themselves to us. We find that we are in turn their angels, for we continue to show that there is hope, faith and love in spite of our insurmountable challenges. We know that being a victim and saying *"why me,"* is the path to self-destruction. We know that we can change our attitude from negative to positive in a heartbeat. We can move from *"why me"* to *"why not me."* From, *"poor me,"* to *"amazing me,"* to *"my life has no meaning"* to *"my life has a deeper purpose."*

So, how can we live a full and meaningful life when our bodies are so tired, so dizzy, unfocused and in pain? We can start by opening up our hearts and understanding that we are not our bodies and we are not our disease. As Eckhard Tolle says, *"When we label ourselves, we limit ourselves."* We begin to believe that we are only capable of just so much. We start believing that we are the disease. The disease becomes our identity. We eradicate ourselves.

Our body is the vessel for the soul within us. Our body will eventually wither and die, but our soul is eternal. It is pure energy and formless. Love has no form, yet we give and receive it all the time. We know that there is a greater power that guides us and nurtures us but we cannot see it, yet we seek its presence.

Because we are human, we feel that we are separate and apart from the divine. We feel isolated and alone. This is our ego talking to us. It wants to have power and seeks all of our attention. It complains, it worries, it brings up hurtful experiences of the past that we regurgitate over and over again. Our ego tends to pull us down, puff us up, make someone wrong, control everything, judge the world, make us the victim and isolate ourselves. All in all, it causes pain and suffering. Once we realize that we are not our egos, we can begin to put space between our *"higher self"* and the *"little me"* which is the ego. If the divine is *"everything,"* how can we also exist separate? We cannot. We are all created in the essence of the divine and therefore connected to every human being. We are part of the whole. We cannot control our ego, just as we cannot control our circulation or our heart beat. We can, however, become the witness to our ego. We can recognize when we are being egocentric and choose to replace those self-centered thoughts with expressions of loving kindness. We can choose, because we have *"free will"* to decide to bring a sense of wholeness and peace into our heart and soul. We can choose to turn a negative thought into a life affirming one. Meditation can help us achieve this. Meditation helps quiet the mind and reduce the static in the brain. Through meditation, we realize that this is the only moment that counts. The last moment is history, the future is a mystery and the present is a *"gift."* That is why it is a called a *"present."* When we are fully engaged in the present moment, in a state of *"being"*, we are connected to the divine, which is "being." The ego does not exist in the present moment. We can find peace within our minds and souls. It is our place of refuge. During meditation, it is possible to find this quiet, sacred space for a few moments. The more we can focus and pay attention in the present moment, the more success we will have. We will begin to experience clarity of mind and spirit. From that happiness immerges within us. It is a manifestation of what is.

Meditation slows down our impulsive reactions to daily stress.

Lizabeth Roemer, Ph.D. a professor of psychology at the University of Massachusetts, Boston writes, *"when we are stressed, we breathe shallowly from our chest which triggers the sympathetic nervous system, the flight reaction. If you inhale and exhale more deeply, that activates the opposite, parasympathetic response."* London-based clinical hypnotherapist Georgia Foster writes, *"Your body physically settles down. This type of relaxation prompts the release of feel-good endorphins which can buffer against the biological response to stress."*

When meditating, one concentrates on their breathing to quiet the mind. We pay attention and set our intention. With every breath, we open our souls. We open to the nameless energy of life that just is, to the power of pure awareness, the light of presence. This helps us experience life with greater ease and a sense of calm. It gives us the tools we need to live in the moment.

When we are present, without ego, we notice that we are not judging others or ourselves. We are totally accepting of what is. Acceptance of our life brings us complete healing. We know that we cannot change or control life, we must allow it to be as it is. This brings a sense of freedom and surrender. The Kabbalists (Jewish mystics) also teaches us that during our darkest moment, if we surrender ourselves to God's *"will,"* we bring in the divine light. We experience a greater wisdom, faith and happiness. We are not alone, we are protected.

As part of the whole, we are governed by a *"higher power"*. When we are in the moment, we sense the oneness, the interconnection of all beings. Our senses become acute and there is a newness and freshness. We are overcome by our sense of awe and gratitude for our lives. Because we are awake to our existence in the world, we feel compelled to reach out to others. What can we do to bring joy and love into the world and show our gratitude? Our lives become a blessing to ourselves and others. We understand that we can make a difference in this world. Our joyful energy lights up a room.

We can change the world with one smile, one kind word, one touch of the hand, one hug, one kiss. We experience a profound awakening that the divine needs more angels to spread the love because, "love is all there is!"

Use these life affirming reminders and ideas throughout your day to fuel your soul:

Life Affirming Reminders

- I am life
- I am a blessing
- I am grateful
- I am okay
- I can
- I accept what is
- I learn from every experience
- I am the light
- I am the knowing
- I know that everything is impermanent
- I am a positive person
- I am empowered to spread goodness and love
- I am inspired by everything
- I find value in myself and others
- I am perfect just the way I am
- I love myself
- I love my life
- I bring love and compassion to everyone I know
- I value everyone's opinion
- I know we are all connected

Ideas to awaken inspiration

- Meditate twice a day

- Put on music that makes you feel good
- Surround yourself with positive people
- Write positive messages on your bedroom mirror
- Keep a journal of your daily thoughts
- In your journal, every day list 4 things you are thankful for
- Treat yourself to a bubble bath
- Treat yourself to a favorite meal
- Always remember to be thankful daily
- Read your favorite book
- Keep a book of inspiring quotes near your bed
- Reference online inspiringstories.com; read about other people's challenges
- Use your talents to help others
- Inspire others by telling your story
- Be creative; write, draw, sing, dance, etc.
- Laugh several times a day
- Find humor in every day experiences
- Give hugs and kisses daily
- Practice compassion and patience daily
- Open your heart to others daily
- Show compassion to strangers
- Volunteer in your community
- Participate in prayer

Meditation Exercise I

Sit in a comfortable chair. Close your eyes. Take in 3 cleansing breathes. Now, focus on your breath. See how long it takes to take in a breath, how long you expand your lungs and rib cage and how slowly you let the breath out, deflating your lungs. Pay attention to everything about your breath and how your body feels as you inhale and exhale. Feel a sense of gratitude that you are capable of breathing. Listen to the sounds your nose and mouth make as you take in and let out the breath. Feel your body relax every time you inhale and exhale. When thoughts come into your mind, go back to paying attention to your breath. Do this exercise for 10 minutes twice a day.

Meditation Exercise II

Concentrating on your breath is important but you can expand this exercise to hearing, breath, body and feelings.

First, listen to the sounds around you for four breaths. Then, take in 4 breaths, paying attention to every inhale and exhale. Then, start with the top of your head and work your way down to your feet, paying attention to every part of your body as you relax each part. Then, see how you are feeling, are you anxious, worried, happy, content, etc. Then start the cycle over. If your thoughts side track you, when you realize you are thinking, go back to the beginning of the cycle.

Chapter 30. Home Workouts - *Dave Warren, personal trainer*

Postural Orthostatic Tachycardia Syndrome and Beginning Home Exercise Programs.

Medical Disclaimer:

This publication contains the opinions and ideas of its authors. It is intended to provide helpful and informative material in the subjects addressed in the publication. It is sold with the understanding that the authors and publisher are not engaged in rendering medical, health, or any other kind of personal and/or professional services in this book. The reader should consult his or her medical, health, alternative or other competent professional before adopting any of the suggestions in this book or drawing inferences from it. The authors and publisher specifically disclaim all responsibility for any liability, loss or risk, personal or otherwise, which is incurred as a consequence, directly or indirectly, of the use and application of any of the contents of this book.

As with any exercise program, it is imperative to seek the advice of your medical team before beginning any exercise program. Many of the following exercises may need the assistance of a personal trainer or other qualified exercise specialist.

It is critical to stay well hydrated before, during and after exercising. Many doctors may also suggest adding extra salt or electrolytes to your diet, following workouts. Seek the advice of your doctor as to how he/she would like you to rehydrate following exercising.

Those who think they have not time for bodily exercise will sooner or later have to find time for illness. - Edward Stanley

I believe that POTS is a gravity issue. Perhaps this is why many astronauts come back from prolonged space flight with this condition (although temporarily). With this theory in mind, I have come up with a very effective home exercise program for patients who have POTS and other forms of Dysautonomia.

In healthy individuals, standing up causes the blood vessels in the lower extremities to compensate by constricting. In individuals with POTS, this autonomic process does not happen efficiently, often resulting in a drastic (30 BPM) increase in heart rate and often accompanied by a sharp drop in blood pressure. This leaves these individuals light headed as not enough blood (oxygen) reaches the brain. It also leaves this population with tachycardia, severe fatigue (as the heart has to work three times harder than that of a healthy individual), and a multitude of other symptoms.

When I met Nikki, a 13-year-old client, who presented with POTS, this was the case. In order to address Nikki's POTS and her contraindicated exercise, I needed to come up with a unique strategy that would address her elevated heart rate, drop in blood pressure and decreased exercise tolerance (ability to exercise). The strategy I came up with was extremely simple yet very effective. I took gravity out of the equation. I gave Nikki kinetic activities (exercises) that she could do in a horizontal position involving mostly lower body, legs, and her core. I used vertical loading (one different exercise after another different exercise, repeating this sequence a couple of times in a row). My goal was to increase muscular hypertrophy, which would maintain rigidity (stiffness) in the blood vessels due to the increased muscle tone and tension in the legs. This would aid in keeping the blood from pooling in her lower extremities, which would allow her to increase her exercise tolerance. By not putting Nikki into a vertical position, her heart rate did not elevate and her blood pressure did not drop. Over time, Nikki's exercise tolerance increased, allowing her to increase the intensity of her workouts. She was then able to progress to more strenuous exercises for longer durations of time.

Even though Nikki still has POTS, she was able to develop enough exercise endurance to resume gymnastics, a sport that she has been passionate about since she was a young girl. Many doctors told Nikki that she would no longer be able to participate in this sport. Together, we were able to prove these physicians wrong.

Although Nikki's situation is atypical, the exercise protocol I used for her can be beneficial in most cases of Dysautonomia. This type of exercise programming can at least be a good starting point. Of course, benefits and results may vary depending on the uniqueness of each case of Dysautonomia.

The exercises that would be most beneficial to those suffering from POTS could easily be done on any flat surface, like a bed or on a floor. The important consideration to be addressed is starting at the fitness level of the individual and their overall exercise tolerance.

Remember that POTS is a gravity disorder, so doing exercises in an upright or vertical position will only cause exacerbation of symptoms. With this in mind, I will provide some examples of basic exercises that can be done to help patients to recondition their muscles and get back on the road to recovery.

Please refer to exercise photos at the end of the chapter.

Stretching (each stretch is to be held for 30 seconds)
- Static piriformis stretch
- Static 90-90 hamstring stretch
- Static Erector spine cross leg stretch

Beginner Exercises:
1) Short Lever Crunches:
2) Pelvic lifts
3) Clam
4) Hip extension (prone)
5) Terminal leg extensions
6) Using your foot, write the letters of the alphabet. You can do small case letters and then do capital letters. You can mix it up further by printing the letter and then doing them

in cursive. Any combination will work.
7) Calf raise with a band.

These exercises should be done in a vertical loading fashion, meaning the individual would start with the first exercise, do it to completion and then go on to the next exercise until completing the entire circuit of exercises. The circuit should include 12-15 repetitions of each exercise, completing two sets of each. This tempo can be done as rapidly as the individual is able to do. The client's heart rate should be monitored during the circuit and should never go above 85% of the Maximal Heart Rate. The Maximal Heart Rate can be found by subtracting your age from 220 and your training Heart Rate Zone should be: 220 (Maximal Heart Rate) – 13 (age) * .85 = 175 (Beats Per Minute). This would be a safe heart range to train at.

For people who don't know how to check their heart rate you can check your radial pulse, which can be found on the inside part of the wrist underneath your thumb. To check your heart rate you can use a heart rate monitor. Don't forget that individuals with POTS are more likely to be deconditioned and may be unable to do even these relatively simple kinetic activities. The road to fitness is not always a straight path, but with perseverance and consistency the goal of fitness is almost always obtainable, like it was for Nikki.

Unfortunately, not everybody will see good results while exercising on their own. It is advised and necessary that individuals diagnosed with any autonomic dysfunction, consult with their medical team before working with a health and fitness professional. It is absolutely imperative that if you decide to do any of the exercise program described in this section, that you first discuss it with your physician that is treating your condition. It is my hope that through exercise you will be on the track to a complete and speedy recovery.

David Warren, NASM-CPT, is available to discuss further individualized programming to help you on the road to recovery. Please contact him at any time for a consultation. You can reach

David at 224-628-1455 or you can email him at home-
workouts@comcast.net

Exercise and POTS: How to conduct a proper intermediate workout

Contributed by David Warren- CPT- Through the National Academy
of Sports Medicine

But first things first!

Specific exercises are suggested, but first there are some
principles and concepts which should be understood and followed
for maximum benefit and minimal risk.

The most important thing to remember is that each person
will handle exercise differently so there is no way to anticipate the
exercise outcome for everyone who has POTS.

Everyone suffering with Dysautonomia should use exercise
to improve their health and their quality of life. As your fitness and
conditioning strengthen, you may notice improvement in daily
symptoms and functional status.

This exercise protocol can be used as a possible treatment
option for people suffering from POTS. This program may not be
suited for all individuals. You should always consult with your physician before starting any exercise program.

You must start with exercising the lower body since building
muscles in the legs will improve circulation to the heart and reduce
symptoms of orthostatic intolerance.

Start the initial exercise program while horizontal (stable
posture, resting on a supportive surface such as an exercise ball) to
remain orthostatically stable and without symptoms. Position your
body horizontally by using a resist-a-ball (exercise ball) in the prone
(facing down) or in the supine (facing up) position, keeping the body
at an angle less than 30 degrees. As in the studies, this will keep
your heart rate and blood pressure relatively stable.

To maintain neuromuscular efficiency, it is essential to

maintain flexibility in the muscles and maintain their functional range of motion. In other words, do not overwork the muscles and cause them to become tight and limited in their movement. You have to keep the proper "length tension" relationship and "force coupling" relationship in your muscles. This is due to the fact that each muscle has different attachment sites, pulls at different angles and creates different forces on the joints" (Clark, Corn, Parracino, 2002, p. 5). If you allow the muscles to shorten and tighten you will change their length tension relationship, which will reduce their functional range of motion. This will inhibit the muscles' normal range of motion as well as decrease or inhibit its normal ability to contract properly. One way we can offset this dysfunction in range of motion is through proper stretching. There are three forms of stretching: static, active, and dynamic. We will focus on the static stretches, which will be the simplest and easiest way towards keeping and increasing flexibility. Thus, adequate warm-up and cool down is important to avoid injury and avoid muscle tightness. Begin and end with stretching exercises.

> Note: See back of this chapter for pictures of all stretches and exercises.

Exersices:
Phase I Stretching
- Static piriformis stretch
- Static 90-90 Hamstring Stretch
- Static Erector Spinae Cross-leg stretch

Phase II Exercises - Performed while sitting or lying on the exercise ball.
- Short Lever Crunchies
- Chest press lying back on a stability ball with both feet on the ground
- YTA on a Stability Ball

- Shoulder abduction while sitting on a stability ball
- Bicep curls sitting on a stability ball with one foot off the ground
- Triceps kick-backs on ball

As you progress, more difficult exercises may be tried to create a "Peripheral Heart Action" workout. This programming uses a sequence of unstable upper body exercises in conjunction with lower body stable core exercises that were done in Phase I and Phase II. This process is referred to as "vertical loading" and requires one exercise using the upper body followed by a lower body exercise. Here is an example of how this might look:

Phase III
- Short lever crunchies
- Chest press on a stability ball
- Hip extensions stable
- YTA on a stability ball
- Hip abduction stable
- Scaption seated on ball one foot of the floor

Start Position:
Lie on your stomach on the stability ball, legs and feet extended with toes on the floor. Hold a light dumbbell in each hand with arms alongside of your body. Draw-in belly button; extend arms in front of body.

Movement:
Raise both arms, thumbs up, in front of body at 45-degree angle to eye level; do not shrug shoulders or arch back. Hold; return arms to side of body.

- Terminal leg extensions stable
- Bicep curls seats on a stability ball with one foot off the ground
- Triceps extensions on a stability ball

The set number of repetitions and sets would be 12-15 reps and 2 to 3 sets per exercise to develop improved levels of neuro-muscular control and functional strength. The Peripheral Heart action piece should also aid in giving cardiovascular benefit. The exercise should be done at 60% of maximal effort in regards to load (weight you lift). As your exercise tolerance increases individuals who suffer no exacerbations or contraindication to exercise can probably go to optimum performance training guidelines following NASM's training principles.

Remember individuals with POTS can unfortunately have some setbacks, so it is always important to keep an optimistic outlook towards life and focus on what you can do and not what you can't do. It is essential to look at exercise as a long-term investment towards overall well-being. This statement is especially true for individuals with POTS or any chronic illness.

What about aerobic cardiovascular training?

Cardio vascular training for individuals who have Dysautonomia most likely will have to be addressed when more exercise tolerance is developed. Here are some suggestions that may be helpful. It is imperative to consult with a doctor, physical therapist, or certified exercise specialist with expertise in working with individuals suffering with POTS. With this in mind, here are some cardiovascular activities you can try, provided there are no contraindications for you. These cardiovascular exercises are recommended because of their risk benefit ratio (there is very little risk compared to the benefit). Except for swimming, there will not be a great deal of expertise required to do these activities. Individuals with Dysautonomia who decide to do cardiovascular training must always check their blood pressure and heart rate. Training should be done at the low-end of your training heart rate zone before you increase resistance, duration, and frequency. Those individuals with POTS should start with 12-15 minute cardiovascular effort and see if they can tolerate this duration. It is important to point out that exercise is cumulative. Therefore, even if your cardio endurance is low during cardio in short durations, it will still cause cardiovascular benefit.

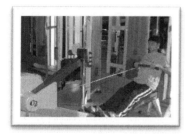

Rowing provides an excellent cardiovascular workout, which integrates your entire body. It is a great piece of equipment for the POTS patient as it enables one to work out in an almost supine position, thus helping to keep blood pressure and heart rate steady.

- **Walking in a pool**. Note: The water temperature should be no warmer than 80 degrees. Water temperature above 80 degrees may cause vascular dilation.
- **Swimming** which allows you to maintain horizontal position which will keep blood pressure and heart rate more constant and lower (Jalisco, 2008, p.575)
- **Stationary exercise bicycle** especially a recumbent bike, which enables your body to be in a reclined position.
- **UB-upper body ergometer**. This is an outstanding piece of equipment, especially for the POTS patient who finds their legs too weak to perform a complete aerobic workout. The UB will allow you to get your heart rate up (while in a sitting position) by just using your upper body.

How to determine your lowest training heart rate zone for cardiovascular exercise:

1) Calculate your maximum heart rate. Subtract your age from 220.

2) Multiple the results by 0.55, or 55%. This is the low end of your training range, and for individuals with Dysautonomia, it is the fastest rate your heart should beat when you

exercise.

Additional leg strengthening exercises.

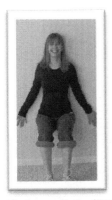

Wall Seat will build your endurance. Stand at a slight angle against the wall, heels twelve inches away, for 30 minutes twice a day. In some people, this results in a complete disappearance of the fainting episodes.

Additional Resources on Exercise:
Clark MA. Corn RJ. Optimum Performance Training for the Fitness Professional. Thousand Oaks, CA: National Academy of Sports Medicine; 2001
For more information concerning Integrative stabilization programming check on the National Academy of Sports Medicine website. (NASM)
How to Calculate and Use Your Training Heart Rate (eHow.com)

Stretching

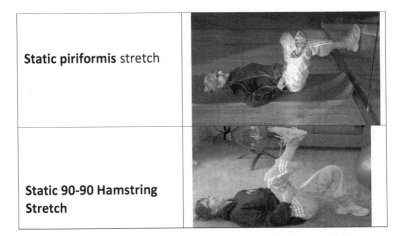

Static piriformis stretch	
Static 90-90 Hamstring Stretch	

Static Erector Spinae Cross-leg stretch	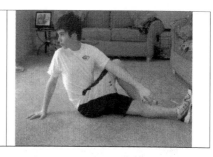

Short Lever Crunchies

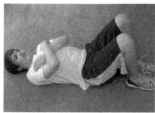   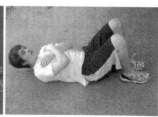

Diagram 1: Start Position   Diagram 2: Finish Position

Chest press *lying back on a stability ball with both feet on the ground*

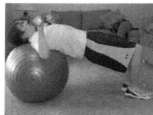   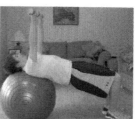

Diagram 1: Start Position   Diagram 2: Finish Position

YTA on a Stability Ball.

Diagram 1: Start – Y	Picture first to the left
Diagram 2: Mid - T	Picture Second to the left
Diagram 3: Finish – A	Picture Third to the left

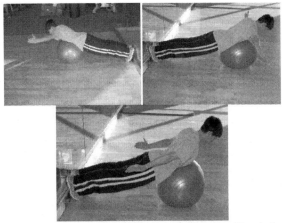

Lie face down on a stability ball with the toes of both feet on the ground. Raise your arms up into a Y shape - hold for a second. Move into a T shape - hold for a second, finally drop your arms into an A shape with your shoulders pulled slightly upward (Cobra) and hold for a second. Then drop your arms toward the floor. That is one repetition.

Shoulder abduction *while sitting on a stability ball*

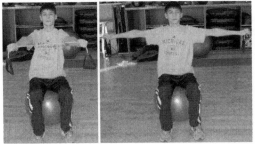

Diagram 1: Start Position Diagram 2: Finish Position

Bicep curls sitting on a stability ball with one foot off the ground.

Bicep curls sitting on a stability ball with one foot off the ground.
Diagram 1: Start Position
Diagram 2: Finish Position

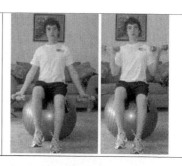

Triceps kick-backs on ball
Diagram 1: Start Position
Diagram 2 Finish Position

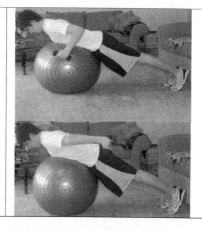

Short lever crunches- Start Position – Finish Position

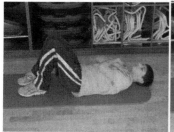 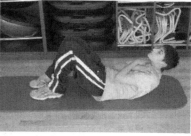

Chest press on a stability ball - *Start Position – Finish Position*

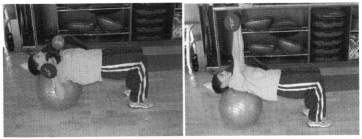

Hip extensions stable- Start Position — Finish Position

Pelvic lifts: Start Position – Finish Position

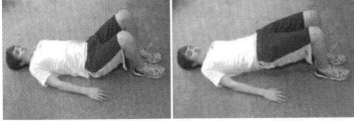

Calf raise with a band: Start Position – Finish Position.

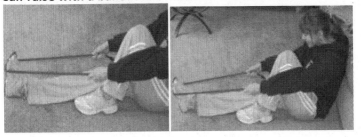

Hip extension (prone) Start Position – Finish Position

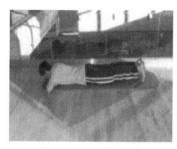
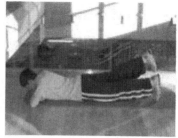

Terminal leg extensions Start Position – Finish Position

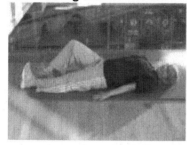
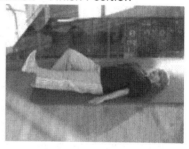

Writing the alphabet with your foot

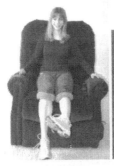
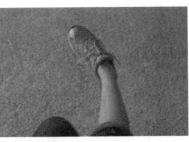

Hip extensions stable Start Position – Finish Position.

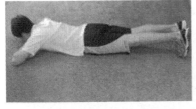
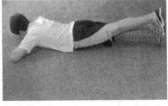

Hip abduction stable Start Position – Finish Position.

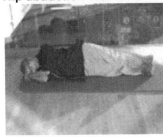
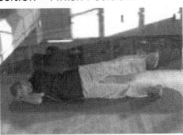

Scaption seated on ball one foot of the floor Start Position – Finish

Position.

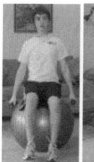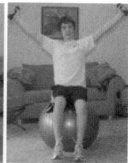

Clam Shells Start Position – Finish Position.

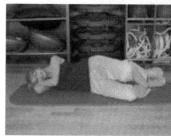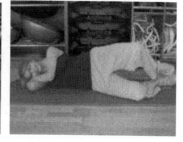

Section 9 - Inspiration

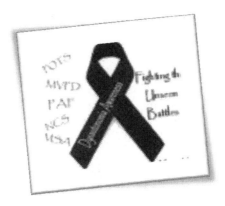

Chapter 31. Spreading Awareness

"If you think you are too small to be effective, you have never been in bed with a mosquito."   ~Betty Reese

Regarding public awareness, POTS may be where autism was twenty years ago – known only to those who were directly affected by it. Only through the efforts of those individuals did autism begin to gain awareness and needed attention. With awareness comes public concern for victims, which eventually leads to a call for research, prevention, treatment and a cure.

It is imperative that we who are affected by Dysautonomia collectively bond TOGETHER and form a UNITED FRONT to help spread awareness. Turning POTS and Dysautonomia into household names will assist in obtaining both federal and private funding that is desperately needed for research.

We must each do our share to help raise awareness. If those of us with Dysautonomia do not share our passion, or do not get active and involved in our communities, how can we expect others who are not directly impacted to care? It is our only hope for eventually defeating Dysautonomia, and providing our loved ones and future loved ones the effective interventions needed to live more active, fulfilling and healthier lives.

Here are some easy ways that you can help spread awareness about Dysautonomia.

Dysautonomia bracelets

You can purchase bracelets at www.dynakids.org.

Give or sell the bracelets to your child's teachers, your friends and family members. Ask them all to wear the bracelet in support of the person with POTS.

Declare a special day at your place of employment or school to wear the bracelets. When you give the bracelets out, include a brief description of Dysautonomia. Laminate the description, punch a hole in it and attach it to each bracelet with a red ribbon.

Schools

Go to your local school and ask if you can provide an informative session on Dysautonomia at a teacher's staff meeting.

Hold a similar session for all of the school nurses in the district.

Ask a speaker (one of your doctors) to come in and do the talking if you do not feel you want to take this on yourself.

Grocery stores

Initiate a "shop and share" where a percentage of the groceries sold on given days will go to any cause you choose, in this case, Dysautonomia.

You can leave handouts and set up posters at the store explaining this syndrome and why you are trying to raise money/awareness.

Newspapers

I have done this in Chicago, so any size market can be done! Your persistence will pay off.

Ask that the newspaper run an article on Dysautonomia. A reporter, such as a medical reporter if they have one, may want to interview you and/or one of your doctors to get information.

This would go perfect in the health section of the newspaper.

Television

Call all of the local TV stations. Ask that the station do a piece on Dysautonomia in their Health Beat or HealthWatch section of the news.

Radio Stations

Some radio stations will give away air time for a good cause.

Look for stations with morning or afternoon talk shows that focus on local issues. They may often conduct on-air interviews for interesting and new topics.

Ask them to do a segment on Dysautonomia. Parents of POTS kids, the kids themselves, and doctors treating Dysautonomia can make great guests for a call-in radio show.

Church or Synagogue

Ask your church or synagogue to help you organize a fundraiser for your cause. Some possible fundraisers include a community rummage sale, book fair, bake-off, Spirit Walk, etc.

Walk for Dysautonomia

Organize a walk! Ask your school, friends, neighbors and colleagues to participate with you.

Call the local newspapers, radio and TV stations to get free media attention. This is a great and inexpensive way to spread awareness.

Organize a Fundraiser

Garage sale, bake sale, lemonade stand, skate-a-thon, bowl-a-thon, dance-a-thon, sing-a-thon, car wash, book fair, raffle, silent auction, Bake and sell pies at Thanksgiving.

YouTube, FaceBook

Make a video with your friends.

Explain what Dysautonomia is and post a link on your FaceBook.

Be creative and make sure the information you are sharing is accurate. You can also share a poem, write a song, do a comedy act, or anything that grabs people's attention.

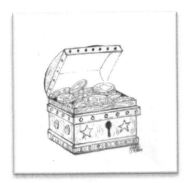

Fabulous and Easy Fundraiser Idea:

A friend of mine, whose son has Familial Dysautonomia, has been very successful with this simple fund-raiser. This idea was taken from FD NOW. (Familial Dysautonomia Now) on the next page is a sample flier.

Digging for Dysautonomia

Turn your gold into gelt (a Jewish word for money with a charitable purpose)!

Gather up your gold scraps, broken chains, mismatched earrings, old watches, gold coins, out-of-style charms, bangles, and bracelets you've thrown in a back drawer, jewelry box or safety deposit box.

Bring your gold to _____and have it immediately appraised for free by our reputable family jeweler. He will test and then weigh your scraps on site. You'll know instantaneously the total value of your gold. Bonus: He will also appraise your platinum!

The Gold Melt for Gelt is a wonderful opportunity to turn outdated jewelry into a tax-deductible donation that will help the lives of those who suffer from Dysautonomia, a debilitating condition that affects the autonomic nervous system and causes a myriad of complicated symptoms including: fainting, dizziness, migraines, fatigue, insomnia, shortness of breath, tachycardia, etc.

For example, if you donate a 14K old-style gold necklace valued at $500, you will receive a tax-deductible acknowledgment for $500; those funds will directly go toward Dysautonomia research/Awareness.

Gold prices are skyrocketing. Ten years ago, gold prices were in the $300 range/ounce. Today, gold prices have more than tripled and are now in the $1,700 range/ounce. In today's gold market, your scraps quickly add up. By collecting and then donating your outdated gold jewelry and spare gold pieces, you make a positive impact on the lives of people who suffer from Dysautonomia.

Your choice! Donate all or a portion of your appraisal.

Note: All you need to do is get a jeweler who will donate his time and help you with this fundraiser. You can arrange a drop off date at your house. Simply send out invitations to your family, friends, coworkers, etc... Make this even more enticing by adding door prizes, food, drinks, desserts, wine and cheese, etc. Add your own personal touches for a fundraiser that is sure to be a real goldmine.

Chapter 32. Poems and More Inspiration

A Ray of Hope

Some days the waves are small
Some days they are enormously tall

Sometimes an under toe takes me away
And sweeps me to the other side of the bay

And I struggle to swim back to shore
Sometime I feel like I can't take it anymore

I wish I could be in San Diego
Where the waves are calm and slow

But here I am in the Midwest
Always having to exercise and rest

I hate it the days when it rains
Because it worsens my joint pains

The waves go up and down so crazy
Just like my blood pressure and people call me lazy

But if a wave knocks me down
I will stand up and will not frown

I look up at the sun, trying to cope
I see in the sun a ray of hope

- Arielle Lobl, age 14

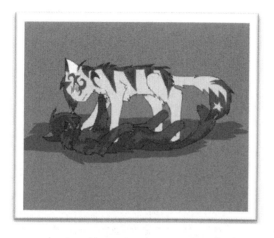

Picture by Sterling Midyett, age thirteen, AKA Meteorstar!
From Versailles, Missouri.

POTS, you will not win.

Section 10. Personal Narratives

Chapter 33. Inspirational Personal Narratives - *A variety of stories of people around the globe with varying degrees and types of Dysautonomia. Their journeys are filled with courage, strength and insurmountable inspiration.*

The following stories were written by POTS patients from around the globe who suffer from varying degrees of Dysautonomia. Their stories are heartwarming, moving and incredibly inspirational.

As each patient's journey with POTS is unique to them, their stories were purposefully not edited in order retain their voice and integrity.

It is my hope that when you read their extraordinary stories, you will be inspired by their strength, courage, determination and perseverance and will come to believe that undeniably "Together We Stand."

Lindsay Junck, 32-year-old female, California, United States of America (lindsayjunck@gmail.com)

In the summer of 2004, after I had completed my first year of law school, I did a six-week study abroad program in Prague, Czech Republic. During the program I became sick. I thought it was just a cold, but since have been told that it was probably a virus. It cleared up in a few days, and I was able to enjoy the rest of my time in Prague. About a month after I returned to the United States, I became ill with severe stomach pain. I couldn't keep food down and dwindled from a healthy weight of 132lbs to a frail 108lbs. I saw many doctors and underwent a plethora of tests, but no one could figure out what was wrong. I had to withdraw from law school, as I was unable to attend classes.

Finally, after about eight months of pain and frustration, I was diagnosed with gastroparesis. Fortunately, I have a mild case that can be controlled through lifestyle changes. I returned to law school the next year and managed to graduate and pass the California bar examination.

Fast forward to May 17, 2009, when I was spending time with friends at an outdoor festival. I began to feel sick and next thing I knew I had fainted on the street. I was taken to the ER and released with a diagnosis of "dehydration". However, in the days, weeks (and now years) that followed, I just didn't feel right. I was dizzy, my heart raced, I had difficulty with balance and suffered from extreme fatigue. I was sent from specialist to specialist who conducted test after test. I was given a diagnosis of iron deficiency anemia, but didn't feel any better a year later when my ferritin iron level returned to normal. A cardiologist to whom I was referred suspected orthostatic intolerance caused by the virus I acquired in Prague and ordered a tilt table test in February 2011. The test results led to a diagnosis of postural orthostatic tachycardia syndrome (POTS). Immediately after the test, the cardiologist came in the exam room, told me I had POTS, that I should drink a lot of water, and that I would never be able to have kids. No other instructions, no follow up appointment.

Fortunately, through the DINET website (www.dinet.org) I was able to meet other POTSies in my area. They recommended a great cardiologist located here in San Diego who is familiar with POTS, Dr. Thomas Ahern. At my first appointment with Dr. Ahern, he informed me that managing POTS involves more than just drinking a lot of water, but also assured me that it would not inhibit my ability to have children. Over the past year and a half, Dr. Ahern has helped me to feel better, but I still experience symptoms constantly. It is difficult for me to work, but I am single and do not have an alternative source of income. My employer does not provide health insurance, so I pay high monthly premiums for private insurance, as my preexisting condition makes me expensive to insure.

At this point I have only been diagnosed with POTS, but more tests may be forthcoming. I worry about whether it will ever be physically possible for me to stand across from the man of my dreams and say "I do", whether I will ever be a productive member of society, or just a drain on its resources. I'm learning to accept my POTS diagnosis; to declare that POTS is what I have, not what I am, but every day is a challenge. However, having POTS has introduced me to a wonderful community of amazing people I never knew existed: the POTS community.   By sharing our experiences, insights, hope and laughter, we are overcoming the challenges together.

Kristen Jakiel's story with Dysautonomia/POTS As seen from her mother's eyes. (Sonjia Jakiel)

This story is from a mother who has had to be a witness to all of this and not be able to do a thing for my daughter except comfort her. My daughter's name is Kristen. She is now 20 years old. I now look back and realize that things that happened with Kristen back when she was grammar school age now make sense.

Back in the summer of 2004, at the age of 14, Kristen got braces put on. She grew a few inches and unfortunately got kidney stones. She lost a lot of weight due to the pain from the stones. She was already having issues with passing out at this point.

Kristen started high school the fall of 2004. She actually made it through freshman and sophomore year without too many episodes of passing out but there were a lot of absences due to being sick and having pain from the kidney stones. In the Fall of Junior year 2006 was when she and I realized that this was more than just being sick with some sort of virus.

One of the classes she was taking was Chorus, which she loved the most. It was her passion. The passing out episodes happened more frequently in this class due to having to continually stand up and sit down. At this point the school had to call 911 for an ambulance several times. Obviously, at this point she couldn't participate in Gym either. She had also passed out during softball while standing out in the field. In February of 2007, she experienced a migraine that lasted for ten days straight. This symptom she had already been having but never this long. During this ten-day episode, she woke up one morning while I was getting ready for work. I made her breakfast. She took a pain reliever for the migraine and went back to bed. I told her to keep her cell and regular phone near her, so I could check on her later from work. I started calling her at about 11:30 A.M., and she was not answering. I kept trying on and off until 1pm and at that time I told my boss that I had to leave because something was not right. When I got home, I tried to wake her up. She would not move. I can't even begin to tell you in words what that felt like as a mother not knowing what was wrong with her. At this point she and I had thought that her body was breaking down or something. This was the scariest experience in my whole life. I can't even speak for her. I ended up having to call 911, because I couldn't get her to wake up. The dispatcher instructed me to check her pulse. I couldn't feel it. He then instructed me to pull her out of her bed onto the floor and put her head back to see if she was breathing. Meanwhile the paramedics were already on their way. Once I got her on the floor and put her head back she came to and grabbed a hold of me, and she was crying. The paramedics arrived and took her to the hospital. I don't know how I did all of this but somehow adrenalin took me over. Somehow as a mother it just happens.

After this episode, her neurologist decided to admit her into the hospital so he could treat her for this migraine. During this stay the cardiologist at the hospital did a tilt table test on her. This is a test that the table quickly tilts up to see how the heart reacts, and she blacked out. She was diagnosed with Postural Orthostatic Tachycardia Syndrome. Needless to say, she had to be tutored at home the remainder of her junior year.

In the fall of 2007, Kristen did go back to school for senior year. She wanted to experience what every other child of her age was able to experience. At this point she was still experiencing chronic fatigue, migraines, digestive issues, passing out, pain in her legs, and brain fog. She was able to stay in school until November and once again she had to be tutored at home until the end of the first semester. At this point she had only one semester left and only had to take one English class to graduate. Her second semester she went to school and took an English class on their computer. She only had to be there 3 days a week for 2 hours a day. She started this class in January of 2008 and finished in February. She did receive her diploma but was not able to walk with her class to receive it.

It breaks my heart that she could never have a real childhood because of this. So many children take for granted that they are able to get up in the morning and go to school and be with other kids. Kristen is not able to get out of bed early. She is only able to get up later in the afternoon. Not to mention how she will be feeling once she is able to get up.

I am very proud of Kristen. She has taken night classes. As of today, she has finished a year of community college. She had 9 credit hours but she still did it. It wasn't easy. Many days she went feeling very weak and sick. But she had to have 9 credit hours. This brings up another subject.

Because of the Dysautonomia/POTS Kristen is not able to work. In order for her to be covered by insurance she has to be attending school full time, which is 12 credit hours. Because of her syndrome, she is registered through the school as disabled and is then able to go to school nine credit hours and that is considered full time for a disabled person. At many points with her chronic fatigue and passing out this has almost been impossible. I as her mother Sonjia or her father John have had to stay at her school and wait for her during each and every one of her classes because of her passing out. I have been told that no one is allowed legally to do anything to help her to bring her to, if she passes out. So the school would have to call 911 every time. I can't afford this. The medical bills have been overwhelming already even with insurance. She will come to when I put an ice pack or something cold on her neck or face. Yet I can't believe that no one in the school can do this? The only other way she would be covered by insurance is if she was declared disabled by the government.

Kristen filed for Social Security in November of 2008. Three doctors provided information and letters stating that she is disabled and is not able to work. She has still received two denial letters stating that they feel she is able to work. I don't understand this. She is not able to drive or take public transportation due to her symptoms. I have to stay at the school with her and she definitely can't live alone at this point. So how is this not being disabled? Since she cannot work her father and I are paying for everything. We are now waiting to attend a hearing in July on this matter. I pray the outcome is good because I don't know how much longer we will be able to afford this without some help from the government.

My name is Lisa Day.

I am 40 years old and live in Northern Texas.

I have a wonderful family that consists of my incredibly smart husband who helped me figure out what was going on with my health and my two amazing children who both have the same condition as I do: POTS, and this is a small tidbit of my rather large story.

As far back as I can remember I dealt with POTS symptoms. Of course, as many do, I had no idea that I was going through was abnormal. I recall thinking that the teachers at my school were cruel for putting all the children through the agony of standing in lines or doing things such as push-ups, sit-ups and jumping jacks. Every time I did these things, I felt dizzy and very weak. I was able to hide my discomfort by leaning on walls or simply enduring the pain, so I assumed that others were hurting right alongside of me.

I also suffered from intense lack of sleep. From the time I was an infant, my sleep patterns had always been off. As long as my mother can remember, I hated naps. My parents were diligent about my bed time, but I often struggled to get a good night's sleep because I would just lie there, staring into the darkness and resenting my parents for forcing me to this hideous isolation. To counter that, there were also many times when I longed to sleep all day, feeling completely exhausted when I had to get up for school. As all parents do, my parents thought I was simply trying to stay home from school and sent me on my way, telling me that I would be better in a bit. They were wrong, as I was always as tired later on that day as I had been when I woke up that morning.

I also had an intense sensitivity to any chemicals, smoke and medications. My mother smoked in our home and in our car, so I was exposed to tobacco on a daily basis, but I never seemed to get used to it. I felt as if someone was strangling me or stealing my air from me whenever I was in direct contact with it. I also loved the way perfumes smelled but hated the way they made my lungs hurt and my head ache almost instantly when I was near them. The same was true for household chemicals and heavy pollution in the air. Other children and even some adults would make fun of me for being so sensitive, telling me that I was just a baby and that I needed to be tougher.

As I matured I started to notice more and more how many things made me feel abnormal. At times I felt like a failure when it came to the physical aspects of life. I subconsciously overcame it by focusing on my academics and making it my goal to be more empathetic to others that seemed to struggle with any kind of handicap or "social difference". I loved being the teacher's pet in my classes, although I would come up with any excuse I could to avoid going to PE, and came close to failing on numerous occasions. I simply could not do what was expected of me in PE, but no matter how hard I tried I often became the brunt of my peer's jokes and the focus of my teacher's frustrations.

The most difficult part was that no one understood or believed me when I tried to explain how I was feeling. Unlike my mother who had a heart problem called PAT all of her life (which caused her heart to race at exceptionally high levels at unpredictable times) doctors didn't see my heart racing when I would go in. It only happened when I stood up, and they never took my blood pressure or heart rate while I was standing. If I complained enough they would just tell me to stand up slower. This drove me crazy as I did get up slowly and it didn't make any sort of difference. When I was 14 I finally got diagnosed with Mitral Valve Prolapse, giving some understanding to the chest pains I was having but not the chronic fatigue, foggy brain and dizziness I experienced quite often, leaving me frustrated and confused.

As I began puberty my POTS (unknown to me) became much more noticeable. I started to black out much more, have small seizures, confusion, very sharp headaches, abnormal bloating when I ate and eventually I started passing out.

The doctors did try me on Corgard, a beta-blocker to see if it would help. I immediately learned that even the smallest dose that they could administer was enough to completely knock me out for hours and leave me to battle with extreme fatigue. Obviously, this was not the answer. Instead, I stopped complaining and started hiding my symptoms even more, leaving me to feel alone in my own reality, which was beginning to feel like my own version of Hell.

When I was 19 I came down with Chicken Pox for the first time. It was also the first time that the doctors registered my heart rate in the 200's. I was sent to the ER. By the time the ER took my heart rate again it was perfectly normal and they looked at me as if I was crazy for coming in. This sadly began years of ER staff treating me as if I was a drug seeker or a hypochondriac, as my symptoms would increase with age.

However, as with any chronic illness, especially one that has no recognition, I went on with life as normal as I could. I had a few jobs in my early twenties, one of which was being a flight attendant. I quickly learned though that whatever was wrong with me did not go hand-in-hand with flying and I had to let that position go. It made me sad as I had to work hard to achieve this long-term goal but the fatigue and illness it brought on, not to mention the tension due to my absences made my decision to quit well worth it. Now I know it would never have worked out.

When I turned 25, I got married and had a baby. To my

amazement my health seemed better than ever while I was pregnant. It was not until the end of my pregnancy that the doctor
picked up on my heart rate being higher than normal and suggested
bed rest. For the most part I didn't feel it. My baby was born
healthy and I felt as if everything had taken a turn for the better.
This was not the case, though. Although he was healthy, he did not
want to sleep nearly as often as most infants do and I began to suffer from what I believed was intense lack of sleep. In reality, it was
the lack of sleep and my own case of POTS flaring up.

For many reasons my son's father and I divorced and by the
time he was three years old I was a single mother. My health became more of a problem than ever. I was beginning to pass out
more often, have seizures and have episodes that would lead me to
the ER in belief that I was having a heart attack on occasion. Of
course I was told each time that there was nothing wrong with me
and that my heart rate and blood pressure seemed perfectly normal
while I was sitting, never having anyone take it while I was standing.
One time I was told that my intense chest pains, numbness in my
left arm and dizziness was all caused by a mild UTI. My frustration
and my fear grew more and more. What was wrong with me? Was I
going crazy? I knew I wasn't, but the doctors all seem to think I was.
How was I to raise my child with these types of health problems?

As life often does, everything continued to work out. I had
good friends around me who thankfully believe me. All they knew
how to do to help me was to take care of my son when I needed
them to and to help me to rest, but this was a huge blessing to me.

When I was 30 I married my husband. He didn't fully understand the magnitude that my health problems had been in my life,
but would soon learn and become very insightful in helping me figure them out. By the time we were married, things had leveled out
a bit and although I had figured out my heart raced some, I was
feeling better until I got pregnant with my daughter when I was 32.
This time my pregnancy was not nearly as easy and my body
seemed in constant need of rest. I was able to do some things. In

fact, I actually took a trip to Colorado in my fourth month where I did very well in the mountains. However by the end of this pregnancy I was extremely exhausted, in a great deal of pain, and had even passed out on occasion. The one thing that had been discovered was that I had no sign of the Mitral Valve Prolapse, confirming in my mind that my issues were not caused by it.

Again, my baby girl was healthy but would not sleep. In fact, her sleeping issues were more severe than her brother's had been. She would often skip her sleeping time in between meals and never got on a napping schedule at all. Of course, I was more exhausted than normal and only through the help of my family was able to take good care of her.

I did recover, and she continue to grow, as did my son, into a wonderful human being and this made me want to have at least one more child. When I turned 37 we started trying again. It wasn't long before I was pregnant with another child. However by my sixth week we learned that I had lost this baby and we would have to try again, which we did.

I knew my health was not perfect and I knew my age was a factor but I really wanted to have at least one more baby. So in a month or so we were once again pregnant. The first few weeks we're fine and at my five week checkup I mentioned my heart issues to my doctor. My heart was not giving me any trouble but She told me to go see a cardiologist just to get a base reading of everything so we would know if anything had changed during my pregnancy. I scheduled my appointment for my sixth week. By the time my appointment came, my heart had become a racing machine. It not only raced when I stood, but when I was sitting as well. I was shaky, weak and in fact I started to feel as if my whole body was completely shutting down. My cardiologist was stumped. She had never seen this reaction to pregnancy in a patient before. She worked with me for a few weeks. We tried everything from Gatorade, to resting, to discussing taking beta-blockers. After some time she realized she could not be of any help. My symptoms were getting worse and I no longer felt safe to be standing. She sent me to another cardiologist. This cardiologist was well respected and experienced with many different and unusual cases.

In the meantime my husband and I had been doing our own research on the Internet. After many hours, he ran across an article about a condition called Postural Orthostatic Tachycardia Syndrome. He was amazed as to how many of the symptoms listed were the same as I was experiencing and had been experiencing my entire life. After much reading on the subject we decided that there was definitely a chance that this was what was causing my problems.

I was so excited. For once I had something to hold onto; something that makes sense that did not leave me feeling as if I was crazy. When my appointment to see this new doctor came about my husband went with me. We were both very anxious to ask her about this condition we had found. When we did, she sent me into tears. She looked at me and told me very rudely that I could not have POTS and then she refused to even test me for it. I was crushed. Why was she refusing to even look into this? I still don't know the answer to that. However, I do know that my husband gave me the courage to move forward and together we found a doctor that would truly look into my condition and after much testing diagnosed me with full-blown POTS.

Sadly, for reasons we may never understand, we found out at 16 weeks that our son had passed away in my womb at around 14 to 15 weeks. At the time they did not contribute this to my health, although that boggled my mind. They told us that there was probably a genetic cause or that after other tests that were performed; it could be because of an issue with blood clotting I had been unaware I had. The doctors felt we had a better understanding of what was going on and in a year's time we were pregnant again, with their approval.

At exactly 5 weeks along, my health fell apart. This time however I was under the care of an excellent Cardiologist, OB/GYN, and also a Prenatal Specialist. I was put on bed rest, received weekly IV's, took blood thinning shots daily and I was as cautious as I could possibly be. After weeks of feeling as if I was physically dying due to the fatigue and overall pain, I emotionally did die. This time, it was when I learned our newest son had also passed away at 14 weeks gestation. We were devastated.

I have spoken with many doctors, have had many tests, and the best that they can tell me is that it could possibly kill me if I became pregnant again. This has been hard to swallow, but I think I feared the same. Of course, it is not certain that POTS played into this but no one is willing to say that is not the cause of what has happened.

I do not say this to scare anyone or to keep young women from trying to have a baby. In fact, I have heard many stories where pregnancy helped patients overcome their POTS, as did it with me temporarily in my first pregnancy. However, being that each case of POTS is unique and each has its own causes, I do want to stress that in my experience and opinion, there might be some benefit in not waiting too long to have children, if you are a woman with POTS.

I am now blessed to be on the Board of Directors for a wonderful non-profit, nationwide POTS support group called TADA. My time in the support group has taught me so much about the similarities that all POTS patients face as well as their differences. The one thing that seems universal is the freedom and self-esteem that floods back into their lives once they learn what they are dealing with and also that they are certainly not alone. Others truly do understand.

With all this being said... If I have learned anything in my 40 years it is that life is precious and every aspect of it has its rewards and its downfalls. Because of my POTS, I have learned to allow myself not only to turn to others for support and understanding through the more difficult days (something many of us seem to resist for so long), but to slow down, relax some (again not an easy task for many people with POTS), smell the roses, to appreciate every breath of life that I breathe and better yet... to appreciate and treasure every breath of life that my family breathes. Each moment is very special and should be cherished! I truly believe there is light at the end of this tunnel. I pray you can too!

Rachel B.

I have had so many people tell me to try so many things, and I am getting about fed up!

Taking my vitamins will not cure me. I already do take vitamins, and yes, they help, but they do not cure!

I do not just need to reduce my stress load, though talking to people who say this certainly makes me more symptomatic as my stress increases!

Just because I'm bloating does not mean that I am about to start my period! In fact, I bloat after almost every meal! I really don't have my period every week of the year! But, thanks for your concern!

I can't just sleep it off! Resting does not "do wonders for me" as it may seem like it should. In fact, I can sleep a whole day, and still feel exhausted! Other days, I lie in bed, only getting a single hour of sleep. So, no, I don't have great confidence that sleeping will cure my problems!

Yes, I really do have headaches, bloating, tachycardia, dizziness, fainting, and heart pains. I know it's a lot, but get over it. I don't like it, and I don't need to hear how you are amazed that one person could have so much "wrong" with them!

Exercise will not make all my symptoms go away! It will help, but I'm already doing about all I can. I could try to step it up a bit, but since I'm already about passing out after every time, it just doesn't seem smart!

I do eat! So my low weight is not a problem. I am gaining weight, but it takes time. It would not be healthy for me to gain weight too dramatically. And honestly, my weight is none of your business!

Just because I'm out and about some days does not mean that I am suddenly cured! How about you tell me you're glad I'm able to get out that day instead of telling me that you expect to see me more often now that I'm "better??"

And finally, IT'S NOT ALL IN MY HEAD!!!! I'm not making it up or exaggerating my symptoms! I really feel this horrible, and yes, almost all the time.

Why does everyone think they have an instant cure-all?! I am so tired of hearing what is the cause of my problems! Even the ER doctor had enough sense to tell me he had no idea, and yet so many non-medical people have decided that I have had this long enough, and it's time to fix the problem! And, of course, they know exactly what that problem is! Ok. Wow. Venting does wonders! I feel better now, especially knowing that I'm talking to people who understand!

Written by: Rachel B

Ana Collins

My name is Ana Collins, and I am from Wisconsin. Before I got POTS, I was involved in everything, and I hardly ever got sick. I participated in gymnastics, volleyball, soccer and many other school activities. When I was not participating in school or sporting activities, I was always out with my friends.

Then in 2006 I got 12-hour stomach flu and my health has never been the same since. I could not eat more than a bit of food at a time and I kept losing weight but the doctors just kept brushing it off and said I was just still getting over the flu. I then passed out for the first time after they drew blood, was hospitalized overnight and sent home the next day with a diagnosis of dehydration. Then I started getting terrible stomach pains, so they took a CT scan and found an abnormal mass on my stomach, so they referred me to Milwaukee Children's Hospital. There my attending doctor said my symptoms did not make sense but assured me that she would figure it out, and she did. The mass in my stomach was food, which led to a diagnosis of gastroperisis and everything else going on (crazy heart rate, low blood pressure, dizziness, etc.) was POTS. I was put on medicine after they figured everything out and my POTS was manageable. After one year, I went back to see my doctors as they wanted to do further testing. They thought my POTS should be gone, but it definitely was not.

I was in denial about my illness and none of my friends understood, so I just kept to myself. I did swim team and the coaches would make me stop and lay on the deck because I looked so pale, but I just ignored all of this. Then in late summer of 2008, I got mono, two cases of strep throat and acute tonsillitis. That made my body go crazy, and I went into a huge POTS crash. I could not sit up for more than a minute at a time, and I was so sound and light sensitive I could not leave my room. My fatigue was terrible. I had a lot of problems at school because I could not concentrate or remember a lot of things. Nobody really knew what was going on with me, so I was sent to Mayo Clinic, which turned out to be a disaster appointment. When I got back home my regular POTS doctor wanted me to do physical therapy and I did and that made me worse. I then developed severe joint pain. We were directed to a geneticist, who diagnosed me with Ehlers-Danlos Syndrome. (EDS) This is probably what caused my POTS in the first place, and perhaps why it is still here.

Another hard part about all of this is having to quit the sports I love; especially gymnastics. Gymnastics was literally my life before I got sick and almost all of my friends were and where I spent most of my time during the week. I would also spend most of my weekends traveling and competing. I absolutely loved gymnastics and miss it so much. Now I can only watch gymnastics on T.V., which makes me miss it even more.

One person outside my family who has been the biggest help in all of this is my boyfriend Zane. We had been dating for 6 months when I got severe and he has stuck with me through everything. He has come over every day since I've been severe and on the days when I have a pillow over my head because I have migraine he just comes and sits with me. Without him this would be a lot harder to deal with. He has truly been a lifesaver for me and my family. When I'm too sick to go anywhere he will just sit with me and when I feel okay he will take me places and piggyback me because I have problems walking. He also helps me write my homework because I cannot write for any length of time. I don't think he realizes how much of a blessing he has been and there is no way to repay him for everything he has done for me.

Today I am still struggling with my symptoms. When I go out of the house, I go in a wheelchair because I cannot walk for any length of time, and I am still having a lot of joint pain that we are still trying to get a handle on. I am starting physical therapy again but this time with someone who really understands POTS. I have lost a lot of my friends through this crash and a lot of my family members do not understand why I look so healthy. It's hard when people stare at you and your family and friends do not think you are truly sick. This is so hurtful. What really helped me was to realize that I was not crazy. The doctors believed me; even if some people around me did not. DYNA (Dysautonomia Youth Network of America) really helped my family and me a lot. They were there to support us, and they helped me to work with my symptoms instead of fighting them.

A lot of people do not understand why I am depressed, because I cannot do anything a 'normal" teen can do but I can focus on everything I can do and that is what keeps me going. I know I will get better and I will not be like this forever. I just do what I can and take everything one day at a time.

Written by: Ana Collins

Section 11. Just For Fun

Chapter 34. You Know You Have POTS When......

"Laughter is medicine with no side effects" Anonymous.

Hope this will make the POTSIES out there laugh. I got this list from fellow POTSIES who posted these on my POTS Awareness Site. (See Facebook -POTS Group: Jodi Epstein Rhum)

You Know you have POTS When.............
1. You spend more time horizontal than vertical.
2. You can always pee on command.
3. You have an excuse for not being able to pass a sobriety test. Pray that a police officer never stops you and asks you to walk a straight.
4. You see more of your doctors than your friends.
5. Your idea of dressing up means matching your socks to your sweatshirt.
6. Your blood actually obeys the laws of gravity.
7. You can use your hands (or feet) for your very own personal ice pack.
8. You can open up a Walgreens with all of the medicines you have to take.
9. You do not need to go to Hollywood to see stars. All you need to do is stand up.
10. You have the medical terminology to pass medical school at 18.
11. You know more about your condition than most of the medical doctors you see. You often have to explain it to them.
12. You can eyeball 8 oz. of fluid without using a measuring cup.
13. You can get your heart rate up, by just standing, to a higher rate than someone who has just run the Boston Marathon.
14. Brain fog allows you to nap with your eyes open.

15. You are the only teenager you know who sits down to take a shower.
16. You have the only 5-year-old sibling who can say Postural, Orthostatic Tachycardia Syndrome.
17. No need to paint your fingernails, they already have such a nice bluish tint!
18. The doctor calls you to see how you are doing because he has not heard from you in a few days.
19. You know the first names of all of the Fireman in your town.
20. You are so tired after putting on your clothes; you need to take a nap.
21. You are finally not fatigued; unfortunately it is now 2:00 A.M.
22. You have enough medical material to be a stand-up comedian; the problem is you cannot stand up.
23. You experience more temperature changes than a mood ring.
24. You get to tell someone in their 90's, whom you are following on a flight of stairs, to slow down because they are going too fast.
25. You have seen every infomercial ever made and have learned at least 100 ways to dice and slice tomatoes.
26. Get to answer 'No" a million times to the question, "Is that all of your meds?" when you go to the doctor.
27. You are a very cheap date. You can barely eat because you always feel bloated, and you already feel too drunk and dizzy to drink alcohol.
28. You never have to go to an amusement park because you always feel like you are on a rollercoaster, anyways.
29. You have your doctors on speed dial.
30. You have your best thoughts at 4:00 in the morning.
31. You get your daily exercise by walking back and forth to the bathroom.
32. You are the youngest person at your cardiologist's office

and yet seem to be breathing the hardest.

33. Have hot flashes even though you are at least 30 years away from menopause.
34. You do not want to kneel at church because you are worried if you do, you may either faint when you stand up or your knee will dislocate.
35. A good day is a day when you only have one doctor's appointment.
36. Your medical file has more pages than the Bible.
37. You have more accommodations than the entire special education population at your school.
38. You are the healthiest looking sick person. You are an oxymoron.
39. You like to wear your Uggs in the summer and short sleeve shirts in the winter.
40. You have to cancel more plans than a politician makes promises.
41. Heat, long lines and fluorescent lights are your worst enemies.
42. You have seen every type of doctor whose name ends in "ologist".
43. You have been to the ER over 5 times and no one can still figure out what is wrong with you or what to do to make you better.
44. You have had every part of your body x-rayed or scanned.
45. You know what a jackhammer would feel like if it were inside your head.
46. You are incredibly strong but often cannot open up your own water bottle.
47. You have too many symptoms to remember them all.
48. People often say to you, "Do you think this could just be stress?"
49. You can sleep for 23 hours and still feel fatigued.
50. You drink more liquids in a day than most people drink in a

week.
51. Your body can gage the weather more accurately than the meteorologist.
52. You feel like you have "morning sickness" all day long.
53. You can sit with the old men at the back of the church/temple and discuss beta-blockers and chest pains.
54. You are the only one in the grocery aisle picking out the foods that have the highest sodium count you can find.
55. You are the only one who can go to Mexico for three weeks and come back looking paler than before you went.
56. You know you have POTS when............ you can laugh at these jokes.

Chapter 35. Interesting Facts about Dysautonomia

"Courage does not always roar. Sometimes courage is the little voice at the end of the day that says I'll try again tomorrow".
- Mary Ann Radmacher

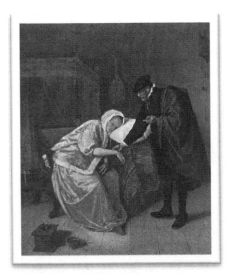

Dysautonomia Found In Art

Doctor and His Patient was painted by Jan Steen in the mid 1600's. This picture was painted during the Dutch Realism period. During this period in history artists were starting to paint real life, even those that were ill. It is postulated that Jan Steen was painting someone with Dysautonomia. Observe the painting closely and see if you can find distinguishing features that support the fact that Jan Steen may have indeed been painting a woman that suffered from this syndrome. There are at least ten traits that I uncovered. See if you can find them all.

Answers can be found on the next page

- Female
- She is pale
- Her body appears flaccid
- Her left hand is bluish in color (venous pooling)
- She appears faint
- A physician is taking her pulse
- She looks fatigued
- She is dressed in heavy clothing and is wearing a hood. This may symbolize body temperature regulation issues.
- Has light hair
- Has light eyes

More Interesting Facts

- Dysautonomia was once called Neurasthenia. This literally means "weak nervous system." It was once treated with bed rest.
- POTS has been referred to by various names, including neurocirculatory asthenia, mitral valve prolapse (MVP) syndrome, irritable heart, soldier's heart, idiopathic orthostatic intolerance, orthostatic tachycardia syndrome, postural tachycardia syndrome, hyperadrenergic orthostatic tachycardia and hyperadrenergic orthostatic hypotension.
- Greg Page, from the famous Australian children's show "The Wiggles" had to quit the show because he has Dysautonomia. See Gregpage.com for more information.
- Mayo Clinic estimates that 1 in 100 people have some form of Dysautonomia.
- Astronauts have been coming back from prolonged space flight with OI, orthostatic intolerance. This is believed to be a result of the deconditioning that occurs in a zero gravity environment.
- Giraffes do not get Orthostatic Intolerance (OI). One of the reasons is that giraffes "have a very tight sheath of thick

skin over their lower limbs which maintains high extravascular pressure in exactly the same way as a pilot's g-suit."

- Dysautonomia seems to affect females 5 to 1 over males.
- Animals, though very rare, can get Dysautonomia.
- Most veterinarians study Dysautonomia in vet school, yet most medical school students do not!
- Many people diagnosed with fibromyalgia and chronic fatigue syndrome may have been misdiagnosed. They may in fact actually have a form of Dysautonomia.
- In some people's opinion, many people who have fainted with no explanation may have Dysautonomia.
- Migraine headaches, according to my research, may one day fall under the category of Dysautonomia.
- Dysautonomia has been reported to occur after some breast implant surgeries (Richard N. Fogoros M.D.) About. Com Heart Disease
- Dysautonomia is often triggered after a period of prolonged bed rest, especially following a virus, surgery, broken bone, etc.
- People with Dysautonomia tend to do better at sea level and in places where there is little change in barometric pressure.
- Mares can get colic from drastic changes in barometric pressure. This can result in death for the animal.
- Caucasians seem to be affected by this illness more often than non-Caucasians.
- Tall people seem to be more affected by POTS.
- A major growth spurt has been shown to be one of the many triggers for POTS.
- POTS has been highlighted on several TV. shows including Mystery Diagnosis Season 5, Episode 3: The Woman Who Kept Falling Down Original Air Date—28 January 2008 and House- Episode 19 (Season 6): "The Choice"
- Diets high in carbohydrates have been connected to im-

paired vasoconstrictive action. Eating foods with lower carbohydrate levels can mildly improve POTS symptoms.

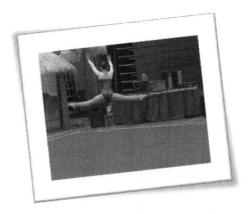

Chapter 36. Poem - "Fly Again"- *Jodi Rhum*

I watched her, motionless from the stands
She floated through the air, she was a gazelle
Sailing, flipping, twisting
Beautiful, flawless, perfection
Her strength, evident in every move of her majestic body
A ballerina, spinning, twirling, flying
Soul defying
Casting to the upper echelons of the heavens
Now the bird has lost its wing, spiraling downward, lost, confused, broken
Too dizzy to fly
Take my strength, breathe my breath, and mend your wing
Use your courage, your determination, and your spirit to fly again
Lift yourself up, dance in the moonlight, and defy gravity once again
Sail, flip and twirl
Look up and soar to limits of the sky, for then you will fly again
Oh, to see you fly again.

Part II - POTS; It's Real - Written by Medical Professionals

Edited for Medical Content by: Svetlana Blitshteyn, MD

POTS; It's Real

Wayne Dyer once said, "I always believed that the highest form of ignorance is when you reject something you don't know anything about," but I came to learn from this syndrome that the worst form of ignorance is actually when you judge someone or something you know nothing about.

Many of us have had similar experiences on our journey to find a diagnosis. Most of us have been told by at least one doctor, family member, friend, teacher, etc. that POTS is not truly a "real" illness. Some are too cowardly to say it to our faces, but we quickly learn who believes and who judges. Many presume it is impossible to have so many symptoms. Surely this POTS "thing" is just all in your head or it is stress or anxiety related. Some of us have even been told that perhaps this illness is just a cry for attention. Of course, we are all tired of hearing this, as it could not be farther from the truth. It is because of this frustration that I wrote this book in the first place and in doing so gathered dozens of medical doctors to contribute chapters to support the fact that POTS is real.

During the process of writing this book, I interviewed a new pediatrician on the phone, in deciding if I should switch to his practice, I asked him point blank if he thought POTS was a real syndrome. He was flabbergasted that I asked the question. He replied in a very strong voice, "Why would doctors prescribe beta-blockers if this was not a real illness? " He was further dumbfounded when I told him how many people, including some doctors, that I had run across were convinced otherwise.

The following section is for those people out there who have had a hard time convincing their friends, family members, spouses or doctors that POTS does exist. It is also for those who want to learn more about the history, physiology, mechanisms and coping techniques as they relate to this syndrome. If after reading the next chapters, the disbeliever still is in denial that POTS is a real diagnosis, then perhaps he/she will always choose to live in the dark.

Truth will always be truth, regardless of lack of understanding, disbelief or ignorance. – W Clement Stone

Chapter 37. Symptoms, Signs and Mechanisms of POTS. *Svetlana Blitshteyn, MD*

Symptoms and signs of POTS

Because the autonomic nervous system regulates the function of many organs of the body, POTS, a form of Dysautonomia, is a disorder that can affect any or all organ systems controlled by the ANS. For some patients, POTS can be manifested as predominantly a dysregulation of the cardiovascular system, with disturbance of the blood pressure and heart rate, while for others, gastrointestinal or genitorurinary system can be involved, in addition to the cardiovascular system.

Symptoms and signs of POTS are numerous and multi-dimensional, reflecting the consequence of the impaired ANS function. Symptoms can vary in number and severity over time, often on a daily and sometimes on an hourly basis. Many patients experience certain symptoms chronically, while for some, symptoms can be recurrent, with symptom-free periods occurring between flare-ups. Chronic or fluctuating symptoms, and their unpredictability, can result in significant impairment in a person's ability to function on a day-to-day basis. Studies have shown that in POTS, degree of disability correlates with symptom severity and that POTS can be as disabling as congestive heart failure or chronic obstructive pulmonary disease [1].

POTS is a disorder of orthostatic intolerance; thus, many symptoms occur in a standing position, and their severity is greater in standing than in sitting position, but some patients may also experience symptoms when laying down. In addition, certain symptoms, such as lightheadedness, dizziness and fatigue, may occur when a patient's blood pressure and heart rate are within the normal limits, a phenomenon which often causes confusion and misunderstanding for some health care providers, who may assume that if vital signs are normal, then symptoms should not occur.

Symptom is a term that describes subjective evidence of a disease that a patient experiences and reports to the doctor, while sign is an objective evidence of a disease that a physician is able to observe without the patient's description. Pain is an example of a symptom while fever is an example of a sign.

In order to better understand the nature of symptoms and signs of POTS, it helps to categorize them on the basis of their possible mechanism. In a series of 152 patients with POTS evaluated at the Mayo Clinic in Rochester, MN, symptoms were grouped by presumed cerebral hypoperfusion, autonomic over activity, sudomotor origin, gastrointestinal, genitorurinary and pupillary dysfunction and generalized symptoms (2). These terms are explained below.

Cerebral hypoperfusion is a term used to describe a state in which not enough blood is distributed to the brain. Cerebral hypoperfusion may occur when a patient with POTS assumes an upright posture. Symptoms can include:

- Lightheadedness or dizziness in 78% of patients
- Presyncope (near-fainting) 60%
- Weakness 50%

Autonomic over activity refers to an increase in function of the autonomic nervous system, more commonly the sympathetic nervous system in POTS. Symptoms can include:

- Palpitations 75%
- Tremulousness (shaking) 38%
- Shortness of breath 28%
- Chest wall pain 24 %

Sudomotor function refers to the component of the autonomic nervous system that controls sweating. Symptoms can include:

- Increase in sweating 9%
- Loss of sweating 5%

Gastrointestinal symptoms:
- Nausea 39%
- Bloating 24%
- Diarrhea 18%
- Constipation 15%
- Abdominal pain 15%
- Bladder dysfunction: 9%

Pupillary dysfunction/eye problems: 3%
- Sensitivity to light
- Excessive glare

Generalized symptoms:
- Fatigue 48%
- Sleep disturbance 32%
- Migraine headache 28%
- Myofascial pain 16%

Other symptoms of POTS can include
- Heat intolerance
- Exercise intolerance
- Flushing
- Anxiety
- Cold hand and feet
- Cognitive complaints, such as poor concentration, memory or word recall
- Neck and shoulder pain
- Numbness and tingling
- Feeling "wired" or "easily overstimulated"
- Increased thirst
- Increased urination
- Dry mouth
- Dry eyes

Symptoms can often get worse or precipitated by the following:
- Exercise 53%
- Heat 53%
- Meals 24%
- Menstrual cycle 15%

Signs of POTS can include
- Tachycardia
- Low or high blood pressure
- Fluctuating heart rate or blood pressure
- Reduced pulse pressure
- Cold and clammy hands
- Paleness
- Hyperventilation
- Bluish discoloration of the legs or arms (possibly due to decreased blood supply to the skin)

Who gets POTS?

POTS can affect anyone at any age, but the most frequently affected population is women between 15 to 50 years of age. It has been observed by various researchers that POTS is more common in women than in men, with women being 5 times more likely to be affected by POTS than men. The reasons for female predominance in POTS have not been clearly defined, but it has been suggested that female hormones may play a possible role in the development of POTS. Furthermore, women are more likely to be affected by the orthostatic stress than men [3]. Women also appear to have a physiologically different sympathetic nervous system activity at rest and in response to low blood pressure than men [4].

The exact prevalence of POTS is unknown, but it was once estimated that approximately 500,000 of Americans were affected by POTS. The number is probably higher now due to the increasing availability of diagnostic labs and improved physicians' education and recognition of POTS in the recent years.

Although less common in adults, POTS can also affect children and teenagers, who are more likely to also have hypotension than adults. [5]

There is currently no data on the prevalence or characteristics of POTS in elderly. This may be due in part to a high prevalence of hypertension, cardiac arrhythmia, cardiovascular disease and orthostatic hypotension, all of which may obscure the features of POTS, thus making the diagnosis extremely difficult.

When can POTS begin?

POTS can present under various circumstances, and its onset may be acute - symptoms began within less than 1 month, subacute - symptoms began within 1-3 months or slow - symptoms began within more than 3 months. Some patients are able to recall the exact day when symptoms appeared, while others are unaware of the symptom onset. Many patients can identify a preceding infectious illness, while for others POTS began slowly, without any identifiable cause. Others contend that they had symptoms as long as they can remember. Some women report symptoms onset at menarche, while others report symptoms appearing during pregnancy, labor and delivery or post-partum. Symptoms onset or worsening is also noted around the time of menopause.

POTS can be precipitated by

- Infection
- Influenza
- Viral gastrointestinal illness
- Viral upper respiratory illnesses
- Pneumonia
- Bronchitis
- Pharyngitis

- Mononucleosis
- Lyme disease
- Surgery
- Pregnancy
- Trauma

POTS is also described in the medical literature in association with autoimmune disorders (eg. Lupus, sarcoidosis, rheumatoid arthritis) anatomical brain malformation (eg. Chiari I malformation) [6] connective tissue disorders (eg. joint hypermobility syndrome, Ehlers Danlos Syndrome, Marfan syndrome), [7] genetic mutation of a norepinephrine reuptake transporter protein,[8] genetic disorders such as Kleinfelter's syndrome.[9] lightning injury,[10] vaccination. [11]

Patients have also reported symptoms occurring after a new medication was introduced, after running a marathon or after another extreme physical activity, or during a period of severe psychological or emotional stress, such as for example, death of a close family member or a divorce. Interestingly, approximately 40% of patients report having some symptoms of orthostatic intolerance or fainting in the past. [2] One possible explanation may be that a physically or psychologically stressful event, such as a viral illness, pregnancy, surgery, or extreme physical activity, may have precipitated POTS in those people who are genetically predisposed to it. However, until more research is done to elucidate the mechanisms of POTS, all considerations remain hypothetical.

POTS may have a familial predisposition, with approximately 14% of patients reporting a family history of orthostatic intolerance disorders [2]. The number of patients with a positive family history of POTS or neurcardiogenic syncope, may be as high as 40% [12]. While there is currently no evidence that POTS is a genetic disorder, mother-child pairs affected by POTS have been observed in clinical settings, raising a possibility that a mitochondrial transmission may be involved in some cases.

Proposed mechanisms of POTS

POTS is a complicated disorder, and, as you recall, POTS is a syndrome and not a disease. This means that POTS may be caused by many different abnormalities in the human physiology, which in turn can produce a collection of symptoms and signs, ultimately resulting in a syndrome called POTS. Simply put, POTS is not one disorder and likely encompasses a spectrum of disorders with different mechanisms, causes and symptom severity, which ultimately lead to the final common pathway, known as POTS.

POTS physiology

Central to POTS, both in definition and symptoms, is the problem of orthostatic tachycardia. Why does it occur? Recall from the previous chapter that as humans evolved, so did the body's mechanisms to counteract the effects of gravity. Normally, when a person stands up, as much as 25-30% of blood volume may pool in the lower body as a result of gravity. When pooling of that much blood volume occurs in the lower body, it reduces the blood volume that is left in the upper body and the blood flow that is needed maintain the function of the heart, lungs and the brain. As blood volume falls, so does the blood pressure, and the fall in blood pressure is immediately sensed by the special sensors of the body, called the baroreceptors. The baroreceptors are located in the arch of the aorta, in the carotid arteries, in the heart and in the lungs. Once a fall in blood pressure is sensed, the baroreceptors activate a complex system of mechanisms, which ultimately result in slight increase in the heart rate (approximately by 10-15 bpm), slight increase in diastolic blood pressure (approximately 10 mmg Hg) and little or no increase in systolic blood pressure. Subsequently, the body normally employs other elaborate mechanisms and processes, many of which are controlled by the autonomic nervous system, in order to restore the blood flow to the heart, lungs and brain. These protective mechanisms are the reasons why humans are able to remain upright for extended periods of time without problems.

In POTS, the protective mechanisms against gravity appear to be abnormal, and as a result, the loss of blood volume in the upper body due to the blood pooling in the lower body, is not counteracted sufficiently. This results in an elevated heart rate on standing, in excess of what is expected normally – i.e. the orthostatic tachycardia. The orthostatic tachycardia appears to be a compensatory mechanisms rather than a primary abnormality. In fact, when this tachycardia is abolished, as seen in patients who have undergone cardiac ablation in an attempt to correct the sinus tachycardia, the symptoms of POTS and orthostatic intolerance may escalate because this compensatory mechanism no longer exists. Cardiac ablation for treatment of sinus tachycardia in POTS is therefore contraindicated.

If orthostatic tachycardia is a compensatory mechanism and not the primary abnormality, then what exactly causes POTS? This question continues to be the central aspect in science and is still under investigation. Nevertheless, as a result of decades of research, a wealth of knowledge uncovering the mysteries of POTS emerged, with many details of POTS mechanisms, pathophysiology and subtypes now coming to light. The main topics summarizing the most current understanding of POTS are outlined below.

POTS and neuropathy

The neuropathic POTS is believed to be the most common type. It is estimated that about half of POTS patients have this type. The word "neuropathic" refers to the abnormalities in the structure or function of the peripheral nerves. Recall that the autonomic nervous system (ANS) includes the sympathetic and the parasympathetic components. The ANS regulates the size of blood vessels in the body, which is an important factor in maintaining blood pressure in an upright posture in response to gravity. In neuropathic POTS, the sympathetic nerves supplying the blood vessels in the lower limbs are dysfunctional, resulting in a lack of expected constriction of blood vessels in an upright posture. The lack of the appropriate constriction then activates a whole range of physiologic compensatory mechanisms, including an increased sympathetic nervous system activity, which then causes a compensatory increase in heart rate in a standing position. Keep in mind that the actual process is much more complex than what is described here, and the details are still being worked out.

POTS and hypovolemia

Many patients with POTS are known to have low blood volume. The normal circulating blood volume in the body is about 70 ml/kg, and thus, a 70-kg person would be expected to have about 4,900 ml of blood, or a little less than 5 L. In POTS, the blood volume is decreased by 10-30% from normal [13].

Normally, when blood volume is low, the kidneys begin to conserve water and salt in an attempt to correct the blood volume deficit. This is accomplished through a system of hormones known as renin-angiotensin-aldosterone system. Unexpectedly, the researchers found that instead of the increased levels of renin and aldosterone in patients with low blood volume, the levels were actually lower in patients with POTS than in people with normal blood volume. This abnormality in renin-angiotensin-aldosterone pathway may be a possible cause or a contributor to the low blood volume in POTS. [13] One explanation as to why the kidneys do not produce an expected level of renin is that renin release is regulated by the sympathetic nervous system. If the sympathetic nerves are dysfunctional in POTS, then the kidneys that are supplied by the sympathetic nerves would be unable to release an adequate amount of renin to counteract the low blood volume state.

POTS and hyperadrenergic state

POTS can be associated with a state where the body produces too much norepinephrine, i.e. the "hypreadrenergic" state. It is believed that anywhere between 10-30% of patients have hyperadrenergic POTS. Increased levels of norepinephrine can occur as a result of a low blood volume or the abnormal sympathetic function, but may also be the primary problem. When a person stands, the sympathetic nervous system activates, releasing the norepinephrine, which in turn constricts the blood vessels in the body to maintain blood pressure against gravity. Normal level of norepinephrine in an upright position is below 600 pg/ml, but in patients with POTS norepinephrine rises to above 600 and sometimes above 1000 pg/ml in response to standing. This can result in an elevated blood pressure, called orthostatic hypertension. It is worth noting that norepinephrine can be also elevated in a supine position in POTS, causing increased heart rate, palpitations, sweating and anxiety, but to a lesser extent than in standing.

POTS and autoimmune antibodies

Recently, ganglionic acetycholine receptor (AchR) antibodies were detected in the blood of approximately 14% of patients with POTS. [2] Antibodies are proteins that the body produces as part of the immunologic defense system against a foreign entity, such as in response to an infection. However, antibodies can also be produced abnormally, against the body's own proteins. When this occurs, an autoimmune disease may result, such as for example, lupus or sarcoidosis. Recall that acetycholine is an essential neurotransmitter of the autonomic nervous system that binds to the receptors in the peripheral ganglia – the collection of the neuronal bodies – of the ANS. It is to these receptors that the antibodies are produced, resulting in the autoimmune type of POTS. Why the antibodies are produced remains unknown. One possibility is that a previous viral illness may have activated the immune system, causing an inappropriate attack on the body's own receptors. The same hypothesis is proposed for many other autoimmune disorders, including multiple sclerosis.

POTS and Norepinephrine Transporter

Norepinephrine transporter (NET) is an important protein that functions to clear out the norepinephrine in the neurons. When this protein is either dysfunctional or deficient, norepinephrine cannot be cleared properly in the nervous system, which results in the hyperadrenergic state.

A family with multiple members affected by POTS was described in the New England Medical Journal. [6] In this family, a genetic mutation was identified in the gene that coded for NET, which resulted in the abnormal NET. The family members had extremely high levels of norepinephrine as a result of dysfunctional NET. While only one family is known with this type of genetic mutation, some researchers propose that patients with POTS, who do not have other family members affected, could also have some type of dysfunction of NET. [14] The results of these studies are currently pending.

Certain medications can also affect the function of NET, which may result in orthostatic tachycardia. These medications include tricyclic antidepressants and some medications used for treatment of attention deficit disorders. Interestingly, some patients with POTS tolerate and have good results when a low dose of tricyclic antidepressants is used for treatment of migraine headache, sleep disturbance or myofascial pain. This illustrates the different underlying mechanisms and different treatment responses in POTS, whereas for some, the medication can cause or exacerbate the orthostatic tachycardia, while for others it may actually be helpful.

POTS and beta 2 adrenergic receptor

Beta 2 adrenergic receptor is another important component of the autonomic nervous system that has been implicated as a possible mechanism in POTS. [15] When norepinephrine is released in response to standing, it may bind to the beta 2 adrenergic receptor in the blood vessels of the lower limbs causing vasodilation.

It has been proposed by some researchers that beta 2 adrenore-ceptor functions abnormally in POTS. Specifically, there may be a decreased vasodilation related to the activation of beta 2 adrenergic receptor and a variation in the structure of the receptor itself in some patients with POTS. [15]

POTS and nitric oxide

Nitric oxide, a molecule that regulates many physiologic processes, including vasodilation, has been studied as a possible culprit in patients with POTS. In addition to causing vasodilation in blood vessels, nitric oxide also modulates the release of norepinephrine from the skeletal muscles and the heart and regulates blood flow to the brain. Circulating nitric oxide is synthesized primarily by an enzyme called endothelial nitric oxide synthase (eNOS). In one study, researchers found that certain variants (genotypes) of eNOS occurred less frequently in patients with POTS compared to the control group. [16, 17] In addition, it has been suggested that elevated levels of eNOS contribute to the development of POTS, but more studies are needed to explore the role of eNOS and nitric oxide in POTS.

POTS and mast cell activation

Mast cells play an important role in the body's immunologic, allergic and inflammatory responses. Produced by a bone marrow, mast cells mature in various tissues of the body and are particularly abundant in the skin, lungs, digestive tract, mouth and nose. Mast cells contain and release histamine – an essential mediator of the immune and allergic responses. Histamine also causes vasodilation, constriction of the airways, pain and itching.

Mast cells appear to be activated in some patients with POTS. These patients experience episodes of flushing, shortness of breath, headache, lightheadedness, diarrhea, nausea, vomiting and excessive urination. These episodes can be triggered by standing, exercise, meals and sexual activity. Orthostatic tachycardia and elevated blood pressure occur in response to standing. Elevated methyhistamine, a breakdown product of histamine, can be found in the urine of patients if collected for 2 hours following the onset of flushing episode. [18] At this time, it is not clear whether mast cell activation is the primary mechanism or if increased sympathetic nervous system activity causes mast cell activation. Patients with POTS and mast cell activation may benefit from treatment with antihistamine medications.

References

1. Benrud-Larson LM, Dewar MS, Sandroni P, et. al. Quality of life in patients with postural tachycardia syndrome. Mayo Clinic Proc 2002; 77: 531-537.

2. Thieben MJ, Sandroni P, Sletten DM, et. al. Postural Orthostatic Tachycardia Syndrome: the Mayo Clinic experience. Mayo Clin Proc 2007; 82: 308-313.

3. Fu Q, Witkowski S, Okazaki K, Levine BD. Effects on gender and hypovolemia on sympathetic neural response to stress. Am J Physiol Regul Integr Comp Physiol 2005; 289: R109-116.

4. Bonyhay R, Freeman R. Sympathetic neural activity, sex dimorphism and postural tachycardia syndrome. Ann Neurol 2007: 332-339.

5. Medow MS, Stewart JM. The postural tachycardia syndrome. Cardiol Rev 2007; 15: 67-75.

6. Prilipko O, Dehdashti AR, Zaim S, Seeck M. Orthostatic intolerance and syncope associated with Chiari type I malformation. J Neurol Neurosurg Psychiatry 2005;76 : 1034-1036.

7. Gazit Y, Nahir AM, Grahame R, Jacob G. Dysautonomia in the joint hypermobility syndrome. Am J Med 2003;115: 33-40.

8. Shannon JR, Flattem NL, Jordan J, Jacob G, Black BK, Biaggioni I, Blakely RD, Robertson D. Orthostatic intolerance and tachycardia associated with norepinephrine-transporter deficiency. N Engl J Med 2000; 342: 541-549.

9. Hainstock MR, Gruchala NE, Fike N, et al. Postural orthostatic tachycardia in a teenager with Klinefelter syndrome. Congenit Heart Dis 2008; 3: 440-442.

10. Grubb BP, Karabin B. New onset postural tachycardia syndrome following lightning injury. Pacing Clin Electrophysiol 2007; 30: 1036-1038.

11. Blitshteyn S. Postural tachycardia syndrome after vaccination with Gardasil. Eur J
Neurol 2010; 17: e52.

12. Blitshteyn S, Bett, GL, Poya H. Pregnancy in Postural Tachycardia Syndrome: clinical course and maternal and fetal outcomes. American Academy of Neurology Scientific Program, 2010.

13. Raj SR, Biaggioni I, Yamhure PC, Black BK, et al. Renin-aldosterone paradox and perturbed blood volume regulation underlying postural tachycardia syndrome. Circulation. 2005;111:1574-1582.

14. Esler M, Alvaregna M, Pier C, et al. The neuronal noradrenaline transporter, anxiety
and cardiovascular disease. J Psychopharmacol 2006; 20: 60-66.

15. Jacob G, Garland EM, Costa F, et al. Beta2-adrenoceptor genotype and function affect hemodynamic profile heterogeneity in postural tachycardia syndrome. Hypertension 2006; 47: 421-427.

16. Medow MS, Minson CT, Stewart JM. Decreased Microvascular Nitric Oxide-Dependent Vasodilation in Postural Tachycardia Syndrome. Circulation 2005; 112:2611-2618.

17. Garland EM, Winker R, Williams SM, et al. Endothelial NO Synthase Polymorphisms and Postural Tachycardia Syndrome. Hypertension 2005; 46:1103-1110.

18. Shibao C, Arzubiaga C, Roberts Ii LJ, Raj S, et al. Hyperadrenergic Postural Tachycardia Syndrome in Mast Cell Activation Disorders. Hypertension 2005; 45: 385-390.

Chapter 38. POTS and Lifestyle - *Svetlana Blitshteyn. MD*

Surviving a POTS Relapse: "This too shall pass..."

Since POTS can often have a fluctuating and an unpredictable course, it may be challenging, both physically and psychologically, to deal with a POTS relapse, in particular after a symptom-free or minimally symptomatic period. While every person may develop their own way of dealing with a relapse of POTS, the following suggestions are generally helpful in surviving the challenges of a POTS exacerbation.

1. Keep a hopeful attitude.

It's easy to get discouraged when symptoms worsen, but keep hope alive that the relapse is likely temporary and that better days are ahead. Reassure yourself that you have survived relapses before, that feeling better is possible and that "this too shall pass."

2. Try to identify the triggers if possible.

It can be informative and empowering to identify the triggers for POTS exacerbation, if possible. These triggers may include a viral illness, bacterial infection, stress, overexertion, anemia, migraine, allergies or lack of sleep. First, you can learn to avoid or prevent your triggers in the future, and second, you can reassure yourself that once a triggering event is addressed or removed, symptomatic improvement will follow. However, if there are no identifiable triggers or precipitating factor discovered, don't be discouraged and don't become obsessed with finding a reason why you feel worse. POTS may often worsen spontaneously, without any identifiable causes, and as such, it may be futile to try to identify the triggering factor where there may be none.

3. Call your doctor and schedule an urgent visit.

Your doctor will examine you, check your vital signs and establish a treatment plan that may include extra fluids and salt loading, medication change or adjustment in dose or infusion therapy with saline solution. In addition, your doctor may treat an underlying cause of POTS relapse if there is one, such as a migraine headache, urinary tract infection, allergies or anemia.

4. Notify your employer or school administrator.

Taking sick days may be optional for some and necessary for others. If you find yourself so symptomatic that you are unable to function despite your best efforts, it is advisable to take time off to recuperate. Notify your employer or school administrator about your absence and provide a note from a physician confirming your illness. By law, you or your physician are not required to disclose the nature of the illness to your employer, and the disclosure of your diagnoses are left to your discretion. It may be a good idea to contact human resources or school administration to discuss details regarding the allowed sick time, work-from-home option, FMLA, long-term disability, completion of missed homework or exams and other job or school accommodations.

5. Keep yourself comfortable.

During POTS flare-up, it's important to keep your mind occupied with quiet activities that are enjoyable, meaningful and distracting. Reading a good book, listening to soothing music, watching an uplifting movie, crocheting, writing in a journal and meditating are among the activities that one can do lying in bed or in a recliner.

6. Move around as much as you can.

Since POTS is a disorder of the orthostatic intolerance, symptoms typically intensify when standing or sitting and lessen when lying down. Naturally, patients with POTS tend to feel better immediately when lying flat. However, while supine rest may be necessary during a flare-up, prolonged bed rest is typically detrimental. Therefore, it is advisable to get up frequently, move around, walk, stretch or sit as much as you are able to withstand since prolonged rest can result in worsening of orthostatic intoler-ance, decreased blood pressure, dehydration, muscle atrophy, de-conditioning and even blood clots. Alternating periods of supine rest with mild physical activity is recommended to avoid the nega-tive impact of inactivity. For those who are more severely affected and are unable to stand, exercising in a supine or sitting position by doing stretches and leg lifts is an option.

7. Avoid feeling guilty.

Guilt is a powerful emotion that can strike anyone with a life-altering chronic illness, and it can be particularly severe during a flare-up. If you concentrate on what you cannot physically accom-plish while feeling ill, you can easily become overwhelmed, frus-trated, and depressed. Feelings of inadequacy, envy, anger and family discord may also surface during a stressful time. When expe-riencing a flare-up, it is best not to dwell on what cannot be done (i.e. go to school or work, clean the house, cook dinner, drive the children to a soccer practice, go out with friends or attend family outings or birthday parties). Instead, convince yourself that you will be able to do some or all of these activities once you are feeling better and look forward to the time when accomplishing what you set out to do is possible.

8. Surround yourself with supportive people.

Recruit family members, friends, neighbors and health care providers to help you get through a POTS relapse. Whether it is help with grocery shopping, preparing meals, doing laundry, driving chil-dren to school or in severe cases, receiving care and assistance from a visiting nurse, it is critical to establish a support system that would allow you and your family to handle the physical, psychological and medical aspects of a POTS flare-up. Don't forget to express your gratitude to those who helped you through the difficult times: the flare-ups are not only a challenge for you, but also to your caregivers, family, employer and your health care team.

9. Give yourself permission to cry or to feel sad.

Dealing with a chronic illness that may take a fluctuating and unpredictable course is difficult and at times overwhelming, so give yourself permission to feel sad or have a good cry if you feel like it. Such moments can be cathartic and therapeutic and should not be viewed as a sign of weakness.

10. Set goals and challenge yourself.

No matter how small and inconsequential the tasks may seem, setting goals and challenging yourself to achieve those goals is important for the psychological well-being and can boost your morale and confidence. Whether it is getting dressed, walking to the mailbox, organizing a closet, preparing a meal or making a phone call, setting goals and achieving those goals can form a schedule, provide motivation, prevent boredom and give a sense of purpose and accomplishment.

11. Live life to the fullest.

After symptoms subside and you are able to return to some or all of your previous activities, enjoy each day and live life to the fullest. Obviously, when you are feeling well, thinking about a possible relapse in the future may be the last thing that goes through your mind. Conversely, some people will find themselves obsessed over a possible relapse, so much so that they may unnecessarily limit their activity in order to avoid symptomatic worsening. While it is important to maintain a positive and hopeful attitude, it is equally important to be aware that flare-ups can occur with or without triggering factors. Finding the right balance between maintaining an active lifestyle while being mindful of your limitations and trigger factors may lessen anxiety over the unpredictability of flare-ups without impacting your day-to-day activities or causing a paralyzing fear of relapses. This unique and delicate balance is the key to living a satisfying life despite chronic illness.

Shop with POTS: How to shop and NOT drop!

A seemingly simple and routine activity, such as shopping, can turn into a huge undertaking for patients with POTS. Imagine driving up to the store, parking your car in the closest possible parking spot, entering and walking around the store, picking out groceries or clothes, standing in line hoping that there are no price check delays from the customers before you, paying for the items and making it back through the parking lot to the car all in under 10-30 minutes or less of standing time before disabling symptoms of orthostatic intolerance or syncope begin!

Since shopping requires the ability to remain upright for prolonged periods of time, it is not surprising that patients with POTS find shopping a difficult and sometimes impossible task. This may be particularly frustrating for teenagers affected with POTS who may feel left out when their friends decide to socialize at the mall. Patients often begin to avoid shopping malls altogether and opt for smaller stores or shopping on line. In fact, a good practical assessment of the patient's orthostatic tolerance is to ask about their estimated shopping time. If you can shop for 60 minutes without significant symptoms and without POTS flare-up or severe fatigue after shopping, then you are certainly in better shape than someone who can only shop for 10 minutes before needing to sit down or lay on the floor of the shopping mall. The question of shopping time can be very useful to a doctor trying to understand the degree of impairment that one experiences from orthostatic intolerance.

Since the advancements of technology permeated all spheres of our lives, including retail, shopping for patients with POTS and other chronic illnesses with limited mobility or stamina is no longer as challenging and as exhausting as it once was when there was no option of purchasing items on-line. Nevertheless, going out to the stores is an inevitable chore for some and an enjoyable activity for others. If you have POTS, you might want to utilize the following tips when venturing out shopping:

1. Schedule your shopping trip during your best time of the day when your symptoms are minimal, which for many patients with POTS would be during afternoon or evening hours.

2. Before leaving the house, prepare a water or Gatorade bottle to take with you, a small snack and medications that you may need to take in the store if you feel symptomatic. These medications may include an extra dose of a beta blocker or Midodrine, depending on what your treatment regimen is.

3. Make sure that you are well-hydrated before the shopping trip. A salty snack or an extra salt tablet along with a bottle of water can provide a quick boost of energy and extra standing time.

4. Take a friend or a family member shopping with you if you are uncomfortable shopping alone or need help standing in line.

5. Go shopping during the days and hours when the stores are less busy and less crowded.

6. If you have a disabled parking permit, don't be ashamed to use it. If you were approved for a disabling parking permit through your doctor's office and city hall, you have a legitimate medical reason to have the permit and to use it as you see fit. Parking at a designated handicap parking spot may allow you to access the store easily and save standing time and energy for the actual shopping rather than reaching the store's entrance.

7. Learn to shop efficiently. Prepare a list of items that you need to purchase and know where and how to locate these items ahead of time in order to minimize time and hassle in

the store. Research if these items are available in the store on line or by calling in the store prior to going there.

8. Use a seat cane, a wheelchair or a scooter for extended shopping time or shopping that requires walking long distance.

9. Ask the store manager for help if you need assistance carrying groceries to your car, finding an item or standing in a long line waiting at the checkout counter.

10. When waiting in line, do counter-maneuvers to increase your standing time and avoid fainting.

11. Wear a medic alert bracelet that lists your diagnoses, allergies and in-case-of emergency contact person if you have one.

12. If you are feeling ill and unable to shop for groceries or other items of necessity, ask family, friends or neighbors for help. In some cities, grocery stores offer an option of ordering groceries on line, which are then delivered to your home – an invaluable service for people with POTS and other chronic illnesses.

Bath, POTS and Beyond: When it comes to POTS, nothing is off limits

Yes, for many patients with POTS, some basic activities of daily living will become challenging. Remember POTS is life-altering and what specifically it alters depends on many factors, not the least of which is the severity of symptoms.

Since one of the mechanisms of POTS is vasodilation, i.e. dilation of the blood vessels in the lower extremities, factors that can cause vasodilation in healthy people can cause increase in symptoms in patients with POTS. Bathing in hot or warm water will result in vasodilation, which subsequently may lead to a decrease in blood pressure and a rise in heart rate. The following are tips that can help with bathing and showering:

1. Avoid soaking in warm bath for any period of time. Hot tubs and saunas may be particularly detrimental to patients with POTS.

2. Take showers with cool or lukewarm water.

3. If you are unable to stand in the shower, use a shower chair, which can be obtained from a medical supply store.

4. Before you are finished showering, turn the water to cool or cold and let it run on your legs for a minute or two. The cold water helps vasoconstrict blood vessels and prevents blood pooling and a drop in blood pressure.

5. Shower during your least symptomatic hours during the day. You may want to shower before bedtime rather than in the morning, when patients with POTS are typically most symptomatic.

6. If you are someone who faints easily, listen to your body: turn the water off and sit down or lay down immediately to prevent loss of consciousness. Consider taking a shower when you are not alone in the house and leave the bathroom door unlocked in case you need help from others.

7. Note that washing your hair with arms raised above the heart level may increase symptoms of POTS because elevating the arms decreases return of the blood to the heart, which results in increased heart rate and decreased blood flow to the brain. Instead wash your hair by holding your arms close to the body.

8. After shower, sit down and rest. Have a rolling stool in your bathroom where you can sit and blow dry your hair or put on makeup.

9. If you feel dizzy or weak after the shower, lie down for a few minutes or drink a glass of Gatorade.

10. If you are very sick on a particular day and are unable to shower, don't. Give yourself permission to shower when you feel less symptomatic.

POTS and Pans: What's for dinner?

Maintaining a household is a full-time job – just ask a healthy stay-at-home mother - and it should come as no surprise that preparing meals for your family requires a great deal of energy for those with a chronic illness. Having a home-cooked meal is the key to a nutritious diet and healthy food choices. However, a chronic illness like POTS can certainly make it difficult to provide these meals consistently, especially during a POTS relapse.

If you are unable to cook because of POTS, take solace in the fact that fast foods, like pizza, hot dogs, canned soups and TV dinners contain high amounts of sodium and may be the type of food that a person with POTS can reliably utilize during a POTS exacerbation or a particularly symptomatic day. Of course, consuming fast food meals and frozen dinners on a regular basis would result in poor diet and unhealthy lifestyle and may eventually lead to high cholesterol, hypertension, and obesity. The following tips can help you manage meal preparation without over-reliance on fast foods:

1. Cook during the time of day that you feel least symptomatic and on days of the week that you do not have to work, attend important events or have planned activities that require a lot of energy.

2. Cook once or twice a week, as your health and time allows, and store leftovers in a freezer in sealed containers or bags. You can easily thaw the frozen home-made food and warm it up before serving.

3. When cooking or baking, try to use the oven rather than the stove. You can put a cooking pot or pan in an oven and let it bake or broil without your further participation while cooking at the stove would require your constant presence in the vicinity of a hot stove.

4. Choose easy recipes that are not too cumbersome to make and that are not time-consuming. Rachel Ray's book, "The 30-minute meals" is an excellent resource for easy-to-make nutritious meals.

5. Use a high rolling chair or stool in the kitchen, which would minimize standing or moving around the kitchen.

6. Chop and mix ingredients at the kitchen counter or table while sitting down.

7. If you can split meal preparation into several tasks that can be accomplished at separate times or days rather than do it all at once. For example, you may consider cutting meat in pieces, mixing it with vegetables, marinating it in olive oil or vinegar and placing it in the refrigerator for a few hours or overnight before baking or barbequing the meat.

8. As with other household chores, enlist the help of family members. Children can help you by bringing utensils and meal ingredients to you so that you can avoid running around the kitchen or getting up frequently from the chair. Children can also help with mixing, placing cookies on a baking sheet, decorating the cake and doing dishes.

9. A dishwasher is an essential appliance in the household of a person with POTS, so consider investing into purchasing a dishwasher if you don't have one. Since it requires bending to load and unload the dishwasher, you may want to delegate the task to your children or significant other.

10. If you are planning to prepare meals or dessert for a birthday party or dinner with friends, consider baking and cooking on the day before the actual event and storing it in the refrigerator. It may not be as fresh as you would like it to be, but it may save you energy and strength for the actual event. The last thing you want is to prepare a scrumptious dish in time for the party and then not feel well enough to enjoy the party, or worse, not being able to attend at all due to POTS.

11. Always have "emergency food" available in the freezer for the days when you may be too symptomatic to cook. The emergency food can consist of a frozen pizza that you

can bake in a toaster oven, TV dinners that are easy to microwave and canned soups that are high in sodium and can quickly boost your blood volume.

12. If all else fails, give yourself a break and call your favorite take-out place for delivery. It would be worth paying for a meal while saving yourself energy and worry over the "what's for dinner" question.

POTS and Spots: Trying To Keep Your House Spotless

It's inevitable that a messy house will require major cleaning at some point, and like other physical activities cleaning can be challenging if you have POTS. Therefore, for those who are still well enough to attempt cleaning, the following tips may help:

1. Learn to accept some degree of mess and do not feel guilty that your house cannot be spotless at all times.

2. Try to tidy up daily in spurts instead of taking on cleaning the entire house all at once.

3. Enlist the help of other family members: remember you can't do it alone and it's important for children to learn to do chores.

4. Divide and conquer: pick chores that are less physical, such as dusting, sorting and organizing closets, and leave more physically-demanding chores, such as vacuuming and scrubbing the floor or a bath tub, to others.

5. Start cleaning when you feel your best and avoid forcing yourself to clean when you're most symptomatic.

6. Plan your day so that you could take a break and rest after cleaning. Cooking dinner after cleaning the house may not be a good idea if you know that doing too much in one day can usually cause a crash the next day.

7. For those with migraine and sensitivities to smells, wearing a mask while cleaning may help avoid triggering a migraine from exposure to the odor of cleaning solutions.

8. If you have allergies, wear a mask and gloves while cleaning to prevent worsening of allergies, which can result in increased POTS symptoms.

9. Whenever possible, sit on the floor while organizing closets, sorting things or folding laundry. Avoid repetitive bending, twisting or reaching with your arms to the top shelves as these may transiently worsen dizziness, light-headedness and palpitations.

10. If you can afford it, hire professional cleaners. Your energy is precious and investing it into more important activities than cleaning may be worth the price of a cleaning service.

POTS and Tots: It takes a village

Whether you have had POTS before pregnancy or developed it after you have had a child, taking care of kids while having POTS is very challenging and can leave you extremely exhausted, symptomatic and frustrated. Any healthy mother would tell you that taking care of an infant or a toddler is no easy task: in the words of Charlotte from "Sex and The City 2", "How do the moms who have no help do it?" It is therefore understandable that a chronic illness would make motherhood even more challenging. Despite the challenges, however, women and men with chronic illness are just as capable, competent and loving parents as their healthy counterparts.

Since POTS affects predominantly women of reproductive age, it is expected that many women with POTS will either have children or have had children despite the diagnosis. The following are useful tips on taking care of children that may help parents with POTS or those who are planning to have children.

1. First and foremost, establish a support system to help you care for an infant, a toddler or a young child. Recruit the help of grandparents, siblings, distant relatives, friends, neighbors and anyone else who is offering help. Remember,

you can't do it alone and it does "take a village" to raise a child, especially when you have a chronic illness.

2. If you do not have any family members or friends to rely on, invest in a full-time or a part-time babysitter, as dictated by your needs. Although finding a good nanny whom you can entrust with the care of your child is not easy and is also quite expensive, having a reliable and trustworthy babysitter is invaluable when you have a chronic illness and no other help.

3. Consider part-time daycare if you are able to drive or if you have a family member or a trusted friend who can drop off and pick up your child so that you can rest during these hours.

4. When caring for an infant, organize your living space to become both infant- and POTS-friendly. Have bottles, formulas and pacifiers available within reach to minimize running around. Set up a changing table to a height that would allow you to sit while changing diapers.

5. Rest when the baby sleeps. This advice is often given to any mother with an infant, and it is even more important for women with a chronic illness. Try not to use the time for cleaning, cooking or other physical activities, but rather maximize the amount of rest and sleep when your baby is napping.

6. Put the crib next to your bed so that you can easily reach for the baby and breastfeed or bottle-feed without getting up and running to the kitchen.

7. If you are breastfeeding, remember to drink extra fluid and consume food high in salt to replenish the fluids in your body. Breastfeeding uses up a lot of energy, nutrients and fluids, so it is important to have adequate fluid, proteins and vitamin intake. Use a prenatal vitamin in addition to a healthy diet with high fluid and sodium intake.

8. Incorporate various fun activities that you can do sitting or lying on the floor as part of the playtime with your toddler. Reading, painting, playing with play dough, and building with blocks are some of the activities that you can enjoy with your toddler.

9. Have your child's favorite DVD available as a back-up plan when you are feeling particularly symptomatic and need some down time. While you are resting nearby, they can be entertained and give you a break that you need.

10. A stroll outside may present a challenge. Have a bottle of water always available when talking a walk with your baby. Many strollers will have a bottle holder attached or a basket on the bottom to place your things. Know your limits and sit down immediately when symptoms of pre-syncope begin so that you could prevent fainting when caring for your baby, especially if you are alone.

11. Have a cell phone with you at all times, especially if you are prone to fainting and have enough warning to call your "in case of emergency" person if you feel pre-syncopal and are taking care of your child alone. It is extremely important to have safety measures in place should you become symptomatic and unable to watch your child. This may include calling your spouse, neighbor or friend who can be available to help you with childcare on a short notice.

12. Enjoy motherhood! Children are a precious gift, so cherish every moment of raising them. Most healthy mothers at some point will experience feelings of guilt and inadequacy in their parenting abilities and with a chronic illness presenting an added challenge, these feelings will invariably intensify for mothers with chronic illness. Allow yourself to experience these feelings as part of the process. However, seek professional help if you feel that your feelings are interfering with taking care of your child or if you are depressed or anxious.

13. Be kind to yourself and proud of your effort, perseverance, strength and courage. Yes, being a parent and having POTS is difficult, but many people are doing it or have done it and survived the challenge, and so can you.

POTS and pregnancy

For any young woman whose life has been changed by a diagnosis of a chronic illness, a question of whether she can have children will invariably become a vital point in the understanding, acceptance and coping with the illness. Since POTS is commonly diagnosed in women of reproductive age, the issues of POTS as related to child-bearing will span from pre-conception to pregnancy to post-partum period. Only a few years ago, limited information existed in literature addressing the topic of pregnancy in patients with POTS. With the absence of research studies examining POTS and pregnancy, it was not uncommon for some autonomic specialists to recommend to their patients that pregnancy should not be attempted unless they have been asymptomatic and on no medications for at least a year. This recommendation, while may be ideal in theory, presented an unrealistic goal for many women whose lives have been affected by chronic symptoms of POTS, without a chance for remission or possibility of discontinuing medications, thus leaving many of them disappointed, frustrated and hopeless.

Fortunately, in the past three years, more information on POTS and pregnancy became available through a few small studies, which demonstrated successful pregnancies in women with pre-existing POTS, some of whom were also taking medications before, during and after pregnancy to control symptoms. [1-6]

Below are the most common questions concerning pregnancy and POTS that are encountered in clinical practice and the answers that are based on the most current medical information from the scientific literature.

Q: Will I be able to have children after a POTS diagnosis?

A: Absolutely. Many women have had successful pregnancies after developing POTS.

Q: Will POTS affect my ability to conceive?

A: As we currently understand it, POTS does not affect fertility based on the limited research available on the topic.

Q: Will I feel worse during pregnancy?

A: It has been once thought that pregnancy improves symptoms of POTS, chronic fatigue syndrome and fibromyalgia. While many women with POTS (60-70%) will experience improved or stable symptoms of POTS compared to before pregnancy, others can expect symptomatic worsening, especially during the first and third trimesters.

Q: Will I feel worse after pregnancy?

A: It has been shown that the course of POTS after pregnancy is variable, meaning that some patients will experience worsening of symptoms, while others will have stable or improved symptoms compared to before pregnancy. In one study, 50% of women reported improved or stable symptoms of POTS six months post-partum compared to before pregnancy. [6]

Q: Will POTS have any effect on the growth and development of the baby in-utero?

A: As far as we know it, POTS does not appear to cause any negative effects on the fetus. It has been shown in four small research studies available to date that there has been no congenital abnormalities noted due to POTS. In one study, the infants had somewhat smaller birth weights than in the general population, which may have been due to medication side effects.

Q: Is POTS genetic and will my child have POTS?

A: POTS is not a genetic disorder in the sense that it does not follow the type of genetic transmission that occurs in cystic fibrosis, for example. Although research in the genetics of POTS is currently lacking, it has been shown in various studies that POTS may run in families, affecting more than one family member. [6,7] Remember POTS is not a uniform disorder; rather it is a heterogeneous entity, meaning that various mechanisms and causes may have led to a collection of symptoms and signs that satisfy the definition of POTS. Therefore, while POTS is not transmissible to children through one particular gene, it is conceivable that children may be predisposed to autonomic dysfunction as adolescents or adults through their general genetic makeup. However, at this time, it is impossible to predict or calculate the likelihood of a child developing POTS if one parent is affected.

Q: Would I be able to continue my medications for POTS throughout pregnancy?

A: Some women will be able to discontinue all medications before pregnancy, while others would have to continue during and after pregnancy. If you rely on a medication to control symptoms of POTS and discontinuing it would result in significant functional impairment, then remaining on your medication throughout pregnancy is an option that you should discuss with your physician. Most medications that are commonly used to manage POTS are Pregnancy Category C, which means that there are no adequate and well-controlled studies in humans, but potential benefits may warrant use of the drug in pregnant women despite potential risks. However, medications, such as beta-blockers are commonly used in pregnant women with hypertension; fludrocortisones use is necessary in pregnant women with Addison's disease, and SSRI's is typically prescribed for pregnant women with depression. Therefore, these medications can be either continued or initiated during pregnancy in women with POTS. As with any medication in pregnancy, the rule for POTS is to use the least number of medications at the lowest dose possible.

Q: Will my pregnancy affect the course of POTS in the long run?

A: While there is currently not enough research data to definitively answer this question, several studies that have been conducted on patients with POTS indicate that pregnancy does not seem to affect the long-term course of POTS. In the study by Blitshteyn et al, which examined 17 pregnancies in 10 women with POTS, 50% of patients felt that their symptoms of POTS were either stable or improved at 6 months and 1-year post-partum compared to before pregnancy. [6] In another study by Low et. al, autonomic testing results were not different between women with POTS who had children compared to women with POTS who never had children. [4]

Q: I developed POTS post-partum and would like to have another child. Will another pregnancy make me even sicker?

A: Unfortunately, to date, there have been no studies examining the course of POTS with subsequent pregnancies in women with post-partum onset of POTS. The several studies that have been done on the topic of POTS and pregnancy have been targeted at women who developed POTS before pregnancy, and thus are not likely applicable to women with post-partum onset of POTS.

Q: Can I breastfeed with POTS?

A: It appears that POTS in itself does not represent a contraindication to breastfeeding. Since breastfeeding is very important to infants, mothers with POTS as any healthy mother would typically be encouraged to breastfeed by their healthcare providers. Several points need to be considered, however, if you have POTS and would like to breastfeed.

1. Breastfeeding contributes to blood volume loss and therefore, fluid consumption will need to be increased appropriately, above the typical fluid intake for a patient with POTS.
2. Breastfeeding is usually tiring even for healthy mothers, both as a physiologic process and because your baby relies on you for feedings around the clock. Consider pumping milk and storing it in the freezer so that someone else can bottle-feed your baby during the night in order to give you a break and much-needed sleep.
3. If you feel symptomatic because of POTS and need to resume taking medications, discuss with the pediatrician whether these medications are safe to take while breastfeeding. You may be allowed to breastfeed while taking certain medications at a low dose, while breastfeeding may not be an option with other medications.

Q: Can I have a vaginal delivery or should I opt for a C-section because of POTS?

A: The first case report published in literature described two women with severe POTS who delivered via a C-section without complications, which were interpreted by some patients and obstetricians that C-section may be a better option for women with POTS. [1] However, contrary to the initial reports, subsequent case reports and studies suggested that most women with POTS had safe and uncomplicated vaginal deliveries and that POTS in itself was typically not an indication for a C-section delivery. In fact, since C-section is considered a surgery with its inherent surgical complications, such as an increased risk of bleeding and infection, it is probably not a desirable method of delivery in women with POTS compared to vaginal delivery. However, if you do need to have a C-section for obstetrical or other reasons, your doctor will likely monitor your vital signs more closely due to POTS and may need to consult other physicians, such as an anesthesiologist and cardiologist, due to your condition.

Q: I heard that an epidural lowers blood pressure. Should I therefore attempt a natural birth?

A: Obviously, it is important for any pregnant woman to discuss with their obstetrician ahead of time the type of pain control desired during labor and delivery. For women with POTS, it is especially important to have effective pain control since pain is a powerful stimulus for the autonomic nervous system activation and may result in tachycardia, hypertension or hypotension. Although epidural anesthesia can lower blood pressure, a slow infusion of the anesthetic can ameliorate hypotension as a side effect. Liberal intravenous hydration with normal saline or lactaid ringer solution and careful monitoring of the blood pressure and heart rate during administration of the epidural anesthesia can also decrease the risk of hypotension associated with the epidural anesthesia.

If you are considering a natural birth without any medications or pain control methods, you should discuss whether it is a viable option for you with your team of physicians, which may consist of an obstetrician, cardiologist, a maternal-fetal specialist and others that you may have received care from during pregnancy. These specialists will determine whether you are healthy enough to undergo natural birth and should guide you through the process, if natural birth is allowed to take place.

References

1. Glatter K, Tuteja D, Chiamvimonvat N, et. al. Pregnancy in postural orthostatic tachycardia syndrome. Pacing Clin Electrophysiol 2005; 28: 591-593.
2. McEvoy MD, Low PA, Hebbar L. Postural orthostatic tachycardia syndrome: anesthetic implications in the obstetric patient. Anesth Analg 2007; 104: 166-167.
3. Kanjwal KK, Karabin B, Grubb BP. Outcomes of pregnancy in patients with Postural Orthostatic Tachycardia Syndrome. PACE 2009; 32:1000-1003.

4. Powless CA, Harms RW, Watson WJ. Postural tachycardia syndrome complicating pregnancy. J Matern Fetal Neonatal Med 2010; 23: 850-853.

5. Kimpinski K, Iodice V, Sandroni P, Low PA. Effect of pregnancy on Postural Tachycardia Syndrome. Mayo Clin Proc 2010; 85: 639-644.

6. Blitshteyn S, Bett, GL, Poya H. Pregnancy in Postural Tachycardia Syndrome: clinical course and maternal and fetal outcomes. Under Review in J Matern Fetal Neonatal Med.

7. Thieben MJ, Sandroni P, Sletten DM, et. al. Postural Orthostatic Tachycardia Syndrome: the Mayo Clinic experience. Mayo Clin Proc 2007; 82: 308-313.

Chapter 39. The Tip of the Iceberg- Overview of Dysautonomia - *William Suarez, Pediatric Cardiologist*

Common Dysautonomias: Syncope is just the tip of the iceberg
Suarez, W., MD., FACC

A Study from the Division of Pediatric Cardiology

NW Ohio Congenital Heart Center and University of Toledo Medical Center
Phone: 419-251-8036
Email: William.Suarez@Utoledo.edu

Introduction:

Dysautonomic conditions in pediatrics are quite common. At one time or another many of us experience symptoms related to imbalances in the autonomic nervous systems. Some can be quite innocent in nature with some people experiencing nausea or head-aches while others experience pallor or even syncope. These patients are able to trigger a dysautonomic reflex but don't necessarily become incapacitated with a flurry of symptoms that leave them unable to do daily activities. The common ability of blood to trigger an episode of syncope in some people while not in others clearly raises questions regarding each person's individual triggers for dysautonomic symptoms.

The problem is that there are many children and young adults out there that experience a group of non-specific symptoms that can clearly incapacitate them for the vast majority of a day and multiple days of a week. These symptoms can start at very young ages, or can develop in late adolescence for the first time. Many times patients are seemingly well until a protracted viral or bacterial infection triggers an underlying predisposition for dysautonomic symptoms. The classic scenario most pediatric physicians see in the office or in the emergency room are the children who experience an "unexplained" syncopal episode. These are classically in the early morning during a hot shower, before breakfast, or while sitting at school during a biology laboratory animal dissection. Some may be standing in line for a prolonged period of time before developing nausea, stomach discomfort, and then syncope. Athletes who don't keep up with fluids on hot days may also predispose themselves to these types of episodes as well.

For practitioners to know how to deal with these patients, they must understand the common historical features, identify the lack of physical findings on examination, and address the predisposing factors or "triggers" that precipitated the event. When we evaluate these patients in a systematic fashion and rule out "red flags", then we can avoid costly emergency room evaluations and diagnostic studies as well as avoid unnecessary aggravation for families. When we identify these patients early by history, we can move quickly into teaching them the importance of taking responsibility for symptom reduction by identifying the prodromal symptoms sooner. The latter will aid them in taking the appropriate steps needed to decrease their symptoms and prevent progression to complete syncope.

History:

Most physicians who are well familiar with the more common type of Dysautonomic pediatric patient feel that a detailed history alone can identify 90% of these types of conditions. The typical patient experiences a classic prodrome of symptoms predominantly when in an upright position however semi-recumbent positions can also elicit the mechanism for symptom initiation. The classic patient will frequently know that they do not feel well and most will become quiet or somewhat withdrawn. Next, they may feel an increase in body temperature and may even become flushed and diaphoretic. Early in the course of this prodrome, patients experience nausea, stomach ache, or gastrointestinal distress and may even vomit. If no change in position occurs, the symptoms will progress to a general sense of overall fatigue and total body weakness. Dizziness soon follows with associated generalized pallor.

The previously mentioned prodrome is what I refer to as "level one" symptoms. If the patient is able to lie down and elevate their legs, they may be able to stop the impending progression of this mechanism. If not, level two symptoms commence. The latter is associated with progressive loss of peripheral vision from the "out-side" in, toward the media aspect of the line of sight. Some will describe this as "tunnel vision". This can be associated with impaired auditory ability with voices that sound muffled or they cannot hear at all. Occasionally, patients have complained about facial numbness or tingling. Once they progress to this level, syncope is almost assured. The total loss of body muscle control is transient with most patients losing consciousness only for seconds. Once in a supine position, they awaken and are typically "clear headed" and answer questions appropriately. They are frequently fatigued and very pale or "grey" with slow heart rates and low blood pressures. From an Autonomic Nervous System perspective, they have just experienced Sympathetic Nervous system in-put withdrawal, leaving an unopposed Parasympathetic Nervous System tone. Once this mechanism leads to a complete syncopal event, they are at risk for recurrent events in that same day.

The above related prodrome is often seen for patients with the cardio-inhibitory type of neurocardiogenic syncope (NCS). In patients with other forms or Dysautonomia, such as postural orthostatic tachycardia syndrome (POTS), patients experience an exaggerated sympathetic response to positional change and prolonged standing that results in an overly excessive heart rate and many can experience a normal, elevated, or gradually decreasing blood pressure over time when assuming an upright posture. If orthostatic blood pressure and heart rate evaluations are performed in these patients, the lack of an immediate drop in blood pressure, may falsely reassure physicians that true orthostasis is not present. These patients increment their heart rate by over 40 beats/minutes when standing. Thus, orthostatic assessment must include heart rate change in addition to blood pressure with change in position.

In my experience, the history in patients with POTS is frequently one involving tachycardia or palpitations with prolonged standing. The primary problem seems to be related to excessive sympathetic activity when patients are upright. This causes increased anxiety, chest discomfort, and shortness of breath. Many patients feel as if they have been exercising and are constantly fatigued and dizzy. These symptoms can mimic a generalized anxiety disorder and frequently these patients are incorrectly diagnosed as such. The latter can lead to years of persistent symptoms and referral to multiple subspecialists due to gastrointestinal symptoms, chronic headache, and chronic musculoskeletal and joint pain. Many of these children are sent to psychiatrists for evaluation for presumed psychosomatic etiology. Unfortunately, these patients experience real symptoms and because most physicians assume that there is no organic basis to their complaints they become depressed and withdrawn.

Patients with orthostatic hypotension appear to be the easiest to uncover. Their symptoms are frequently associated with postural change and are frequently reproducible. They tend to increase their heart rate by over 20 beats/minute or drop their blood pressure by 20 mmHg or more upon assuming and upright posture. The latter is frequently caused by diminished intravascular volume or inadequate response by the peripheral vascular resistance vessels with standing. They may not have the same prodrome of symptoms as NCS and POTS and some may manifest an increase in heart rate and maintain a normal blood pressure for a short period of time before losing peripheral vasomotor tone and developing the characteristic hypotension associated with dizziness, presyncope, or syncope.

Looking for the trigger

One thing is certain in the management of patients with the most common versions of the Dysautonomias; patients must be able to identify their specific "triggers". For some, a noxious smell or image of blood can elicit a "neuro-cardiac" reflex resulting in a variety of clinical symptoms. For others it is far more encompassing.

Patients who are plagued by these chronic syndromes tend to know what sets them off. The most frequent trigger universally shared is "stress". Stress comes in many forms, emotional, personal, environmental, social, familial, academic, athletic, and medical. We and our patients are constantly bombarded by stress, but they are more adversely impacted by it. The total body stress imposed by a systemic illness is enough to make, a relatively stable patient, experience daily symptoms for weeks. Athletes who are always pushing themselves to the brink of exhaustion due to their competitive nature may quickly find out that they are incapacitated for days.

At times the offending stress can be avoided, but often they cannot. Patients must find ways to use conservative and/or medical therapies to successfully navigate through difficult challenges. Learning how to modify behaviors or goals may help. Placing one's "best foot" forward is extremely helpful. If one maximizes rest and nutrition this may provide added support to deal with the many stresses life can deal out. If a patient is ill, then they should not try to take on added responsibilities or try to push their performance in sporting events.

It's not all about syncope

The most common reason for most dysautonomic patients to seek medical attention is after a syncopal episode. Syncope tends to conjure thoughts of sudden death and frequently patients will have a very expensive evaluation to reassure family members that this patient is not going to die. Although syncope gets the headlines with these patients, many experience more debilitating symptoms but never pass out. Many will have gastrointestinal distress, nausea, and alternating bowel patterns for years. They may be worked up for eating disorders, lactose or gluten intolerance, enuresis, or ulcer disease. The lack of restful sleep leads to excessive missed school time, fatigue and difficulties in concentration. Some children and adolescents may start to feel that they are unintelligent due to the difficulties in learning and following through with assignments. The exact basis for many of these symptoms is still predominantly unknown. Many of the gastrointestinal symptoms may be due to significant venous pooling in the mesenteric circulation. It Is well known that patients experiencing hypotension, may first complain of gastrointestinal symptoms such as nausea and abdominal pain and if they lie down this may quickly improve. Some gastrointestinal manifestations such as difficulty swallowing, early satiety, constipation, diarrhea, and cramping are extremely common and sometimes progressive. These symptoms frequently cause patients to be referred to gastroenterologists for a myriad of tests.

Chronic headaches frequently prompt head CT and MRI scans but are later diagnosed and treated as Migraine disorder. In many cases the latter occur when the patient experiences "low blood" pressure. In all fairness, it is well known that Migraine disorders are commonly seen in Dysautonomic patients and this should be kept in mind when treating them. Severe headaches can in fact trigger full-blown neurocardiac response; thus patients with Dysautonomia and associated Migraine disorder should be treated as quickly as possible. One should document a blood pressure at the time of the headache and if low, guide therapy aimed at improving the blood pressure first before moving to anti-migraine medication. Dr. Blair Grubb has shown that there is an association between Dysautonomia and Epilepsy so one must use the history to help guide diagnostic evaluations.

Chronic musculoskeletal pain can be seen in all Dysautonomic patients but is more frequently seen in the POTS patient. This may in fact be Fibromyalgia or a variant of Fibromyalgia (FBM) as well as due to reflex sympathetic dystrophy (RSD). In patients with Hypermobility Syndrome and POTS the pain can involve large joints, neck and rest of the spine. At times spinal manipulation has been of benefit for some of our patients. The medication Pregabalin has been approved for use of FBM in adults but not pediatrics. I have used this in some of my non-pediatric patients with varied success. Muscle strengthening via mild graded exercise helps patients maintain tone and strength; the latter is helpful as patients work to increase slowly the scope and duration of exercise as symptoms allow. This must however be done slowly since in some patients exercise can frequently trigger symptoms.

Constant fatigue is frequently at the top of most if not all Dysautonomic patients list of symptoms. The latter is extremely similar to chronic fatigue syndrome in general. Many times we have seen patients develop post-viral Dysautonomia with chronic fatigue such as what is seen with Epstein Barr Virus and Cytomegaloviral infections. To date there is no specific remedy for this symptom. We do our best to educate patients regarding the prompt recognition of symptoms to prevent progression to syncope which can help prevent the worsening of fatigue. Adequate sleep and nutrition are extremely important to help one's body deal with the multitude of stresses that can trigger significant events. The fatigue however can be bad enough to cause patients to sleep throughout the daytime, leading to an inability to fall asleep at a normal hour. This causes their sleep cycle to be altered perpetuating a problem of insomnia and late morning or early afternoon awakenings. If the patient is school age, they frequently find it difficult to attend class leading to significant missed school days.

An interesting problem shared by a large percentage of Dysautonomic patients is what they term "brain fog". The latter is an inability to comprehend material in school being taught to them despite them focusing on the instructor and trying to pay special attention to the material. This can be extremely frustrating for students, especially for those who may already have any form of pre-existing learning difficulties. Although extremely bright students can overcome this problem, it takes a significant amount of their time and effort. The latter can be frustrating for them as well. It is not uncommon for grades to fall after the onset of symptoms; however patients who respond to therapy tend to improve their grades over time especially if they are compliant with their treatment regimen. There are times when patients will need specialized help with their curriculum or extra time with their assignments and a school 504 Plan or an IEP can really make a difference. For more severe patients, stimulants have shown promise in certain patient subsets to help with focus, concentration, and organization. Plans must be individualized and constantly reassessed with input from the patients and their educators.

Behavior

The many different faces of Dysautonomia can bring about a number of different emotions and attitudes in patients. In those who are quickly identified and respond to therapy, attitudes are usually quite good since they feel better and their lifestyle is not significantly compromised. However for patients who are not diagnosed for years, are told that they are faking symptoms for secondary gain, have severe enough symptoms to compromise their health and lifestyle or don't respond well to therapy, they face an even more dangerous problem. Hopelessness can set in at any time in Dysautonomic patients and can undermine the best laid-out medical plans. The feeling of hopelessness forces patients to focus on the worst of their symptoms and can cause them to isolate themselves from others. Symptoms of depression can soon set in and exacerbate all symptoms and allow suicidal thoughts to occur. These patients must be identified and be brought to the attention of a trained social worker, Psychologist, or Psychiatrist. Keep in mind that some medications for behavioral issues can be helpful in dysautonomic patients such as SSRIs or TCAs, although supportive studies are not clear regarding their alleged efficacy.

Menses and oral contraceptives

It is clearly known from experience that many females will experience an increased sensitivity to their symptoms either during or shortly after their menses. The frequent stress of intense symptoms, blood loss, poor fluid intake and vomiting can really destabilize the best of patients. Regulating their hormonal surges may provide added stability in blood pressure and help with some patients who have prolonged or excessive bleeding during their cycles. For females of an appropriate age, oral contraceptives may provide an additive therapy for Dysautonomic symptoms. However before beginning to discuss some thoughts about oral contraceptives and Dysautonomia, one should seriously determine the risk-benefit ratio before embarking on this journey. A family history of stroke or clotting disorders may make starting these medications just too risky. Also the many different preparations may cause side effects in patients such as headaches, mood swings, weight gain, or gastrointestinal distress that make medical compliance highly doubtful. The commonly known side-effect of high blood pressure could be very much welcomed in individuals with persistently low resting and standing blood pressures. Some oral contraceptives can regulate the menses well enough to decrease heavy flows and thus preserve intravascular blood volume or decrease the number of periods so that the stress of menstruation is not experienced every 28 days.

In a study looking at Familial Dysautonomia, Maayan et al. was found that 81% of women had significant premenstrual syndrome which frequently triggered their dysautonomic symptoms. Two-thirds had their menses regularly. Women who started oral contraceptives frequently saw a drop in the severity of the premenstrual symptoms and lack of dysautonomic crisis.

Conclusion

This chapter was written to explain to the vast population who have, care for, know, or treat patients with Dysautonomia, that these patients can be very complex. If we are to help them, we need to take time to ask about how Dysautonomia is affecting their entire life, not just whether they are dizzy and passing out. Keeping in mind that the many stresses faced by patients can exacerbate symptoms, we must work to identify each trigger and devise a game plan aimed at minimizing the stress.

Chapter 40. When to see a Gastroenterologist (GI Specialist) and what to expect- *John Fortunato, M.D.*

Autononic Instability and Chronic Unexplained Nausea in Children

John E. Fortunato, M.D.

Correspondence

John E. Fortunato, M.D.Wake Forest University School of Medicine

Department of Pediatrics, Division of Pediatric Gastroenterology

Medical Center Blvd Winston-Salem, NC 27157

TEL: 336-716-3009; FAX: 336-716-9699 jfortuna@wfubmc.edu

Many patients who have POTS or other autonomic dysfunctions, often initially present with nausea, stomachaches and other GI Complaints of unknown ideology. Often these patients end up at the neurologist's office and are diagnosed with abdominal migraines. John E. Fortunato, a pediatric gastroenterologist from Wake Forest University in North Carolina, addresses some of these GI symptoms typically seen in POTS patients and offers many possible treatment options.

Jodi Rhum

Pediatric Gastrointestinal Motility Center at Wake Forest University

As the field of pediatric gastroenterology (GI) advances, there are many new treatment options available for children suffering from motility disorders. Children with motility disorders are a continually increasing percentage of the patients seen by pediatric gastroenterologists and the complexity of their needs is requiring more specialized care. The GI motility center at Wake Forest University provides a specialized level of care for children with both neurogastrointestinal and functional disorders including swallowing problems, gastroparesis, intestinal failure, refractory constipation, as well as chronic abdominal pain, vomiting, and nausea. The team is directed by Dr. John Fortunato and consists of two pediatric GI motility faculty, three nurses, and an administrator. A close collaborative relationship exists between the pediatric and adult GI motility teams including joint research projects and weekly clinical meetings to discuss patient care. The connection between these teams also greatly facilitates the transition of pediatric patients to adult providers as children grow.

Chronic Nausea and Orthostatic Intolerance

Chronic unexplained nausea is a specific focus of the pediatric motility group. Nausea is a serious health problem disruptive to daily life that occurs in up to 10% of children in the community. Childhood nausea affects as many as 80% of those evaluated for gastrointestinal symptoms such as abdominal pain. Nausea leads to frequent absence from school, sleep disturbances, and eating problems in over 50% of children with unexplained gastrointestinal symptoms including chronic nausea and pain. [1-3] Chronic symptoms may result in complications such as malnutrition as well as psychological consequences to patients and economic impact to families. [4] Chronic nausea represents a very diverse phenotype, and its mechanism is often not known. There are limited tools available to better define the cause of chronic unexplained nausea; therefore, treatments have been empirical and less effective than desired. [5,6] One of the objectives of the pediatric motility program at the Wake Forest University School of Medicine is to identify specific biological mechanisms of unexplained childhood nausea.

To address the significant gap in understanding clinically relevant nausea, we have described a group of pediatric patients presenting to our clinic with chronic unexplained nausea and orthostatic intolerance (e.g., postural orthostatic tachycardia syndrome [POTS] or neurally mediated hypotension [NMH]) most of whom also demonstrated gastric dysrhythmias (abnormalities in the electrical activity of the stomach) before treatment (manuscript under review). If these patients met criteria for POTS or NMH based on an abnormal tilt table test, they were treated with fludrocortisone acetate as well as recommended to increase their water and salt intake. There was symptomatic improvement of nausea in these patients when treated with fludrocortisone acetate, a standard therapy for orthostatic intolerance.

Our initial findings raised concern about problems with the autonomic nervous system, a condition sometime referred to as Dysautonomia. The autonomic nervous system is closely tied to regulating the cardiovascular system including heart rate and blood pressure, but also plays an important role in gastrointestinal motility. Dysautonomia manifesting as orthostatic intolerance is found in nearly 500,000 Americans with approximately 15% of all children experiencing syncope before the end of adolescence. [7,8] While fludrocortisone treatment in our patients resulted in symptomatic relief for many patients, it may not be the optimal agent for all patients with orthostatic intolerance, and future research is needed to determine the mechanism between Dysautonomia and gastrointestinal symptoms such as nausea. [9] In addition, while fludrocortisone proved to be helpful in some patients with orthostatic intolerance and nausea, its use to treat nausea alone has not been established, and thus, fludrocortisone should not be used unless conditions such as POTS or NMH have been defined.

Autonomic Problems Defining

Based on these early data, we have begun a more extensive analysis of autonomic function both at rest and during the tilt table testing to better characterize the relationship between the sympathetic and vagal balance in these subjects. The testing is simple to perform consisting of a standard 70 degree tilt table test for 45 minutes in conjunction with continuous measurements of blood pressure, heart rate and electrocardiogram (ECG) tracings using a noninvasive device connected to a patient's finger and wrist. All symptoms including nausea, lightheadedness, and pain are recorded every 10 minutes after tilt to determine if tilting acts as a precipitant.

Fluctuations in blood pressure and heart rate reflect the dynamic interplay of diverse physiological processes [10] and are acceptable measures for cardiovascular autonomic balance. Increased blood pressure variability (BPV) and reduced heart rate variability (HRV) are predictors for many disease conditions. [11-15] Analysis of arterial blood pressure and heart rate has provided new insight into the autonomic vascular and cardiac regulation. [16] BPV and HRV are useful tools for the study of the mechanisms involved in cardiovascular regulation in both normal and diseased conditions. [17] Baroreflex sensitivity (BRS) provides a measure of the gain of the reflex arc which modulates heart period in response to changes in blood pressure. Assessment of the BRS function and BPV in our subjects provides more information about the sympathetic nervous system and its balance with the parasympathetic system.

Better understanding of the specific autonomic disturbances in patients with nausea may allow more timely and better selection of drugs such as vasoconstrictors and beta blockers both of which have also been empirically used to treat orthostatic intolerance. [18] The combination of tilt table and continuous autonomic assessment in our study provides data on baroreflex sensitivity for control of heart rate (BRS), heart rate variability (HRV) and blood pressure at rest and during the tilt mimicking a daily life stressor (upright posture/standing) and the response pattern may provide additional diagnostic information important for patient management.

Initial Approach to Chronic Nausea

Chronic unexplained or "idiopathic" nausea is a diagnosis of exclusion and can only be reached after careful consideration of metabolic, mechanical, or mucosal inflammatory causes. The causes may include, for example, a diagnosis of inflammatory bowel disease, celiac disease, liver or pancreatic disease, hiatal hernia, or bowel obstruction. Particularly in the context of chronic headaches, central nervous system malignancies should always be considered.

Thus, depending on the clinical symptoms and signs, initial testing may include upper endoscopic evaluation, upper gastrointestinal series, or gastric emptying scans. Basic laboratory testing including a complete blood count and metabolic panel along with assessment of amylase and lipase levels may be appropriate if liver/pancreatic disease or chronic blood loss is suspected. Collaboration with a genetics/metabolic team is often advisable for symptoms from birth or if a specific metabolic disorder is suspected. In addition, imaging of the brain (CT scan or MRI) is necessary for unexplained headaches or any signs of neurological impairment. This often takes place after consultation with neurologists.

Because our current routine diagnostic tests such as endoscopy and radiographic tests often fail to uncover any abnormalities to explain these symptoms, patients are frequently denied a diagnosis and a focused treatment plan. Children are often subjected to multiple additional endoscopic procedures including repeat upper endoscopies and colonoscopies intended to identify a potentially subtle finding that may have been missed on earlier evaluation. In addition, routine questions involving symptoms outside the GI tract including dizziness particularly when upright, debilitating fatigue, increased perspiration, and feeling of one's heart racing when standing for prolonged periods are often omitted during a gastroenterology assessment. These symptoms may suggest dysfunction of the autonomic nervous system and have been observed in some cases after an upper respiratory or GI illness.

Some pediatric patients may be labeled as having "behavioral issues" or psychological problems. While psychological concerns must always remain a consideration particularly in patients with a chronic illness, it remains unclear whether symptoms such as anxiety or depression are the primary cause of GI symptoms or a consequence of longstanding symptoms. Thus, psychological evaluation may be necessary in some children to address this concern.

Motility Disorders and the Electrogastrogram (EGG)

When chronic nausea remains unexplained, gastroenterologists may consider the possibility of a motility problem. Gastrointestinal motility disorders may play a role in the pathogenesis of unexplained nausea. [19] Gastric motility is regulated by myoelectrical activity originating from a pacemaker region along the greater curvature of the stomach. Due to the invasive nature of most motility tests such as antroduodenal manometry, there is a lack of control data in healthy children. Thus, in pediatric motility disorders, drug and surgical therapeutic decisions are made with limited data obtained either from retrospective studies and case series or "norms" extrapolated from adult studies rather than comparisons with true pediatric control data.

Electrogastrography has been used in both adult and pediatric studies to determine if gastroparesis and symptoms such as nausea and vomiting are associated with abnormal gastric rhythms. [20-25] Gastric slow waves coordinate normal 3 per minute gastric peristaltic contractions. [26] In contrast to the normal three cycles per minute (cpm) slow waves, gastric dysrhythmias are defined by abnormally rapid or slow gastric electrical events, respectively termed tachygastrias and bradygastrias. The gastric dysrhythmias disrupt normal gastric peristalsis and have a role in the generation of nausea and postprandial symptoms. [19-25]

Unlike most motility studies, electrogastrograms (EGG) are minimally invasive and can be readily performed in children as young as infants with minimal discomfort (27). For this reason normative data in healthy children have been far easier to obtain than in other types of motility testing. [28-34] Despite the technical ease of performing EGG in children, there is a lack of consistency in hardware settings, analysis software, and test conditions including the optimal provocative test. These issues may in part explain why the use of EGG is not widely accepted in children. [35] Nevertheless, several studies have demonstrated that abnormal gastric myoelectrical activity in pediatric patients may play a role in the pathophysiology of functional symptoms such as nausea and pain. [19,23-25,35] Electro-gastrography can also be used as an objective measure of the therapeutic effect of medications. [36]

Conclusion

The association between HRV and orthostatic intolerance defined by the tilt table test may allow more widespread use of HRV in assessing the autonomic nervous system and EGG in assessing gastric electrical activity in patients with nausea and provide a basis of determining the effect of therapy. Better definition of the mechanism of orthostatic intolerance and chronic nausea in children opens the possibility of extending this diagnostic technology to a broader age range of children with GI symptoms, including those with neurological impairment and developmental disabilities.

In the future, we will attempt to define the mechanism for orthostatic intolerance as it relates to nausea by exploring not only heart rate changes, but differences in BRS, blood pressure and heart rate variability, thereby, potentially elucidating the specific role of the sympathetic versus parasympathetic nervous system. Thus, we are at the early stages of characterization of a newly recognized phenotype of chronic nausea in children: autonomic instability associated with orthostatic intolerance, gastric dysrhythmia and nausea.

REFERENCES

1. Sullivan, S.D., et al., Gastrointestinal symptoms associated with orthostatic intolerance. J Pediatr Gastroenterol Nutr, 2005. 40(4): p. 425-8.
2. Roth-Isigkeit, A., et al., Pain among children and adolescents: restrictions in daily living and triggering factors. Pediatrics, 2005. 115(2): p. e152-62.
3. Rask, C.U., et al., Functional somatic symptoms and associated impairment in 5-7-year-old children: the Copenhagen Child Cohort 2000. Eur J Epidemiol, 2009. 24(10): p. 625-34.
4. Hyams, J.S., et al., Dyspepsia in children and adolescents: a prospective study. J Pediatr Gastroenterol Nutr, 2000. 30(4): p. 413-8.
5. Functional Gastrointestinal Disorders. 3rd ed. Rome III: The Functional Gastrointestinal Disorders, ed. D.A. Drossman, E. Corrassiari, and M. Delvaux. 2006, Lawrence, KS: Allen Press, Inc. 419-486.

6. Perez, M.E. and N.N. Youssef, Dyspepsia in childhood and adolescence: insights and treatment considerations. Curr Gastroenterol Rep, 2007. 9(6): p. 447-55.

7. Robertson, D., The epidemic of orthostatic tachycardia and orthostatic intolerance. Am J Med Sci, 1999. 317(2): p. 75-7.

8. Ruckman, R.N., Cardiac causes of syncope. Pediatr Rev, 1987. 9(4): p. 101-8.

9. Riezzo, G., et al., Comparison of gastric electrical activity and gastric emptying in healthy and dyspeptic children. Dig Dis Sci, 2000. 45(3): p. 517-24.

10. Akselrod, S., et al., Hemodynamic regulation: investigation by spectral analysis. Am J Physiol, 1985. 249(4 Pt 2): p. H867-75.

11. Palatini, P. and S. Julius, Heart rate and the cardiovascular risk. J Hypertens, 1997. 15(1): p. 3-17.

12. Lombardi, F., et al., Heart rate variability and its sympatho-vagal modulation. Cardiovasc Res, 1996. 32(2): p. 208-16.

13. Malliani, A. and N. Montano, Heart rate variability as a clinical tool. Ital Heart J, 2002. 3(8): p. 439-45.

14. Stein, P.K., et al., Heart rate variability: a measure of cardiac autonomic tone. Am Heart J, 1994. 127(5): p. 1376-81.

15. Task, F., Heart rate variability: standards of measurement, physiological interpretation and clinical use. Task Force of the European Society of Cardiology and the North American Society of Pacing and Electrophysiology. Circulation, 1996. 93(5): p. 1043-65.

16. Cerutti, C., C. Barres, and C. Paultre, Baroreflex modulation of blood pressure and heart rate variabilities in rats: assessment by spectral analysis. Am J Physiol Heart Circ Physiol, 1994. 266(5): p. H1993-2000.

17. Parati, G., et al., Spectral Analysis of Blood Pressure and Heart Rate Variability in Evaluating Cardiovascular Regulation: A Critical Appraisal. Hypertension, 1995. 25(6): p. 1276-1286.

18. Grubb, B.P., Y. Kanjwal, and D.J. Kosinski, The postural tachycardia syndrome: a concise guide to diagnosis and management. J Cardiovasc Electrophysiol, 2006. 17(1): p. 108-12.

19. Chen JDZ, Lin X, Zhang M, et al. Gastric myoelectrical activity in healthy children and children with functional dyspepsia. Dig Dis Sci 1998;43:2384-91.

20. Lin Z, Eaker EY, Sarosick I, et al. Gastric myoelectrical activity and gastric emptying in patients with functional dyspepsia. Am J Gastroenterol 1999;94:2384-90.

21. Parkman HP, Miller MA, Trate D. Electrogastrography and gastric emptying scintigraphy are complementary for assessment of dyspepsia. J Clin Gastroenterol 1997;24:214-9.

22. Koch KL, Hong SP, Xu L. Reproducibility of gastric myoelectrical activity and the water load test in patients with dysmotility-like dyspepsia symptoms and in control subjects. J Clin Gastroenterol 2000;31:125-9.

23. Friesen CA, Lin Z, Hymen PE, et al. Electrogastrography in pediatric functional dyspepsia: relationship to gastric emptying and symptom severity. J Pediatr Gastroenterol Nutr 2006;42:265-9.

24. Diamanti A, Bracci R, Gambarara M, et al. Gastric electrical activity assessed by electrogastrography and gastric emptying scintigraphy in adolescents with eating disorders. J Pediatr Gastroenterol Nutr 2003;37:35-41.

25. Riezzo G, Chiloiro M, Guerra V, et al. Comparison of gastric electrical activity and gastric emptying in healthy and dyspeptic children. Dig Dis Sci 2000;45:517-24.

26. Physiological basis of electrogastrography. Handbook of Electrogastrography. Eds. KL Koch and RM Stern. Oxford Press, New York, 2003, pp37-67.

27. Koch KL, Tran TN, Stern RM, et al. Gastric myoelectrical activity in premature and term infants. J Gastrointest Mot 1993;5:41-47.

28. Levy J, Harris J, Chen J, et al. Electrogastrographic norms in children: Towards the development of standard methods, reproducible results, and reliable normative data. J Pediatr Gastroenterol Nutr 2001;33:455-61.

29. Friesen CA, Lin Z, Schurman JV, et al. Autonomic nervous system response to a solid meal and water loading in healthy children: its relation to gastric my-oelectrical activity. Neurogastroenterol Motil 2007;19:376-82.

30. Riezzo G, Chiloiro M, Guerra V. Electrogastrography in healthy children. Evaluation of normal values, influence of age, gender, and obesity. Dig Dis Sci 1998;43:1646-51.

31. Hoffman I, Vos R, Tack J. Normal values for the satiety drinking test in healthy children between 5 and 15 years. Neurogastroenterol Motil 2009;21:517-20.

32. Cheng W, Tam PK. Gastric electrical activity normalizes in the first decade of life. Eur J Pediatr Surg 2000;10:295-9.

33. Riezzo G, Castellana RM, De Bellis T, et al. Gastric electrical activity in normal neonates during the first year of life: effect of feeding with breast milk and formula. J Gastroenterol 2003;38:836-43.

34. Patterson M, Rintala R, Lloyd DA. A longitudinal study of electrogastrography in normal neonates. J Pediatr Surg 2000;35:59-61.

35. Cucchiara S, Riezzo G, Minella R, et al. Electrogastrography in non-ulcer dys-pepsia. Arch Dis Child 1992:67:613-7.

36. Cucchiara S, Minella R, Riezzo G, et al. Reversal of gastric electrical dysrhythmia by cisapride with functional dyspepsia. Report of three cases. Dig Dis Sci 1992;37:1136-40.

Chapter 41. POTS; Clinical, Pathophysiological Aspects and Treatment- *Raffaello Furlan- University of Milan*

POSTURAL ORTHOSTATIC TACHYCARDIA SYNDROME (POTS) Clinical, pathophysiological aspects and treatment.

Raffaello Furlan, Franca Dipaola* and Franca Barbic *Internal Medicine, "Bolognini" Hospital, Seriate (Bg); University of Milan; *Internal Medicine, Sesto S. Giovanni Hospital, Sesto S. Giovanni, Milan; Italy.*

Postural Orthostatic Tachycardia Syndrome (POTS), also described as chronic orthostatic intolerance (COI), is a chronic disorder that has been estimated to affect more than 500,000 Americans. Its prevalence is higher in young women (female to male ratio 4:1). (Mayo Clinic believes this number is 5:1) It is characterized by exaggerated tachycardia without hypotension and by symptoms such as: lightheadedness, dizziness, fatigue, palpitations, pre-syncope and occasionally syncope [1] during the assumption of the up-right position.

POTS diagnosis is based on the criteria indicated in table 1

Table 1.

Postural orthostatic tachycardia syndrome (1)

1. Sustained increase of heart rate (HR) of at least 30 beats/min or HR > 120 bpm during standing.

2. Absence of orthostatic hypotension.

3. Duration of symptoms longer than 6 months.

4. Daily occurrence of two or more of the following symptoms of orthostatic intolerance (i.e. symptoms of inadequate cerebral perfusion) including lightheadedness, fatigue, palpitations, headache, nausea, pre-syncope or syncope during upright posture.

Physiology and pathophysiology during up-right position

In healthy individuals, orthostasis results in an increase of venous blood in the lower limbs and splanchnic district with a consequent reduction in venous return to the heart, cardiac output and blood pressure. Arterial baroreceptors (from the carotid sinus and aortic arch) and cardiopulmonary mechanoreceptors (from the heart and lung) detect blood pressure reduction and trigger compensatory neural reflexes resulting in an increased sympathetic vasoconstriction and reduced parasympathetic activity to the heart with cardio-acceleration.

In healthy subjects, standing is associated with an increase of heart rate of about 10-15 beats per minute, of diastolic blood pressure of about 10 mmHg, while systolic blood pressure remains stable. In subjects suffering from POTS, heart rate may rise as high as 130 beats per minutes without major changes in arterial pressure.

Several pathophysiologic mechanisms have been proposed to underlie POTS, including beta-adrenergic hypersensitivity [2], a decreased plasma volume [3,4], inappropriate venous pooling [5], and possible autonomic dysfunction [6,7,8]. In a group of POTS patients, the response to a gravitational stimulus was found to be characterized by an abnormal functional distribution of the central neural sympathetic tone to the heart and vasculature. In particular, there was a reduced capability of increasing the sympathetic vasomotor control during standing in the presence of an excessive cardiac sympathetic drive resulting in an exaggerated tachycardia [9]. Also, it was suggested that the exaggerated postural tachycardia may be due to reflex compensatory mechanisms because of a non-uniform denervation of the legs (patchy Dysautonomia) resulting in a cardiac sympathetic overactivity [10].

Of interest, a mutation of a gene encoding for the norepinephrine transporter protein (NET) has been described in a subject with a POTS phenotype and her relatives. NET promotes the reuptake of norepinephrine from the synaptic cleft. In POTS, NET deficiency may result in a reduced synaptic norepinephrine clearance leading to excessive norepinephrine plasma levels, concomitant tachycardia and symptoms of orthostatic intolerance during gravitational stress. [11]

POTS as a part of a spectrum of cardiovascular orthostatic omeostasis dysfunctions.

It must be emphasized that most of the long lasting symptoms and some of the pathophysiological features characterizing POTS are similar to those observed in healthy humans shortly after return from space [12,13] or following prolonged bed rest [12,13]. The latter are clinical models of both gravitational and physical deconditioning. For instance, an increased orthostatic tachycardia with reduced orthostatic stability, fatigue and lightheadedness have been described in healthy subjects following bed rest confinement. A fall of more than 200 ml of plasma volume, [14] leading to a possible compensatory increase of sympathetic activity and related symptoms, has been reported in healthy volunteers 48 hours after they were lying in bed. A similar reduction in the vascular volume has been observed in primary hypovolemia [3] and confirmed in a subset of patients with orthostatic intolerance [15]. However, in these syndromes a chronic sympathetic over-activity may contribute to sustain the contraction of the vascular space.

There is an overlap between the clinical manifestations of POTS and those observed in the Chronic Fatigue Syndrome (CFS) and Inappropriate Sinus Tachycardia (IST).

CSF is characterized by persistent or relapsing debilitating fatigue [16]. The cause of this syndrome is unknown. Of interest, a hemodynamic profile analogous to the one observed in POTS has been described also in patients with CFS. [17] Indeed, in these subjects HR was found to be constantly higher than in controls despite blood pressure values were similar in both groups. The fact that HR was higher even during the night, that is in the absence of environmental stimuli, highlights the possible role of an abnormality in the central distribution of the sympathetic modulation to the cardiovascular system as pathophysiological mechanism, similarly to what has been hypothesized for POTS. [9].

IST is a disorder characterized by high HR at rest with an exaggerated increase of HR to minimal exertion (18). Various underlying mechanisms have been described for IST, including augmented sinus node automaticity, neural autonomic dysregulation or both. Recently, it has been suggested that the presence of a primary alteration of the sinus node characterized by an increased intrinsic heart rate and by a beta-adrenergic hypersensitivity associated with reduced vagal efferent activity.

Features common to the three conditions are: higher prevalence in young/middle aged females (20-40 years); symptoms lasting for more than 6 months; symptoms (such as palpitations, chest pain, fatigue, pre-syncope) mostly on standing with diminished exercise tolerance; excessive tachycardia with minimal changes in blood pressure on standing; poor quality of life with reactive anxiety, depression and panic attacks.

CFS [19] and IST diagnostic criteria [18] are summarized in table 2.

Table 2.

Chronic fatigue syndrome (CFS) [19]

1. Disabling fatigue (loss of physical and social function)

2. Four or more of the following symptoms: post exertional exacerbation of fatigue, sore throat, tender lymph nodes, muscle pain, multijoint pain, headache, concentration impairment and sleep disturbances. Impaired orthostatic tolerance and anxiety disorders.

3. Symptoms lasting for at least 6 months

Inappropriate sinus tachycardia [18]

1. Resting HR > 100 bpm or increase of HR from sitting to standing (or during minimal exertion) ≥130 bpm

2. Normal P wave axis and morphology at ECG (sinus tachycardia)

3. Absence of secondary causes of sinus tachycardia (anemia, dehydration, hyperthyroidism)

4. Symptoms (palpitations, pre-syncope) clinically attributable to excessive tachycardia

Therapy

Both non-pharmacological and pharmacological interventions may be useful in the management of POTS. However, levels of evidence for each therapeutic option are poor.

POTS induces a progressive physical deconditioning, which in turn tends to perpetuate orthostatic tachycardia and other symptoms following a vicious circle.

Given the well-established effects of physical training in increasing cardiac vagal modulation and reducing resting and submaximal HR, exercise should be recommended to patients. Swimming and other activities in water, where gravity has less impact (1), should be considered as a first choice.

As already reported, hypovolemia may characterize patients with POTS. Water and salt intake should be increased whenever circulating volume is likely to be further depleted such as during hot days in summer or after infectious diseases leading to diarrhea and vomit. Fludrocortisone, a compound which promotes sodium and fluid retention and increases the sensitivity of peripheral alpha-adrenergic receptors may be added.

In some patients the use of alpha-adrenergic drugs such as midodrine (5-10 mg daily) may help to control the lack of vasoconstriction on standing. In patients with significant orthostatic tachycardia, low dose beta-blockers (propranolol 10 mg two or three times a day) or clonidine may improve palpitation and chest discomfort.

Ivabradine, a new sinus node blocker, reduces the firing rate of the sinus node without major effects on blood pressure. A case study showed the benefits of ivabradine (titrated to 5 mg twice daily) in a 15-year-old female with typical POTS, who did not respond to volume expansion and did not tolerate beta-blockers. [20]

Options for POTS treatment with the corresponding levels of scientific evidence are summarized in Table 3.

Rationale	Treatment	Level of evidence (*)
Deconditioning	Physical exercise	Ib
Volume depletion	Water and salt Fludrocortisone Elastic support hosiery	III III IV
Lack of peripheral vasoconstriction	Midodrine	IIb
Hyperadrenergic state	Beta-blockers Clonidine	III III

(*) Ib, at least one randomized controlled trials (RCT). IIb, at least one well-designed quasi-experimental study. III, well-designed non-experimental descriptive studies (case-control or cohort studies). IV, expert opinion.

References

1. Furlan R et al. Am J Med Sports 2002; 4:19-24.
2. Frohlich ED et al. Arch Intern Med 1969; 123:1-7.
3. Fouad FM et al. Arch Intern Med 1986; 104: 298-303.
4. Jacob G et al. Circulation 1997; 96:575-80.
5. Streeten DHP et al. J Lab Clin Med 1988; 111: 326-35.
6. Low PA et al. Neurology 1995; 45: S19-S25.

7. Mosqueda Garcia R et al. Circulation 1995; 92 (Suppl I): I-90.

8. Low PA et al. J Auton Nerv Syst 1994; 50: 181-8.

9. Furlan R et al. Circulation 1998; 98: 2154-9.

10. Jacob G et al. N Engl J Med 2000: 1008-14.

11. Shannon JR et al. N Engl J Med 2000; 342: 541-9.

12. Convertino VA, Robertson RM. In Robertson D, Biaggioni I (eds): Disorders of the autonomic nervous system, Nashville, Tn, USA, 1995: 311-33.

13. Biaggioni I. In Robertson D, Biaggioni I (eds): Disorders of the autonomic nervous system, Nashville, Tn, USA, 1995: 271-85.

14. Fortey SM et al. Aviat Space Environ Med 1991; 62: 97-104.

15. Jacob G et al. Circulation 1996; 94: 627 (abstract).

16. Schondorf R et al. Am j Med Sci 1999; 317: 117-23.

17. Duprez DA et al. Clin Sci 1998; 94:57-63.

18. Lee RJ. Cardiol Clin 1997; 15: 599-605.

19. Fukuda K et al. Ann Intern Med 1994; 121: 953-9.

20. Ewan V et al. Europace 2007; 9: 1202.

Address for correspondence:

Raffaello Furlan, M.D.
Unità Sincopi e Disturbi della Postura
Medicina Generale, Ospedale Bolognini
Via Paderno, 24
Seriate (Bg), Italy
Università degli Studi di Milano, Milano, Italy
Tel: +39 035 3063614
Fax: +39 035 3063601
E-mail: raffaello.furlan@unimi.it

Chapter 42. How to Know When to Seek Professional Help- *Dr. Neil Gordon, Licensed Clinical Psychologist, Harvard*

Neal J. Gordon, Ed.D. Licensed Clinical Psychologist

As a practicing clinical psychologist I meet children, adolescents and adults to talk about and listen to whatever is on their minds. The meetings occur after someone decides, for whatever reasons, that conversing with a professional is advisable. But, what if you are a parent wondering if it is appropriate to arrange meetings between a psychotherapist and your son or daughter has not indicated any willingness to meet with a counselor, therapist, or "shrink"? What are the signs that psychotherapy is advisable? How do you present the issue? How do you overcome resistance to meeting with a mental health professional? How do you find the best possible resource? These are the issues we address in this chapter.

For those who develop a chronic illness there is much to learn, for their lives are hugely impacted by the disease and its consequences. For example, many of those who have POTS were once high achievers both academically and athletically. With the onset of POTS their grades will usually fall and their athletic participation will be affected. These changes bring about a need for a re-definition of self, for the student who previously self-defined, for example, as an athlete, now needs to address the loss of that self-definition. They need to formulate a new concept of who he or she is. And if they also are coping with an illness, then the task before them is daunting. Coupled with the normal identity issues of adolescence, there is much to work through, and the assistance of a mental health professional is a great assist.

Sometimes, there is so much redefining of self-required that the child or adolescent feels it isn't worth the effort. Thoughts of suicide, massive depression, listlessness, and despondency are obvious indicators that psychotherapy is advised. But for some gathering the momentum to find a therapist or to get out of bed to meet with one are great impediments. Parents need to be aware that their encouragement to meet with a psychotherapist and their assistance in arranging an initial meeting are essential.

Many times people with chronic illnesses fall into depressive periods. Some consider taking their life for they live in terrible pain (joint pain, stomach aches, migraines, and dizziness). It is difficult going through the day. Hope is also often in short supply. They feel that the pain will be unrelenting. They feel that they have been robbed of childhood. But, to make matters worse, many try to hide their illness. Furthermore, sometimes teachers, friends, and other associates have never heard of POTS. The illness is nearly invisible to the general public. Schools do not have the programs to cope with students afflicted with POTS. The family is further estranged due to financial and emotional issues associated with coming to terms with the syndrome. These are significant road-blocks.

Children and adolescents with POTS often feel that no one understands what they are going through. They doubt that a counselor could grasp their situation. Many have been told by doctors, unable to find the proper diagnosis that the illness is all in their heads. Some have been told that what they are experiencing is anxiety and the anxiety is causing somatic complaints. The child who has POTS may believe that seeking help from a mental health expert will merely confirm that everything is "all in their heads".

Adolescents who have great resistance to psychotherapy are plentiful. They came to my office, sit slumped in a chair, and declare verbally and non-verbally that they didn't want to be there. They add that if it weren't for their mother (or father) making them attend this meeting, they would be elsewhere. I ask, "Where would you be?" Sometimes they won't respond. I am often assisted in a first meeting with a child by having had a prior meeting with the parents. In any case, their clothing often reveals occasions for discussion. Perhaps they have a shirt or hoodie with a logo on it, the name of a school, or a rock band, or perhaps they are wearing skate-boarding shoes, or athletic attire. I turn the talk to something relevant to the clue. For example, "I know some students who have attended Indiana (because the person is wearing an Indiana University sweatshirt). Is that where you are thinking of applying to school?"

But if none of my prompts elicits a response I declare, "It seems as if you would rather be anywhere in the world but here." This will usually get a nod. I then follow with "Even jail?   Doing hard time in prison?" A shaking of the head follows this, as if I must be out of my head. "Okay not jail. But perhaps you feel you are in a jail from which there is no escape. Something must have caused your parent to be concerned enough about you to make this appointment. Perhaps I can help you escape from whatever pain you are in. What was it that your mother was seeing that so disturbed her?"

In any case, a calm demeanor, a respectful attitude, a willingness to listen, and a touch of humor do much to lubricate a situation. Gentle indications that the therapist can put into words how the child or adolescent feels also do much to increase the chances that the person will conclude that as long as they are there, they may as well use the time well. I declare that I am an emotional ventriloquist attempting to put into words what others feel. Let me try to put into words what you are feeling, I suggest.

I ask if they use the computer or have a cell phone. I ask them to show me their cell phone and let me know their e-mail address and phone number. Usually I will follow up with a text or an email a few days after the meeting. Often, with luck and the right combination of ingredients a return visit is arranged.

Somatic and Emotional Indicators

The signs that something is bothering your child are numerous, even when the child does not verbally express any problem. Two general categories of indicators that psychotherapy could be appropriate are somatic and emotional. All somatic indicators are bodily markers. If your child has headaches, stomach aches, trouble sleeping, bed-wetting, trouble sitting still, bags under the eyes, weight gain or weight loss, problems waking in the morning, frequent and long naps, rapid eye-blinks, trouble making eye contact, then your child is sending some type of signal that something is going on worth noting. The emotional indicators are frequent temper tantrums, volcanic expressions of emotion, drops in grades, shyness, lengthy silences, nervousness, incessant talking, frequent tearful outbursts, or unwillingness to participate in family activities (especially in pre-pubescent children). None of these indicators automatically indicate that psychotherapy is warranted, but all suggest that parents attempt to understand what is behind their display.

If your son or daughter evidences any of these somatic or emotional indicators, it is advisable to find a quiet time (often late on Sunday afternoons) when no one else is present and say, "*I wonder if everything that we need to talk about has been discussed. Is there something going on with you that has been on your mind and we haven't had a chance to review?*" If they respond, "*No, not anything, what makes you say that?*" Respond with reference to the somatic or emotional marker. Say, "*Well, I notice that you have trouble lately looking me in the eyes,*" or "*It seems as if you have been rather annoyed with your sister,*" or "*You have been taking quite a few naps lately.*"

If your child has POTS you can declare, "It is so hard to be feeling as you are. It is disappointing not to be able to do what you once did. Shouldn't those difficulties be discussed?" Be prepared for them to avoid discussing the matter or dismissing your concern. Simply because you are ready to hear them talk about whatever is on their mind there is no necessary probability that they will be ready to present it. So, end that conversation with something like, "Well, I just want you to know I love you and am willing to hear whatever is on your mind. But, if you would rather present your concerns to someone else, I can help arrange it. In any case, we will give it a few days and see what happens."

Since the reference in the suggested response is oblique, it is likely the child or adolescent will ask for clarification, saying something like, "What do you mean 'presenting my concerns' to someone else? Who?" If they do ask for the clarification, that is a good sign. It means they listened carefully to you and are curious about your meaning. If they do not ask, then perhaps they did not grasp what you were saying, suggesting that their defensiveness is high. You may have to repeat your conversation the following week. In those instances where the question was asked, respond with "I mean with a counselor or psychotherapist."

Often, when adolescents hear parents declare that a mental health professional could be advisable, they react angrily. "If any-one needs to see a shrink, it's you," they may shout. Calmly re-spond, "I would be willing to go with you, or even alone, if you tell me what it is I need help with." That will lead to some revelations on the part of the adolescent. React non-defensively. Try to take in all your son or daughter is saying, for it is at that time that you can learn what is on their mind. End the conversation with, "Thank you for talking with me. I learned a great deal from what you said. Let me think about your words."

For most children and adolescents hearing their parent re-spond as just indicated is a shock. It quiets the son or daughter. Sometimes they may add, sarcastically, "Well, it's about time you heard what I have to say." Let it go, or respond, "I'm sorry that I have conveyed to you that I don't hear you. I'm trying to follow all that you say."

Children and Adolescents with Chronic Illnesses

When children or adolescents have POTS, or any chronic illness, they not only have to confront the issues associated with the illness, but also the psychological implications of being different. Especially as children approach adolescence they want not to be completely different, but a part of some peer group. Who wants to be part of the "sick group"? Even fewer want to be part not only of the "sick group," but also the "psychologically disturbed" group. Getting them to agree to psychotherapy, or even presenting the possibility of meeting with a psychotherapist, are sometimes arduous tasks indeed.

The need to address those tasks, however, is strong, for a chronic illness brings with it not only its own symptoms, but also emotional and psychological consequences. So, what needs to be done?

First, of course, parents need to locate the best psychotherapist. If they feel comfortable asking friends for a referral, that is a great initial option, albeit as previously mentioned, some parents are hesitant to let anyone know that someone from their family is seeking psychotherapy. Another option is the state psychological association for whatever state is your residence. If one googles, for example, Illinois Psychological Association, references will be listed who are geographically close to you. Once you know the names of some psychologists in your area you can Google the name and find out background information on the psychologist. Advanced degrees, such as doctoral degrees, are helpful, but so, too, is the area of specific focus that the psychologist emphasizes. Is the therapist a specialist in working with children, or adolescents, or families, or couples? Often, you can have an initial conversation with the mental health professional prior to an initial meeting. You can ask about fees, insurance reimbursements, therapeutic model, schedule, and any other concern prior to a first meeting. You also can indicate why you are thinking about seeing a psychotherapist for yourself or your son or daughter.

It is debatable which therapeutic model is best because there are advocates of a behavioral, Freudian, psychodynamic, cognitive, neo-Freudian, solution-oriented and humanistic models. Generally speaking, however, patients appreciate therapists who are open, non-judgmental, experienced, focused, systematic, and efficient. Patients or clients in psychotherapy appreciate a person who can translate what is going on in the client's life into easily understandable English and who can assist clients in being able to accomplish goals. They also like it when the therapist is around and not planning soon to retire or take frequent trips away from his or her practice. And, it is helpful to have a therapist who while in charge of the therapeutic endeavor is not over-powering or omnipotent in demeanor.

Schedule a first meeting without bringing your son or daughter. Present your situation honestly, saying, for example, "My daughter has POTS. She is extremely bright, hard-working, and kind, but she also is struggling with her adolescence more than those without the syndrome, for she is often alone, has a school schedule specific to her, and cannot always be available to do what is required. She is reluctant to see a psychotherapist because it will take time from her day and because she feels it will make her feel even more special and different from other teen-agers. On the other hand, we love her and are concerned for her. We don't know what to do."

Often an approach that works well is to have the focus of the therapy not be on the son or daughter, but rather on the family. If the therapist suggests having the daughter/son come in with her parents, or having the whole family come in for an initial visit, then that can be a useful way to discover family dynamics while also allowing everyone in the family to see who the therapist is and how they react to him or her. A subsequent meeting with the parents alone can then work toward a plan of action. Parents should ask each of their children individually how they reacted to the therapist. Ask for what they specifically liked or didn't like.

It is difficult to say whether all children and adolescents with a chronic illness should see a therapist, because there is no "one size fits all" response. However, coping with a chronic illness is a continuing struggle, sometimes visible, sometimes not. Periodic visits with a mental health professional for the entire family are useful means of discussing how life is going in the family, releasing pent-up emotions, and working on goal-setting and goal-assessment. They are well worth considering and exploring. If they seem not worth the time, effort, and expense after some initial explorations, then ask if another therapist might be a better match, or consider waiting six months to a year for another exploration of the viability of the process.

Summary

In short, speaking from the perspective of a clinical psychologist (and therefore biased in favor of the process), I recommend that parents consider seriously the possibility of psychotherapy when they see evidence of any of the somatic or emotional indicators suggesting that something is being communicated by your son or daughter that requires attention. Especially in those situations where a chronic illness is present, periodic assessments with a mental health professional are advisable, often with the focus on the entire family rather than only on the child with the illness.

If you have more questions or want to make an appointment, feel free to contact me at:
nealgordon@post.harvard.edu
Phone number: 708.383.4671, 847.668.11

Chapter 43. Coping with POTS - *Svetlana Blitsht-eyn, MD.*

Coping with POTS, like with other chronic medical conditions, can be a difficult task. It requires understanding the illness and its aggravating factors, awareness of the capabilities and limitations of your body, support from family and friends, a team of competent and compassionate physicians and a positive and hopeful attitude.

If you have been just diagnosed with POTS, you may be feeling overwhelmed, frustrated, helpless and fearful about what the future holds. Add daily disturbing symptoms to the mix, and one can easily fall into the pits of depression. Although as mentioned before, POTS is not a life-threatening condition, it is undoubtedly life-altering. Learning how to live with POTS and how to avoid or minimize the symptoms is a process that does not happen overnight. It takes time and a trial-and-error approach to learn what things or activities make your symptoms better or worse. Whether you keep a written diary or make a mental note, figuring out what helps and hurts your symptoms is the key to allowing you to lead a healthier and more productive life.

Many patients with POTS find that becoming disciplined about their lifestyle allows them to function fairly well, whether at work or at home. They have learned from experience the aggravating and alleviating factors for their symptoms and have become aware of how much they are able to accomplish on a given day. These patients have noticed consistently that going beyond the limits of their physical capabilities results in a flare-up of symptoms and inability to function for days following the overexertion. They are then forced to rest and recharge in order to regain their baseline energy and return to their previous level of functioning.

While it would be logical to want to avoid such "crashes", it may be impossible to do so in some situations. After all, life is unpredictable! In the cases where flare-ups are unavoidable, try not to stress about the consequences. Enjoy what you are doing at the moment and do not anticipate the worst. You may be surprised to find out that the anticipated worsening of symptoms is not as severe as you thought it would be, or, if it is exactly what you have anticipated it to be, remind yourself that it would pass as it always had in the past. Such approach will help minimize anxiety about a possibility of flare-up and provide a more positive outlook even if an anticipated flare-up occurs.

Furthermore, leading a regimental and disciplined lifestyle may sometimes result in the lack of spontaneity and avoidance of activities or situations that have predictably increased your symptoms. As stated previously, POTS is life-altering, but how much it alters your life lies in a delicate balance of how severe your symptoms are versus how you manage to function given the severity of symptoms.

Clearly, will-power alone will not make your heart rate slow down or your blood pressure to change, although those who are trained in biofeedback, may be able to achieve both. Mind over matter would not be enough if your symptoms are not controlled, whether by medications and/or nonmedication approach. However, if your symptoms are fairly well-controlled in general, do not be afraid to start pushing your limits gently and carefully by undertaking activities and tasks that you fear would result in worsening. For example, if bicycling in the park has been your activity prior to becoming ill, you may want to start bicycling around your house first during the hours that you feel best. Then add more time and greater area of bicycling every week to gradually move toward bicycling in the park.

For some patients with POTS, avoidance of things, places or situations that increase symptoms has narrowed their ability to function and limited their life just as much or more than POTS itself. Since reclining or lying down minimizes or completely abolishes the symptoms, it is easy to fall into the trap of rest and reclining as a way of symptomatic relief or even a form of "false" therapy. While this method seems a plausible, and often necessary, approach short-term, prolonged rest or reclining is detrimental and should be avoided. Numerous studies have shown the negative effects of deconditioning on healthy people and those with autonomic disorders. Deconditioning affects not only the muscles of the legs or the heart, but also the blood vessels and the entire autonomic nervous system. Thus, avoiding every and all precipitating factors or situations where symptoms could potentially flare-up can cause significant physical and psychological limitations.

The goal of every person living with a chronic medical condition is to live a happy and productive life. For many patients with POTS, the goal can be achieved through a combination of medication and nonmedication therapy, while for others, with more severe and disabling symptoms despite treatment, it may not be possible to return to the previous level of functioning.

It can be extremely difficult for patients, family members and physicians to accept the fact that some patients with POTS do not improve over time and with treatment, and that some actually become worse. These patients often describe undergoing a period of mourning with all the stages of grief as if mourning a loss of loved one. They are faced with a daunting task of figuring out how to live their life to the fullest, given the disabling symptoms and the limitations. For them, finding a new life, with the goal of maintaining physical, psychological, financial and social aspects of living, is a process that often requires soul-searching, faith, support from family and friends, reassurance from physicians and counseling with a therapist specializing in treating patients with lifelong chronic illnesses.

Whether your symptoms have improved, are improving, or are getting worse over the years, living with POTS means learning to manage your symptoms while maintaining the activities of daily living. As many POTS sufferers correctly attest, living with POTS is like "being on a rollercoaster ride". Symptoms can significantly fluctuate in severity over the course of the day or even hours resulting in patients being completely asymptomatic at one time of the day or entirely disabled and bedridden at other times. Moreover, the onset and offset of symptoms can be unpredictable, with triggering factors not always identifiable. This unpredictability and uncertainty can make keeping a daily schedule difficult, if not impossible sometimes.

The following suggestions would help you minimize the impact of the unpredictability of POTS on your daily life while maximizing your productivity and sense of accomplishment.

- Set up goals that you wish to accomplish for the day, whether it is as basic as getting dressed in the morning or as complicated as going grocery shopping.
- Strive to achieve the goals that you set for that day, yet allow yourself to re-schedule these goals for another day or time when you feel better.
- Use the hours that you feel best to accomplish the most important tasks.
- Be flexible: re-scheduling because you are not feeling well is not a sign of weakness.
- Be kind to yourself: you are not a failure because you could not complete a task that you planned out to do
- Prioritize on what activities are important.
- Eliminate activities that are non-essential or that are not worth spending your precious energy.
- Delegate what can be delegated to others; it will save your energy for the most important tasks of the day.
- Don't feel ashamed to ask for help: you can't do it yourself all the time, especially when you are dealing with chronic illness.
- Take pride in what you are able to accomplish for the day: it may not be what you used to do before you became ill, but it is what you set out as your goals for the day.
- Surround yourself with family and friends who are sup-

portive and encouraging.

- Try to stay away from people who look down on you because of the chronic illness, who take pity or who do not believe that you have a chronic illness.
- Be honest with people about your illness if they ask
- Do not use POTS as an excuse to avoid responsibilities.
- Spend your energy and standing time wisely.

Coping With the Diagnosis The Secret in My Life – One Patient's Story

They say that honesty is in the best policy, but I've kept a secret about having POTS for as long as I could. Perhaps I have kept it a secret from myself, as much as from other people, especially at times when my symptoms were minimal. I lied to myself that maybe I don't have POTS anymore, that the fact that I could never spend a day shopping or hiking or just walking around was just a variation of normal and not the subtle signs of illness. At school and at work, I would always try to hide my inability to stand by trying to avoid it as much as I could or alternating standing with sitting down where it was impossible to avoid it. When no one else seemed to have a problem with standing, I would fidget, feel dizzy, contract my muscles, drink water to counteract the effect of gravity on my body, and by the end of standing would feel exhausted, drained and weak. None of my friends knew that I had POTS, and probably almost no one suspected that anything was wrong.

When POTS hit me full force, I no longer had the luxury of mild symptoms that I could hide or compensate for, so keeping a secret became much more difficult; yet, I still managed to continue. I've isolated myself from many friends, avoided making plans or commitments out of fear of not being able to keep them due to symptoms and stayed in touch mostly over the phone or E-mail, where I continued to pretend that my life is fine. I was afraid to share with anyone other than my immediate family the turmoil and the suffering that became my life, and I did not want their pity, or even sympathy.

It was a different story keeping my secret at work. When I could no longer push through the fatigue and pain to maintain my schedule with long work hours, I was forced to "come out" to my boss, an experience that was traumatizing and extremely unpleasant, once again justifying my desire to keep my illness a secret. After POTS was no longer a secret at work, I had to find a way to keep my professional relationships with co-workers while keeping communications about my illness to a minimum. If someone at work asked me how I was feeling, I would reply with "fine, thank you." If someone commented on how pale I looked that day, I would put more make up to mask my face the next day. If I felt that a colleague was more sincere and wanted to know if I am getting better, I would allow myself to reply with a neutral response, "I have good days and bad days." I would pretend to be cheerful and energetic at the time when I felt like I am near passing out. If I felt that I could no longer hide my symptoms through acting, I would find an empty room and close the door and wait for the symptoms to pass.

Yes, I've become a great actress as a result of having and hiding POTS. I wonder what it would have been like if I had been open and honest about my illness from the start, but I dreaded having to explain a mysterious illness to others and wondering whether they are making their own judgment of me or my illness. Since POTS is unknown to the general public, I feared that it would not be taken seriously and perhaps would be thought of as "stress", or "anxiety", or "hysteria". I did not want to explain my symptoms of profound fatigue, racing heart and difficulty standing even for a few minutes to healthy people, who may have reacted with "oh, I have that sometimes", or "I am always tired" as a way to imply that my illness was just no big deal.

So, I continue to keep my illness a secret. I keep it to myself as I much as I can because this is my struggle, my suffering, my life. Perhaps one day when POTS is more recognizable, like diabetes or asthma, I may become brave enough to tell the world about my ill-

ness, but for now I will keep living with a secret: it may be easier this way.

If you had been diagnosed recently with POTS, you have probably experienced symptoms for a while. Observations show that a patient with POTS may go undiagnosed for years. These observations also demonstrate that a patient with POTS may see up to 10 or more doctors before getting a correct diagnosis. You may feel relieved to finally have a name to your multitude of symptoms and validated that these are not "all in your head."   A majority of patients with POTS have been misdiagnosed with a psychiatric condition, typically from the spectrum of anxiety disorders, at some point in the course of the illness. Thus, a diagnosis of POTS may be liberating in a sense that it may confirm what you had suspected already: that you did not make up your symptoms and that you did not cause the physiological dysfunction of your body.

As a newly diagnosed POTS patient, you are probably feeling overwhelmed, or even frightened. The following suggestions can be helpful to the newly diagnosed patient with POTS:

- If you have just received a diagnosis of POTS from a physician, ask whether you can establish a long-term relationship with her/him. If it is not possible for you to continue seeing this physician, whether because of the geographic location of the clinic, or because that physician acts as a consultant only, ask whether this physician can communicate with your local physician regarding your care.
- Obtain copies of all medical records pertaining to your diagnostic workup and keep these organized in a folder or a binder. You can later share these records with your other treating physicians.
- If a treatment plan has been made between yourself and your treating physician, make sure to follow through all of the recommendations in the plan, including medication and

non-medication treatment.

- As much as possible, avoid negative thinking, such as, for example "my life is over", "it will never be better", etc.
- Stay hopeful that with treatment and time, improvement in your health is probable.
- Educate yourself about all aspects of POTS and stay current on the latest research, if at all possible.
- Avoid obsessing over symptoms and illness, in general. This may be particularly difficult for all patients with POTS, both newly diagnosed and those who have had it for many years. As you learn what to avoid and how to manage your symptoms, you will find that implementing different things to keep POTS at bay becomes less time and energy consuming and more automatic than when you just received the diagnosis.

Coping with Disability

POTS can be very disabling. A study by Dr. Low and colleagues revealed that patients with POTS had the same disability scores as patients with congestive heart failure and chronic obstructive pulmonary disease [1]. Disability varies greatly among patients and for each patient at different times in their life. As stated in previous chapters, employment and education can be significantly affected. With proper treatment, some patients are able to maintain full-time employment, while others discover that part-time work is more manageable. Still, some patients are unable to maintain any type of employment, despite maximum medication and nonmedication therapy.

Perceived disability correlates with severity of symptoms [1], and those with milder illness may have less functional impairment, and thus able to cope better with POTS, compared to those who are more severely affected. At times, however, some patients with severe POTS are able to function better than those with milder illness. What allows some patients to cope better than others may be due to a combination of various factors, such as their personality traits, adaptability to adversity, tolerability of bothersome symptoms and attitude toward chronic illness. Additionally, support system, spirituality and faith are important factors in influencing a patient's ability to cope with chronic illness.

Chronic Illness and Depression

Many studies have shown that chronic illness places major stress on patients and their family. Furthermore, those with a chronic medical condition have a greater risk of suffering from depression. The more severe the condition is, the more likely a patient will experience depression [2].

By itself, depression can be incapacitating, but if a patient also has a medical illness, it can make outcomes worse for both conditions.

Depression can accompany medical conditions for a number of reasons:

- Medical disorders may contribute biologically to depression by altering hormones and neurotransmitters in the brain. [3]
- Patients with chronic medical conditions may become clinically depressed as a psychological reaction to the pain, fatigue and/or disability caused by the illness or its treatment, or difficulties coping with a medical condition. [2,3]
- Some medications that are used to treat POTS, like beta blockers, can also cause or worsen depression.

Symptoms and Signs of Depression

Depressed mood   Feeling hopeless, sad, discouraged, or empty.

Loss of interest or pleasure	Inability to experience pleasure. Nothing seems to interest you anymore, including former hobbies, social activities, and sex.
Appetite or weight changes	Significant weight loss or weight gain—a change of more than 5% of body weight in a month.
Sleep changes	Insomnia or oversleeping (also known as hypersomnia).
Psychomotor agitation or retardation	"Keyed up," unable to sit still, anxious, restless or sluggish, slow speech and body movements, lack of responsiveness.
Fatigue or loss of energy	Physically drained. Even small tasks are exhausting. Can't do things as quickly as you used to.
Self-loathing	Strong feelings of worthlessness or guilt. Harsh criticism of perceived faults and mistakes.
Concentration problems	Inability to focus. Difficulty making decisions. Can't "think straight." Memory problems.
Irritability	Grouchy, easily annoyed, and frustrated by little things. Angry outbursts.
Aches and pains	Depression can cause or exacerbate many physical symptoms, including headaches,

backaches, diarrhea or constipation, abdominal pain, and aching joints.

Chronic Illness and Anxiety

Anxiety can be a major part of any chronic condition, including POTS. It is important to be aware that physical symptoms of anxiety disorder can be identical to the manifestations of POTS (4,5). This similarity may account, in part, why many health care professionals misdiagnose POTS patients with anxiety disorders. Furthermore, some patients who have both conditions are sometimes confused whether symptoms are due to POTS, anxiety or a combination of both. Interestingly, for some patients, as the symptoms of POTS are alleviated with proper treatment, anxiety also diminishes.

Psychological Symptoms of Anxiety

- Apprehension, uneasiness, and dread
- Impaired concentration or selective attention
- Feeling restless or on edge
- Avoidance
- Hypervigilance
- Irritability
- Confusion
- Behavioral problems (especially in children and adolescents)
- Nervousness and jumpiness
- Self-consciousness and insecurity
- Fear that you are dying or going crazy
- Strong desire to escape

Physical Symptoms of Anxiety

- Heart palpitations or racing heartbeat
- Chest pain

- Hot flashes or chills
- Cold and clammy hands
- Stomach upset or queasiness
- Frequent urination or diarrhea
- Shortness of breath
- Sweating
- Dizziness
- Tremors, twitches, and jitters
- Muscle tension or aches
- Headaches
- Fatigue
- Insomnia

Coping with Depression and Anxiety

If you think that you are experiencing symptoms of depression or anxiety, you need to see your primary care physician, who may refer you to a mental health provider. You may think that by being aware of the symptoms of anxiety or depression, you may be able to recognize these conditions yourself, but self-diagnosis is not reliable and only a licensed health professional can make a diagnosis. Medications and cognitive-behavioral therapy are effective treatment options for depression or anxiety. Below are helpful tips that you can implement in your life to help lessen the symptoms of anxiety:

Exercise regularly	Exercise is an effective treatment for anxiety. Yoga and aerobic activities are particularly calming.
Get enough sleep	Lack of sleep can exacerbate anxiety.
Eat a healthy diet	Healthy eating can help you in your battle against anxiety and stress. Make sure your diet includes plenty of fruits and vegetables.
Meditate	Many types of meditation have been shown to

	reduce anxiety. Common types of meditation include mindfulness, walking meditation, and transcendental meditation.
Practice relaxation techniques	Relaxation techniques such as deep breathing and visualization can help reduce anxiety.
Avoid alcohol and drugs	Don't use substances to cope with your anxiety. They can make the problem worse, and eventually will cause problems of their own.
Reduce caffeine intake	If you're consuming caffeinated beverages, including soda, coffee, and tea, in order to increase blood pressure or improve stamina, consider cutting back. Caffeine can increase anxiety, cause insomnia, and even provoke panic attacks.
Cultivate a support system	Spend as much time as possible with people who make you feel good and are emotionally supportive. The more social support you have from friends and family, the less vulnerable you will be to anxiety and stress.

Family Members Coping with POTS

If you are a family member of someone who has POTS, you are probably aware of the many frustrations this illness has caused for them and your family. The scope of this illness is so wide that it can impact many aspects of life not only for those who suffer from POTS, but also for their spouses, partners, children, parents and friends. Fatigue and unpredictable flare-ups of symptoms are usually the main factors that could limit what your loved one can do on a given day. Coping with illness for patients with POTS relies heavily on the support system at home. Conversely, family members of those with POTS may find themselves overwhelmed and stressed with new responsibilities, and sometimes unable to cope with the illness.

A chronic illness can place a major strain on a marriage, but it can also reveal and strengthen the many aspects of your relationship that, otherwise, may have gone unnoticed. Compassion, selflessness, mutual respect and communication are all but a few qualities that constitute a strong relationship and that affirm the "in sickness and in health" promise.

The following are important points shared by the patients and their family members that can help you cope with the chronic illness of your loved one, while providing them with support and care.

- Help with the physical tasks as much as you can. You may have to completely take over certain household chores that are particularly physically demanding for someone with POTS, such as, for example, grocery shopping, vacuum cleaning, or mopping the floors.
- Understand that your partner has a chronic illness and that because of the fatigue and other symptoms, they may not be able to function as well or as much as they did when they were healthy.
- Do not keep score as to who does what. During the most symptomatic periods, you may have to do all housework temporarily.
- Be supportive and encouraging. Remember that your partner needs your support to get through the rough times as well as to get better.
- Avoid being over-protective and allow independency. People with chronic illness want to be independent as much as possible. They do not want to feel like they are "a burden" to others.
- Treat your spouse as equal, even at times when you carry more household responsibilities.
- Be flexible and accommodating. If you are going out and your partner doesn't feel well, you may have to cut your outing short. Instead of being upset or sad about it, be glad that you were able to spend that time, even if not as long as

you planned, away from home.

• Stay hopeful. At times when the illness is worse, your partner may feel particularly down and hopeless and may look to you for a source of hope and comfort.

• Try not to let POTS to become the main focus for you or your loved one affected with it.

• Do not use POTS as a source of confrontation, arguments or blame.

• Take care of yourself. Family members often forget their own needs when taking care of others.

References

1. Benrud-Larson LM, Dewar MS, Sandroni P, et. al. Quality of life in patients with postural tachycardia syndrome. Mayo Clinic Proc 2002; 77: 531-537.
2. National Mental Health Association Fact Sheet. Co-occurrence of depression with medical, psychiatric, and substance abuse disorders; 2000.
3. Goodwin GM. Depression and associated physical diseases and symptoms. Dialogues Clin Neurosci. 2006; 8: 259-265.
4. Raj V, Haman KL, Raj SR, et al. Psyhiatric profile and attention deficits in postural tachycardia syndrome. JNNP 2009; 80: 339-344.
5. Blitshteyn S. Postural tachycardia syndrome and anxiety disorders. Letter. JNNP, April 8, 2009.

Part III – Patients' Experiences about Treatment Options that have Worked for them

Chapter 44. Patient Story – *POTS Treatment Center – Dallas, Texas- Nikki Rhum*

In October of 2011, my then 16-year-old daughter, Nikki, who had been diagnosed with POTS and Ehlers Danlos Syndrome type III four years earlier, came down with Strep throat.   From there on in, it was a downward spiral for her. Her symptoms became exacerbated; on top of her other debilitating symptoms of low blood pressure, tachycardia, joint pain, headaches, nausea, etc., she began to now also have a chronic migraine. She also developed vertigo, extreme light sensitivity and was unable to walk unattended from her bedroom to the bathroom due to severe dizziness and weakness. She missed four months of high school and was in and out of local hospitals. Nikki was feeling so ill that she could no longer even text her friends, use the computer or even watch television, because it hurt her head more to do so. She began wearing sunglasses (sometimes one pair on top of another) in the house, hoping that it would minimize her migraine. I feared she would quickly fall into a deep depression, and we might lose our daughter to her syndrome.

I had almost lost all optimism, when I got a phone call in January from a friend of mine, who has two children that also have POTS. She told me about the POTS Treatment Center in Dallas, Texas. We both believed it was too good to be true. A few months later and no relief of my daughter's symptoms, I decided to call Dr. Mary Kyprianou of the POTS Treatment Center and find out more information about the biofeedback program she was offering for POTS patients. It was a call that would change our lives.

Dr. Kyprianou called me back herself and talked to me for almost an hour. She explained that she had a 100% cure rate with migraines and encouraged me to give her program a chance. I expressed to her my apprehensions, (expenses, time away from work, more missed school for my daughter, etc.) and she explained to me that sometimes you just have to take a leap of faith. I was incredibly impressed by Dr. Kyprianou's knowledge and compassion on the phone that day, and I decided to take that leap.

From the moment my daughter and I walked into the POTS Treatment Center, I knew I had found gold. From the calming Zen-like atmosphere of the office to the friendly staff and incredibly warm disposition of Dr. Kyprianou, I immediately began to feel a renewed sense of hope. Dr. K. greeted us with open arms and explained the program thoroughly to my daughter and me. She then asked Nikki if she understood the physiology of her syndrome. No doctor, of the dozens we had seen, had ever thought to do this. Dr. K. showed my daughter a diagram and explained the sympathetic and parasympathetic nervous system to her, and she explained to her how her health and wellness program could help to make her symptoms better. Dr. K. also explained to us both that the POTS Treatment Program would also incorporate stress management, nutrition counseling, vitamins, supplements, sleep enhancement and exercise protocol specifically designed for POTS patients, like my daughter. She was confident that the combination of these would help my daughter to get back on her feet. She told Nikki that it was not a choice, that she would recover and that she was now in the driver's seat. Dr. K. enforced to her how she would gain control over her own symptoms and how she would teach her to do just that. As she spoke gently to my daughter, I felt a large burden lifted from my shoulders, and I began to relax for the first time in many years. My skepticism began to fade, and I felt strongly that this treatment after years of healers; chiropractors, acupuncturists, herbalists, Eastern and Western doctors, (we had tried it all) etc. would finally be the one that would make a difference.

Dr. K. told Nikki how she would train her to control her muscle tension, blood flow, heart rate, etc. through an integrative approach of neuro biofeedback and health and behavior procedures. My daughter and I were a bit cynical but listened intently as she further explained the process. Dr. K. then placed sensors on Nikki's skin and explained to her that she would be able to see many of her own physiological processes such as: breathing, blood flow, temperature regulation, heart rate, etc. on the computer screen in front of her. Using this technique, she would be trained how to monitor these responses and how to make adjustments to alter them. Dr. K. expounded on the fact that Nikki would receive instant auditory and visual reinforcements every time a positive change in one of the aforementioned areas was made. The brain wanting to continue receiving this instant gratification would continue making these positive changes until eventuality it would become second nature. I sat back in my chair, still questioning this whole process, yet now starting to think to myself that this was making more sense.

The first several days at the Treatment Center were uneventful, and I was not seeing much progress. I watched from the sidelines as Nikki's heart rate went from 90 beats per minute to well over 130 beats per minute (bpm) when she made the slightest of postural changes. I was not too encouraged. Over the next several days and more therapy, Nikki was trained how to keep her pulse rate at a more stable rate. I did not think this was possible, but I watched it on the screen with my own eyes. Nikki could now keep her heart rate at about 80 bpm while remaining in a sitting position. Now the real test would come later in the week when they would teach her to keep her pulse rate down and stable, while standing.

During the first week in Dallas, Nikki and I would go to the POTS Treatment Center, she would do her biofeedback session, the doctors would speak with me and come up with a plan of action for the next day and then I would take Nikki to one of the many upscale shopping malls in the area. My daughter, being a typical teenage girl, loves to shop and I thought this would not only be a great distraction but would also be an excuse for her to exercise. The first three days of shopping, my daughter could not walk through the mall without my support. By day four of treatment, she broke away from my hold and began to walk on her own. I asked her if she was feeling any better, and she said that she had not noticed any changes. I decided to take a step back and simply watch for improvements rather than to ask her directly. She seemed very nervous about getting her hopes up too high and once again being disappointed; she was guarded about her chances of recovery.

By the end of the first week, Nikki was able to stabilize her heart rate during her biofeedback sessions to around 80 bpm while standing. She was now talking to her friends on her cell phone, watching TV with me, and she even did a handstand (she was a former gymnast) in the hallway of the hotel; still she reported to me that there was no change in her condition.

By the second week of treatment, she was now able to out shop me, and she began to leave her sunglasses back at the hotel. Her endurance was much better, and she was now waking up easier for her appointments and could be on the run for a few extra hours each day. Nikki finally admitted that she was feeling less fatigued.

The POTS Treatment Center gave my daughter back to us, and we will forever be grateful. Nikki continues to do biofeedback every day from a portable machine that we were given through the center. She started her junior year of high school and has only missed two days due to illness. Since she has been back from Dallas: she has gone on long walks, has gone extreme trampolining, is constantly going out to dinner and to the mall with her friends and even danced the night away at Homecoming. Nikki is not yet 100% better, but she is at least functioning 90% better and now has more good days than bad.

Last March of 2012, we decided to take a leap of faith, and we landed on angel's wings. My daughter continues to soar to new heights every day. Thank you to the POTS Treatment Center for teaching my daughter and giving her the confidence to fly again.

Jodi Epstein Rhum

For more information on The POTS Treatment Center, please view their website at
http://www.potstreatmentcenter.com

POTS Treatment Center-
7515 Greenville Ave. Suite 1005 Dallas, Texas, 75231
Phone - 214-369-8717

Chapter 45. Mayo Clinic's Pediatric Pain Rehab Center - *Ellen Kessler*

There are other options available to help your child manage and even recover from POTS. After going through a particularly difficult winter last year, 2 ½ years into my daughter's POTS diagnosis (and 1 ½ years after my son's), we learned of a rehab program at the Mayo Clinic in Rochester, Minnesota, that was having great success with POTS patients. The Pediatric Pain Rehabilitation Center (PPRC) runs a three week program for adolescents, ages 13-21, who are suffering from chronic pain, autonomic dysfunction or other chronic symptoms.   PPRC applies a multi-disciplinary approach to rehabilitating teens with chronic POTS and chronic pain, with the goal of getting them back to a fully functional life. The change in my kids has been amazing. After participating in this program both of my children are now back in school full time, participating in extra-curricular sports, and having full and happy social lives.

This program is not just for the chronically ill teens; parent participation is required which is one aspect of this program that sets it apart from any other and I believe what makes it so successful. As parents and primary caregivers, our child's success depends on our ability to learn, change and regain control of our family dynamic. In many cases, especially my own, the family dynamic gets completely turned upside down when you have a chronically ill child.

When we arrived at Mayo, the level of knowledge, compassion and understanding among the professional staff caught my attention right away. The staff understood completely that up until this point this illness was controlling our lives – running from doctor to doctor seeking answers and waiting for a cure. They knew that by the time we decided to come to Mayo we had taken our kids to every specialist, had every test and had ruled out every life threatening illness.   What they made us understand was that our children wouldn't be cured but they could and would learn to live with

POTS.   They would teach my kids how to control their symptoms instead of having those symptoms control them. They would teach them to push past their pain and fatigue to get back to living their lives. They would empower my children to take control of and take responsibility for their illness and their symptoms. And the most surprising thing, they assured me that my kids would return to school full-time after graduating from PPRC!

The stated goals of the program are for each teen to return to school and regular daily activities; to increase their physical strength and stamina; to reducing pain (POTS) behaviors; to reduce stress utilizing stress management techniques; to re-establish social relationships; and to reduce reliance on health care professionals. These goals are met through a variety of therapies and educational sessions including: physical therapy, occupational therapy, cognitive behavioral therapy, biofeedback, stress management and deep breathing techniques.   One of the first steps in rehabilitating the kids is physical therapy to increase their strength and begin to re-condition their bodies. After spending so much time inactive and lying in bed, my kids were weak and had very little muscle tone. The physical therapists assess each child individually and start the PT at each child's level when they arrive. My daughter could only walk on the treadmill for five minutes the first few days. Through daily cardio, toning and resistance exercises my kids were able to rebuild their strength very quickly. In fact, by the time we were ready to leave at the end of the three weeks, my daughter was running two miles! We left with a plan for the kids to continue their physical activities on their own, no need for physical therapy at home. They are aware of what they need to stay conditioned and can be like normal teenagers - workout at a gym with their friends or participate in sports at school.

Reducing pain and POTS behaviors is the next step in rehabilitation. Pain (POTS) behaviors are any actions or behaviors that draw attention to symptoms. This can include complaining, whining, limping, talking about their illness, going to the school nurse,

avoiding activities and irritability. These behaviors need to be discouraged because anytime our kids are reminded of their symptoms; the symptoms can increase in severity. We are supposed to
ignore these behaviors when our kids exhibit them and not com-
ment or draw attention to any symptoms when we notice them. By
distracting our kids and diverting their attention elsewhere they will
forget about the symptoms and eventually this helps reduce the
severity of their symptoms. It sounds so basic, and also sounds well
and good except we all believe our kids symptoms are different, this
may work for others but not for OUR kid.....I can only say that, in
combination with all the other strategies, I saw it work for every
child in the program, and they each had different illnesses and different sets of symptoms. And I see that it still works with my own
children, even after we've been home for three months.   In fact, I
was asking my son the other day about fire drills at school, and if
they trigger his symptoms – he responded by asking me to stop
talking about it and to stop making him think about it, because being reminded of it made him feel worse!

Reducing stress, this is a difficult topic for us because so
many of us have become ultra-sensitive to this issue. We have spent
years arguing with doctors, well-meaning family members and
friends who have said or implied that POTS is just anxiety or stress,
it's psychological, etc. when we knew it was not; It's not.   Our kids'
symptoms are physiological and very real but stress does have a
significant effect on their symptoms. At PPRC the kids are taught
many strategies to reduce their stress. There are things like relaxation therapy or deep breathing techniques that can (and should) be
practiced several times each day, and then there are longer term
strategies like advance planning of schedules, practicing moderation
in terms of academic course work and in the number of extracurric-
ular activities, and balancing school work with fun activities and
physical activities. When our POTSy kids know what they have to do
each day, are not worried about falling behind or catching up, and
are not worried about doing too much and crashing afterwards,

they have a much easier time keeping their symptoms under control and living their lives.

Before going to Mayo, my kids had gotten to the point where their social interaction was extremely limited. Over time, as they stopped going to school, they lost touch with most of their friends and mainly just spent time with each other and our immediate family. As young teens, they missed out on years at school when they should have been developing and practicing their social skills. It is very isolating spending so much time at home and my kids were completely out of practice socializing with other teens. One part of the curriculum at PPRC is preparing the kids for reentry into school and into social circles. Because the program is a group setting, and all the kids have been in similar situations, they have ample opportunity to develop and practice all their social skills. Significant time is spent in the educational sessions preparing the kids to go home and to resume their lives. It is scary for them to go back to a full life when they have been out for so long! When we came home, both of my kids started new schools (one in high school and the other middle school) where they knew no one, and they both were totally and completely prepared. The transition was seamless and they settled in, made friends and joined activities with complete confidence, all due to the hard work and preparation they received at PPRC.

The parents spend a lot of time learning how to take back control as parents and how to start treating our children like "normal" kids. We all love our kids and we have spent years feeling helpless as our children have been so sick. The professionals at Mayo understand what we have been through and encourage us to be more balanced and consistent in our parenting. They help us individually to develop realistic rules for our kids and our families and then make sure we know how to enforce those rules, consistently. The most important skills I brought home were relearned skills — that we can and should have rules and apply consequences for behavior we don't like.   Just because our kids are going through a difficult situation does not mean we can or should relax our values and household rules. And, we have to give our kids praise and positive reinforcement for behaviors we admire and want to encourage. We have to communicate our expectations and then follow through with consequences if they are not met. Lowering our expectations because they have POTS or are feeling fatigued sends them the signal that they can't do something just when we should be making sure they know that they can. Really, basic Parenting 101 skills, but skills we all let slip away as we fell into the black hole of chronic illness. Three weeks with the staff at PPRC will give anyone the knowledge and courage needed to regain control of your household and your family! I am still amazed that changing my behavior has such a huge impact on my children's behavior. And when my kids change their behavior, there is such a positive effect on reducing their symptoms.

I have to admit, I didn't know much about the Mayo program before we went to Minnesota. I just knew that I had to do something drastic, none of us wanted to go through another year like we had just gone through, and I was reaching the end of my rope after three years. If I had known what was involved, I'm not sure we would have gone, because I didn't have the confidence that my kids could do this. I did not think that my daughter would make it through the first day! But they both did, and they made it back the next day and then the next. At some point during the first week, the peer support and pressure kept them going and kept them upright and moving forward. By the second week they were supporting and encouraging the new kids that had arrived. I am in awe of how hard my kids worked and what they were able to accomplish in just three weeks, and even more so of what they have achieved since coming home.   I am constantly surprised and proud that they have remained committed to their recovery and have continued to get stronger and happier since returning home. I can confidently say that life has somewhat returned to normal. It feels like PPRC pushed a reset button on both of my kids, or as my daughter likes to say when the true story of what was accomplished at Mayo sounds too good to be true: "They sprinkled me with magic dust!"

My son and daughter still have POTS, we don't know why, and it no longer matters. They still need to take medication, have to exercise regularly, drink 2-3 liters of fluids per day and eat a high sodium diet. But after completing Mayo's PPRC they are stronger, smarter and healthier - their symptoms are under control for the first time, and they have been able to resume leading happy, active and busy teenage lives!

*Patients can contact Mayo directly and do not need a physician referral. Mayo will need outside medical records once families have contacted them, but they do take direct calls from parents for admission to the program. Right now their wait list is two to three months, on average.

Chapter 46. When POTS is More than Just POTS

A Successful Quest to Find and Treat the Root Cause

I was a healthy, athletic, 30-something. I had a great career and a happy marriage. I developed POTS symptoms out of the blue while on a snowboarding trip. Of course, I didn't know what POTS was at first, and unfortunately, neither did my doctors. I was misdiagnosed with everything from neuroendocrine cancer, to Addison's Disease, to croup, to "you're just looking for attention." It would be nine months of horrendous symptoms, endless testing, and scary and sometimes ridiculous misdiagnoses before a team of neurologists and cardiologists at Cornell diagnosed me with POTS and autonomic neuropathy. They diagnosed the autonomic neuropathy with a 3 mm punch skin biopsy taken from the side of my left calf.

At first, I was very relieved to finally have a diagnosis that seemed to match my symptoms. But the more I learned about autonomic neuropathy, which is seen in about 50% of POTS patients according to Mayo Clinic's research,[1, 2] the more I realized that POTS was really just a list of symptoms that are sometimes seen together. That's why the "S" in POTS stands for "syndrome." POTS didn't explain *why* I had autonomic neuropathy.   Something had caused my autonomic nerves to die off, and I wanted to know what that was. My original neurologist ran some blood work ruling out diabetes, heavy metal poisoning, and certain infections that are known to be associated with neuropathy. All of those tests came back normal, and shortly thereafter he retired.

After that, I saw six different neurologists at major New York City hospitals. The first two passed me off to more senior neurologists. At least they were honest and admitted that they didn't know what to do. The next four were highly respected researchers in their respective fields. Two of them were the head of their hospitals' autonomic department and one had written a medical textbook on autonomic disorders. I was sure one of these experts would figure out what was causing my autonomic neuropathy. I was wrong.

The first neurologist told me to come back to his office when I could walk two miles. This was not helpful, since I was in a reclining wheelchair at the time and could not even walk from my couch to the bathroom. I had a chest port so that I could receive one liter of IV saline daily, just to keep myself from fainting when I sat upright in my wheelchair. If I could walk two miles, I wouldn't need a doctor.

The second senior neurologist said I was an interesting case. Everyone likes to be interesting, but not when it comes to your health. He was very nice and very intelligent, but he didn't know what was causing my autonomic neuropathy.

The third senior neurologist ran one blood test, which came back normal. He didn't want to run any other tests to look for the cause of my autonomic neuropathy when I asked him to. He acted like I was being unreasonable for even asking.

Then, the fourth neurologist didn't even examine me. He told me to "just get some exercise and see a psychiatrist so you can get used to being sick." He literally waved his hand in the air at me, as if to say, I could not be bothered with you. He said, "There is nothing we can do for you people." YOU PEOPLE? Who talks to a patient like that? All I wanted him to do was test me for the known causes of autonomic neuropathy that I had not been tested for yet, of which there were many. I thought it was unfair to label me with an "idiopathic" diagnosis, without crossing off all of the known causes of autonomic neuropathy off the list. I wanted to turn over every stone until there were no stones left. I was not ready to give in or give up.

After exhausting my options in New York City, I made an appointment at Cleveland Clinic. I had a very positive experience with the cardiology department at Cleveland Clinic. They provided me with a letter of recommendations that included possible medicines to try, lifestyle adaptations, exercises, compression stockings, etc. I was already doing all of those things, and all of that combined simply wasn't enough to get me functioning again.   However, it was good information and it was nice to have it written in one easy to read letter for my doctors back home.   After finishing up with cardiology, I requested a neurology consult, because my main motivation in going to Cleveland Clinic was to find out the cause of my autonomic neuropathy.

I was fortunate to receive an appointment with Dr. Kamal Chemali, an autonomic neurologist who specializes in POTS and autonomic neuropathies.   He was working at the Cleveland Clinic when I saw him, but as of March 2013 he has opened up a new autonomic lab at Sentara Neurosciences in Norfolk, Virginia.   He took his time asking me questions, listening to my concerns, and reviewing my voluminous records. At the end of my visit, he said he was going to test me for many different things, but he thought I might have Sjogren's or amyloidosis. Having done my homework, I knew that these were both possible causes of autonomic neuropathy. Sjogren's is an autoimmune disease that can damage any tissue in the body, although typical Sjogren's is associated with dry eyes and dry mouth, which I did not have obvious signs of.   Amyloidosis is a usually fatal disease that occurs when harmful amyloid proteins build up in your heart, kidneys, brain and/or other parts of your body.   I didn't want to have either of these conditions, but Sjogren's was definitely the lesser of two evils.

Dr. Chemali ordered tons of blood work that I had never had done before, along with some repeat autonomic tests. He also ordered a minor salivary gland lip biopsy to check for Sjogren's, a stomach fat pad biopsy to check for amyloidosis, and three more 3 mm punch skin biopsies taken from my leg (ankle, knee and upper thigh areas) to check for small fiber neuropathy. The small fiber nerves in your legs include sensory and autonomic nerve fibers. The lip biopsy is considered the "gold standard" test for Sjogren's. The Sjogren's blood tests, SS-A and SS-B, are negative in about 60% and 75% of Sjogren's patients, respectively,[3] which is why it's so important to get a lip biopsy if you suspect you have Sjogren's and your blood work is normal. The lip biopsy site felt like a bad canker sore inside my lip for a week or two, but sore throat numbing spray from the drug store kept it clean and numb until it healed.   The stomach fat biopsy was taken from a tiny incision made within my belly button, so there is no visible scar.   The 3 mm punch skin biopsies are no big deal at all.   They offer you a lidocaine injection before taking the 3 mm punch, but having had the biopsies done with and without lidocaine, I think the needle hurts more than the biopsy itself, so I do them without any lidocaine injection.   They simply put some ointment and a Band-Aid over the skin biopsy site and you're done.

My 17 vials of blood work were pretty much normal. I had no abnormal antibodies for Sjogren's or anything else. The amyloidosis stomach fat biopsy was negative.   But, the Sjogren's lip biopsy was positive. JACKPOT! I greeted this news with relief, because we finally had an answer as to why I had autonomic neuropathy and POTS, but also with some trepidation, because I was now facing the reality that I would have this disease for the rest of my life.

Sjogren's is a lifelong autoimmune disease. Unlike some other autoimmune conditions, it does not go into remission. On the bright side, it is somewhat treatable. Rather than throwing symptom-masking POTS medications at the wall and hoping something would stick, we could now treat the root cause of my POTS.   There is another reason I was happy to be diagnosed with Sjogren's; if you have Sjogren's and don't know it, you *will* get worse over time. It is a chronic, progressive disease. The earlier you are diagnosed, the better you can prevent complications and minimize your symptoms in the future. I viewed my diagnosis as an opportunity to better protect my health in the future.

Dr. Chemali recommended that I begin Intravenous Immunoglobulin (IVIG) right away. IVIG is not something you can get at your local pharmacy. IVIG is made up of Immunoglobulin G (IgG) proteins that are pooled from human blood. IgG is the most common antibody type found in the human body. In order to make one dose of IVIG, blood has to be collected from thousands of donors, purified, heat-treated, acid washed, cold fractionated and then some.   Many steps are taken to remove impurities and pathogens, since IVIG is a human blood product. The result is a small jar of clear IVIG liquid that can cost as much as $10,000 to $20,000 per dose. But that tiny jar packs a strong punch.

After three monthly IVIG infusions, I went from being practically bedridden and stuck in a reclining wheelchair for two years, to ice skating again. Yes, ice-skating! I was able to stop my regular IV saline infusions after my first dose of IVIG. Each month, I continued to feel stronger and I noticed my POTS symptoms improving.   One of my local doctors mentioned that my improvement could just be the placebo effect at work. The placebo effect is an important concept in medicine. Research studies in virtually all fields of medicine show that a certain percentage of people, no matter what their disease, will report feeling better or feeling cured, even if the medication they were given was a placebo (just a fake pill and not the real medication). At this point, I didn't care if I was feeling better due to a placebo effect or not.   I was feeling better, and that is all that mattered.   But since IVIG is extremely expensive, I thought it would be good to investigate whether my recovery was something we could objectively document, or whether my IVIG infusions had been the world's most expensive placebo.   After a year of IVIG infusions, my doctors repeated my skin biopsies to check on the density of my small fiber sensory and autonomic nerves.   Sure enough, they had grown back to normal densities.   In fact, they were even on the high end of normal.   Welcome back small fiber nerves, so nice to see you again!.

We also repeated my tilt testing, cardiac exercise stress testing and various breathing tests.   All of the tests showed objective improvement. Technically I still meet the criteria for POTS (30 bpm increase or over 120 bpm within the first ten minutes of standing in the absence of hypotension), but just barely.   Before the IVIG, I was seeing a 70 bpm or more increase in my heart rate during tilt.   Now I barely make it across the 30 bpm threshold. Some doctors might say that I don't have POTS because I have a known underlying cause of my autonomic neuropathy.   Other doctors might say that I have Secondary POTS – that means POTS caused by an underlying condition. The name of my illness is not important to me. I don't need a label. But I do think doctors need recognize that some people diagnosed with POTS do have serious underlying diseases that are the root cause of their symptoms, and that those underlying diseases can often be difficult to diagnose or easy to miss.

I can only imagine how much sicker I would have become had I not pushed for answers.   Once Sjogren's begins attacking your nervous system, it can cause severe irreversible damage, and it is sometimes confused for primary progressive Multiple Sclerosis when it attacks the nervous system[4]   It also causes a 44 fold increased risk for lymphoma[5]   Sjogren's does not get better over time.   It usually gets worse as you age.   You cannot grow out of it.

Even though many of us have never heard of it, Sjogren's is the second most common autoimmune disease in the United States, right behind Rheumatoid Arthritis.[6]   There are an estimated four million American's suffering from Sjogren's, but experts believe that only about 25% of them have been diagnosed.[7]   The average time to obtain a Sjogren's diagnosis from the onset of symptoms to the time of diagnosis is currently over five years.[8] About 90% of Sjogren's patients are female.[7]   This is similar to the 80-85% female predominance we see in POTS.[2]   I know POTS is a very heterogeneous condition, but it does make me wonder whether there are more POTS patients like me who happen to have a hard to diagnose case of Sjogren's causing their illness.

I get a little nervous when I hear doctors telling POTS patients that they will be fine if they just exercise and take their medications, before they have given them a very thorough workup to rule out any underlying causes. I hope they will be fine, but if you have autonomic neuropathy involved with your POTS, it seems to me that your doctors should be giving you a very careful look for a possible underlying cause of that neuropathy. Nerves don't just spontaneously combust. Something has caused damage to them if you have neuropathy. It could be a one-time damaging event, or it could be an ongoing process that is continuing to damage your nerves. If it took me beating down the doors of six highly skilled neurologists before we found my cause, and multitudes of other specialists before that, that makes me think that there are probably other people diagnosed with POTS who have an underlying cause that has yet to be diagnosed.

I shared my story, because I want other patients to realize how important it is to push for the best medical care you can get. If you think your doctor has done a half-baked job to figure you out, go somewhere else. Do not look back. Do not waste time being angry. Just keep pushing forward. Most importantly, do not give up hope.

References:

1.   Kimpinski, K, et al., A Prospective, 1-Year Follow-up Study of Postural Tachycardia Syndrome. Mayo Clinic Proceedings; Vol. 87, Issue 8 (746-752); August 2012.

2.   Thieben, MJ, et al., Postural Orthostatic Tachycardia Syndrome: The Mayo Clinic Experience. Mayo Clinic Proceedings; Vol. 82, Issue 3 (308-313): March 2007.

3.   Shiboski SC, et al., American College of Rheumatology Classification Criteria for Sjogren's Syndrome: A Data-Driven, Expert Consensus Approach in the Sjogren's International Collaborative Clinical Alliance Cohort.   Arthritis Care & Research; Vol. 64, No. 4, (475–487); April 2012.

4.   Birnbam, J., A primer on the neurological complications of Sjogren's. Website of the Johns Hopkins Neurology Rheumatology Clinic. (available at http://www.hopkinssjogrens.org/disease-information/sjogrens-syndrome/neurologic-complications, last viewed February 25, 2013)

5.   Konstantinidis, et al., Bilateral multiple sialolithiasis of the parotid gland in a patient with Sjögren's syndrome. Acta Otorhinolaryngol Ital. 2007 February; 27(1): 41–44.

6.   Kim, L., New Standards to Improve Diagnosis of Sjögren's Syndrome. Website of the University of California, San Francisco. April 9, 2012. (available at, http://www.ucsf.edu/news/2012/08/12521/new-standards-improve-diagnosis-sjogrens-syndrome, last viewed February 25, 2013).

7.   About Sjogren's, Website of the Sjogren's Syndrome Foundation (available at http://www.sjogrens.org/home/about-sjogrens-syndrome, last visited February 25, 2013)8.   SSF Launches 5-Year Breakthrough Goal, Website of the Sjogren's Syndrome Foundation (available at http://www.sjogrens.org/home/about-the-foundation/breakthrough-goal-, last visited February 25, 2013)

About Dysautonomia International

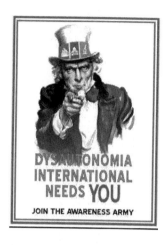

Dysautonomia International is the first global charity dedicated to finding the causes and cures for all forms of Dysautonomia, including POTS. Dysautonomia International actively raises funds for medical research, physician training, patient empowerment and public outreach.

I have served as Vice President and as a member of the Board of Directors of Dysautonomia International since its founding in 2012, along with many other parents and patients impacted by autonomic disorders. We are an all-volunteer organization. Our main office is in New York, but we are global in scope. We also have regional offices in Washington, D.C., Chicago and Los Angeles.

Dysautonomia International is blessed to have a Medical Advisory Board containing some of the world's best autonomic clinicians and researchers from Mayo Clinic, Vanderbilt University, and beyond. Our Patient Advisory Board is an outstanding group of talented people who happen to have an autonomic disorder. They are nurses, lawyers, medical students, public relations professionals, caregivers and college kids, and they bring the patient perspective to all of the work we do. Perhaps most important of all is our Awareness Army. None of the work we do would be possible without the help of our Awareness Army. The Awareness Army consists of volunteers just like you. Members of the Awareness Army help us run local fundraisers, reach out to local media, plan awareness events and projects, help us with social media promotion, and more.

Since our launch in 2012, Dysautonomia International's volunteers have been hard at work. They started the first global Dysautonomia patient mapping project, kicked off the first Global Dysautonomia Awareness Month campaign (October), organized the 2013 Dysautonomia Patient Conference & Lobby Day in Washington, DC, created a website with comprehensive and medically accurate information on autonomic disorders, gave presentations at several physician conferences to help raise awareness of autonomic disorders within the medical community, helped researchers design what may be the largest POTS study ever conducted, we helped other researchers recruit patients for studies on POTS and Chronic Fatigue Syndrome, raised enough funds to issue our first autonomic research grants in 2013 and so much more. Our volunteers accomplished all of that in just our first year.

I cannot wait to see what Dysautonomia International will be able to accomplish as we connect with more patients and families, and continue to grow in the years ahead. *Together we stand* and working together, we *will* conquer POTS and other autonomic disorders!

Jodi Epstein Rhum

If you would like to volunteer for the Awareness Army or learn more about it, please visit: www.dysautonomiainternational.org/volunteer.

If you would like to donate to Dysautonomia International, you can visit our website: www.dysautonomiainternational.org/donate.

If you would like to participate in our patient-mapping project, visit:

www.dysautonomiainternational.org/map.php.

Our Facebook page is a great way to stay up to date on the latest research on autonomic disorders, and also to find out about events going on around the globe pertaining to autonomic disorders. "Like" us at:

www.facebook.com/dysautonomiainternational.

Wrapping Up........

The journey with POTS is not only challenging but frustrating, as well. The only thing that is predictable about this syndrome is that it is unpredictable. Missed school days, work days and debilitating symptoms that interfere with every day of life, make this syndrome even more difficult to deal with. The person with POTS is left to lead a very different lifestyle than before their illness and often has to "redefine" themselves. This coupled with the fact that so few people have heard of this illness and may ignorantly believe that your symptoms are "all in your head"; make living with POTS even more disparaging.

As with many invisible illnesses, in particular those dealing with the autonomic nervous system, although not life threatening, they are none the less, still life altering and may in many cases be debilitating.

Even though presently there is no cure for POTS, there are still many ways in which one can help lesson symptoms, albeit trial and error, and help one to lead a more "pain-free" and fruitful existence. As time goes on, more doctors will be aware of this syndrome, and they will be able to diagnose and treat this disorder more effectively. Additionally, it is encouraging that NASA and top-notch teaching facilities like Mayo Clinic, Vanderbilt and UCLA are researching this illness. It is very likely because of this, new treatments and protocols will soon be available to patients around the globe.

As a patient and or caregiver, it is important to never give up hope and to realize you are not alone in fighting this battle. POTS is undeniably a very complicated syndrome, but always remember you are not your illness. Never ever give up and you will win the war- for together we are strong and "Together we Will Stand."

Wishing you strength, good health and brighter days ahead.

Jodi Rhum.

5

504 Plan · *147, 148, 149, 150,* 156, *157, 158, 163, 164, 166, 186, 188, 192, 199*

A

Accommodations · *147, 149, 150, 192, 208, 227, 230, 231, 232, 233, 234, 237*
acetylcholine · *284, 285*
acupressure · *252*
adolescents · *425, 434, 445, 447, 455, 456, 459, 460, 461, 473*
Adrenaline · *285*
alcohol · *32, 49, 50, 77, 253, 306, 316, 384, 475*
allergies · *32, 223, 268, 286, 312, 321, 322, 409, 410, 415, 420*
anemia · *26, 317, 409, 410, 452*
antibody · *78, 271*
anxiety · *32, 33, 34, 35, 46, 50, 56, 58, 62, 71, 77, 88, 137, 138, 146, 190, 211, 233, 236, 261, 262, 268, 269, 270, 306, 319, 404, 408, 412, 433, 443, 451, 456, 464, 468, 469, 473, 474, 475, 477*
Arnica · *257, 310*
arrhythmia · *25, 29, 114, 399*
arteries · *27, 72, 401*
autonomic nervous system · *19, 20, 22, 28, 29, 33, 34, 68, 72, 74, 84, 88, 127, 135, 142, 204, 284, 285, 286, 288, 362, 395, 396, 401, 402, 404, 405, 428, 441, 443, 445, 447, 454, 465, 501*

B

Baroreflex · *442, 446*
Beighton scale · *118*
beta 2 adrenergic receptor · 405
blood clots · *249, 312, 411*
blood pooling · *54, 64, 222, 313, 402, 416*
blood pressure · *22, 23, 24, 25, 27, 28, 29, 42, 46, 48, 53, 55, 56, 59, 61, 62, 63, 65, 67, 70, 71, 74, 75, 77, 79, 81, 82, 83, 96, 127, 128, 135, 136, 137, 146, 154,* 204, *205, 224, 230, 232, 233, 234, 247, 252, 254, 261, 263, 267, 280, 281, 285, 286, 287, 307, 309, 312, 314, 315, 316, 320, 321, 341, 344, 347, 348, 363, 372, 374, 380, 395, 398, 401, 402, 404, 407, 411, 415, 416, 428, 432, 433, 435, 438, 441, 442, 445, 446, 449, 450, 451, 452, 464, 475*
Blood Pressure · *446*
brain · *22, 24, 26, 28, 32, 50, 52, 53, 56, 59, 64, 66, 67, 70, 72, 73, 77, 79, 82, 83, 154, 160, 231, 246, 251, 282, 286, 305, 307, 308, 311, 317, 318, 319, 322, 335, 341, 369, 373, 396, 400, 401, 406, 416, 436, 443, 471*
Butcher's Broom · *311, 312*

C

Caffeine · *48, 62, 313*
carbohydrates · *62, 282, 283, 288, 290, 321, 389*
Cardio vascular training · *347*
carpal tunnel syndrome · *114*
catecholamine · *69*
Chamomile · *311, 316*
Chiari · 69, 400, 407
Chronic Fatigue Syndrome · *231, 237*
Clonidine · *453*
Collagen · *112*
common faint · *24, 53*
constipation · *309, 319, 435, 439, 472*
cortisol · *48*
Cranio-Sacral Therapy · *317*

D

dehydration · 29, 54, 61, 62, 63, 64, 77, 82, 379, 411, 452
depression · *32, 71, 312, 425, 437, 443, 451, 455, 463, 471, 474, 477*
Depression · *231*
digestion · *22, 23, 50, 79, 127, 128, 135, 141, 204, 311*
Digestion · *24, 49*
Dizziness · *234, 237, 307, 431*
Dysautonomia · *1, 2, 14, 18, 46, 49, 52, 61, 62, 65, 66, 68, 70, 71, 72, 73, 74, 75, 76, 77, 78, 79, 82, 92, 114, 127, 129, 131, 145, 146,*
148, 149, 150, 154, 155, 156, 157, 190, 200, 203, 206, 228, 229, 230, 231, 232, 233, 234, 235, 265, 284, 304, 305, 310, 311, 313, 315, 319, 320, 323, 341, 342, 344, 347, 348, 358, 359, 360, 361, 362, 366, 368, 370, 387, 388, 389, 435, 437, 438, 441

E

Ehlers · *14, 69, 112, 113, 115, 120, 121, 224, 262, 268, 321, 322, 380, 400*
Electrolytes · *314*
endoscopy · *443*
Epilepsy · *56, 237, 435*
Epinephrine · *63*
Ergo meter · *443*
estrogen · *75*
Exercise · *76, 338, 339, 340, 349, 378*

F

fatigue · 31, 33, 34, 40, 61, 64, 70, 71, 72, 144, 146, 147, 160, 204, 211, 219, 233, 236, 254, 286, 290, 308, 318, 341, 362, 369, 370, 373, 377, 389, 395, 413, 424, 431, 434, 436, 443, 448, 450, 451, 468, 471, 476
Feverfew · *312*
Fibromyalgia · *435*

Flat feet · 113
frequent urination · 71

G

gabapentin · 115
gastroparesis · 439, 444
Ginger · 294, 298, 299, 307, 309, 311
Glucosamine · 116
glucose · 24, 62, 79
Glutamine · 306, 316, 319, 320
Gluten · 64
gravity · 17, 20, 22, 28, 39, 64, 82, 340, 341, 342, 383, 388, 391, 401, 402, 404, 452, 467

H

heart · 20, 21, 22, 23, 24, 25, 26, 27, 28, 29, 30, 31, 34, 41, 45, 46, 50, 53, 55, 56, 59, 61, 62, 63, 64, 70, 71, 76, 78, 82, 83, 92, 114, 127, 128, 203, 204, 222, 224, 245, 267, 268, 280, 284, 285, 287, 306, 307, 308, 309, 311, 313, 314, 315, 317, 319, 320, 335, 338, 341, 343, 344, 347, 348, 369, 370, 372, 373, 374, 375, 378, 383, 388, 395, 398, 401, 402, 403, 404, 406, 415, 416, 428, 432, 433, 441, 442, 443, 445, 446, 448, 449, 451, 464, 465, 468, 470
Heart Monitor · 59

histamine · 283, 286, 288, 406, 407
hormones · 48, 68, 80, 117, 398, 403, 471
hydrotherapy · 115
hyperadrenergic POTS · 404
Hypermoblity · 112
hyperthyroidism · 452
hypoperfusion · 396

I

IEP · 3, 139, 147, 149, 157, 158, 160, 161, 163, 165, 166, 171, 173, 174, 175, 176, 177, 178, 179, 180, 181, 184, 186, 188, 192, 193, 197, 198, 199
Implantable Loop Recorder · 59
Individualized Education · 147
Insomnia · 46, 316
Intolerance · 83, 284, 321, 388, 440

J

Joint Pain · 317

K

kidneys · 50, 314, 319, 320, 403

L

Low blood volume · 83
Lucidal · 309

M

Magnesium · 50, 313, 320
Manganese · 307, 320
mast cell · 406, 407
Melatonin · 47, 48, 316, 323
Menses · 437
Midodrine · 83, 453
migraine · 26
Migraines · 54, 230, 237
Mitral Valve Prolapse · 321, 373, 375
Mononucleosis · 400
Motility Disorders · 444
MRI · 38, 59, 435, 443
muscle tone · 222, 250, 341

N

NASA · 81, 82, 84, 501
NASM · 343, 347, 349
nausea · 32, 138, 204, 252, 253, 298, 311, 312, 406, 430, 431, 434, 439, 440, 441, 442, 444, 445, 448
neurally mediated hypotension · 440
Norepinephrine transporter deficiency · 69
nutrition · 3, 128, 283, 434, 436

O

oral contraceptives · 75, 437, 438

orthostatic hypotension · 19, 28, 29, 31, 81, 82, 312, 315, 388, 399, 433, 448
orthostatic intolerance · 20, 21, 22, 82, 83, 84, 114, 136, 219, 225, 315, 321, 344, 388, 395, 400, 402, 410, 413, 440, 441, 442, 445, 446, 448, 450
orthostatic stress · 22, 46, 73, 76, 398
orthostatic tolerance · 317, 413, 451
osteoarthritis · 113, 224

P

palpitation · 452
Parasympathetic Nervous System · 432
Pilates · 115
Plan/Program · 147, 157, 192
Pregabalin · 435
pregnancy · 80, 117, 131, 374, 375, 377, 399, 400, 420, 423, 424, 425, 426, 428, 429
Pregnancy · 68
premature atrial contractions · 114
Premature ventricular contractions · 114
Probiotics · 271, 311
prognosis · 79, 132
propranolol · 452

S

Salt · *66, 74, 280, 290, 291, 292, 294, 295, 296, 297, 298, 300, 301, 302, 315*
Seizures · *55*
sinus node · *451, 452*
Sjogren's · *277, 492, 493, 495, 496, 497*
spondylolisthesis · 113
SSRI · *310*
strep throat · *68*
Stressors · *194*
stroke volume · 307
subluxations · *113*
swimming · *255, 347*
sympathetic nervous system · *23, 83, 336, 396, 398, 403, 404, 407, 442*
syncope · *24, 25, 26, 28, 52, 53, 55, 57, 58, 59, 66, 67, 72, 73, 204, 205, 223, 225, 236, 246, 249, 268, 315, 400, 407, 413, 422, 430, 431, 432, 433, 434, 436, 441, 446, 448, 451, 452*

T

tachycardia · *18, 21, 35, 63, 64, 203, 211, 224, 249, 284, 341, 362,*
378, 388, 401, 402, 405, 406, 407, 408, 428, 429, 432, 440, 446, 448, 449, 450, 451, 452, 477
Tachycardia · *18, 207, 323, 340, 369, 376, 384*
Tai Chi · *115*
Temperomandibular Joint Syndrome · *113*
tendinitis · *113*
tilt table · *21, 369, 440, 441, 442, 445*
Tilt Table Testing · *59*
Tramadol · *115*
Triggers · *53*

V

Vagus nerve damage · *69*
Valerian · *306, 316*
veins · *69, 77, 82, 312*
vertigo · *71, 235, 247, 249, 307*
Vitamin A · *130*
Vitamin C · *309, 321, 322*
Vitamin D · *322, 323*

Y

Yoga · *334, 474*

Made in the USA
San Bernardino, CA
05 October 2018